TEXTBOOK OF IMMUNOLOGY

Second Edition

TEXTBOOK OF IMMUNOLOGY

Second Edition

Emil R. Unanue, M.D.

Department of Pathology
Washington University School of Medicine
St. Louis, Missouri

Baruj Benacerraf, M.D.

Department of Pathology
Harvard Medical School
Dana-Farber Cancer Institute
Boston, Massachusetts

WILLIAMS & WILKINS
Baltimore • London • Los Angeles • Sydney

Editor: George Stamathis
Associate Editor: Victoria M. Vaughn
Design: JoAnne Janowiak
Illustration Planning: Joseph P. Cummings
Production: Anne G. Seitz

Williams & Wilkins
428 East Preston Street
Baltimore MD 21202, U.S.A.

Accurate indications, adverse reactions, and dosage schedules for drugs are provided in this book, but it is possible that they may change. The reader is urged to review the package information data of the manufacturers of the medications mentioned.

Made in the United States of America

First Edition 1979

Library of Congress Cataloging in Publication Data

Main entry under title:

Benacerraf, Baruj, 1920–
Textbook of immunology.

Authors' names reversed on t.p. of earlier ed. Includes bibliographies and index.
1. Immunology. I. Unanue, Emil R., 1934–0000 II. Title. [DNLM: 1. Allergy and Immunology. QW 504 B456t]
QR181.B394 1984 616.07'9 84–7332
ISBN 0-683-08504-2

Composed and printed at the
Waverly Press, Inc. 85 86 87 88 89 10 9 8 7 6 5 4 3 2

Preface to the Second Edition

We have made a series of changes in order to accommodate the mass of new information that became available during the last four years. As before, this book has been designed as an introductory textbook with heavy emphasis on basic immunological phenomena. The major revisions concern the new information on immunoglobulin genes, the analysis of histocompatibility and the function of T cells. The latter two, probably the most difficult topics for the students, are presented, gradually, in four chapters. First, we present a general description of the histocompatibility molecules and their genes (in Chapter 6), followed by their function in transplantation and physiological cellular interactions (in Chapters 6, 7, and 8). Lastly, in Chapter 10, we describe the function of immune response genes as originally discovered.

We are grateful to our many colleagues who helped us with their advice and comments. To note is that Dr. Kurt J. Bloch revised all of Chapter 3, and, with Dr. Susan Canelosi, a great part of Chapter 4. Dr. K. F. Austen revised the complement chapter. Dr. F. S. Rosen revised Chapter 15. Dr. Ronald N. Germain wrote parts of Chapter 11. We also acknowledge the help, in this second edition, of Drs. Martin E. Dorf, Edmond J. Yunis, and Elvin Kabat. Both George F. Schreiner and F. S. Rosen read most of the chapters and provided considerable help on editorial and scientific matters. We are grateful to Pamela Battaglino, who drew all the new graphs of this edition. Finally, we owe a great deal to Barbara K. Gricus, who typed the whole book and also helped us with editorial matters.

Emil R. Unanue

Baruj Benacerraf

Boston, Massachusetts
November, 1983

Preface to the First Edition

The knowledge of immunology has become essential to students of medicine and biology. The applications of its methodology to many fields in the biological sciences are widely recognized and extensively utilized. Furthermore, immunology has been highly successful in applying a variety of fundamental technologies derived from biochemistry, genetics, cell biology, and pathology to the analysis of highly complex phenomena which constitute the immune response. The study of modern immunology has provided us with critical information applicable to other fields of biology and medicine. The differentiation of the lymphoid system and the functions of its component lymphocytes offer to the cell biologists the best analysis of complex cellular systems. The intricate interactions among these cells and the genetics which govern these phenomena are models for other differentiating systems. Furthermore, the genetic problems presented by the generation of diversity in immunoglobulin-combining sites have important applications to molecular biology and genetics. Likewise, the study of complement and anaphylaxis has provided information essential for our understanding of inflammation and tissue pathology.

This textbook is designed to provide information which will permit a medical student, a college student, or a graduate student in the biological sciences to have a basic understanding of the rapidly expanding and complex discipline of immunology. The various chapters cover the entire field describing the basic immunological phenomena, the biochemistry of antibodies and antigens, the immunological techniques, the cellular and genetic components of the immune response, and, finally, immunopathology. The material presented is sufficiently complete to permit an in-depth understanding of immunological phenomena, as well as to serve as an introduction to more extensive studies.

This textbook was originally organized from teaching materials prepared for first-year medical students at Harvard Medical School and provided to them as part of the introductory course in immunology of the Harvard Medical School curriculum. The chapters follow the same sequence as the lectures in the course and cover the same material.

TEXTBOOK OF IMMUNOLOGY

Several chapters were written by colleagues at Harvard Medical School. Dr. Kurt J. Bloch wrote the chapters on antibody structure and with Dr. Susan Canelosi wrote the method chapter; Dr. K. Frank Austen wrote the chapter on complement; Dr. Fred S. Rosen wrote the chapter on immunodeficiency; and Dr. Ronald N. Germain wrote the chapter on tumor immunity. Other colleages helped us by editing certain sections or providing us with their advice and opinion. For this we thank Drs. Kenneth A. Ault, Martin E. Dorf, Eric Martz, and Edmond J. Yunis. Lastly, we thank the first-year Harvard Medical students who, by giving us their criticisms, involuntarily, have taught us how to teach immunology.

Baruj Benacerraf

Emil R. Unanue

Boston, Massachusetts
September, 1979

Contents

CHAPTER 1

Immunology: Principles and Phenomenology

This chapter is an overview of some of the most important immunological phenomena placed in a historical context. This overview is needed as an initial step preceding the detailed analysis of immune cells and molecules and their interactions.

Early History of Immunology: The roots of immunological phenomena are very old. They reside in ancient observations, recorded in disparate cultures, that patients who survived infectious diseases seldom contracted that disease again. Immunology as a science did not emerge until relatively recent. Indeed, one can date it to eighteenth-century England, a time of recurrent epidemics of smallpox. Smallpox was a serious viral disease characterized by infective lesions in internal organs and skin. In the skin, the lesions consists of fluid-containing blebs in the epidermis that break, ulcerate, and scar. At that time, one way to avoid smallpox was through the practice of "variolation", which had its origins in the Middle East. The infective fluid from the pox lesions was inoculated into an individual for the purpose of producing a limited infection. Such individuals were then protected from acquiring the severe disease during the epidemics. Variolation had a limited success since it was difficult to control the extent of infectivity, and frequently, a severe disease would develop. We owe to Edward Jenner the first attempt to "immunize" deliberately against an infectious disease, using an attenuated non-infectious form of the microorganism. At the time that these studies were done, however, there was no knowledge of microbes as the cause of infection. When Jenner was an assistant in practice, delivering "primary care", a young country woman told him that she could not have smallpox since she had already contracted cowpox. Cowpox was a pox virus disease, endemic in cattle, frequently observed in milkmaids. The viruses of cowpox and smallpox share antigens. Jenner first inoculated James Phipps with cowpox infectious crusts and, later in time, practiced variolation on him with small amounts of smallpox infective material. Phipps had developed immunity to the smallpox by the inoculation with cowpox, and no infective lesions developed. Thus, Jenner's attempts were successful, and he concluded that the mild infection with cowpox protected against the severe infection with smallpox. He published his classical memoir: "An inquiry into the causes and effects of the variolae vacciniae" in 1798. Less than two centuries later, the World Health Organization would declare smallpox extinct as a disease, as a result of a worldwide vaccination program.

Our understanding of Jenner's experiment did not come until years later with the formulation of the germ theory of disease, based to a major extent on the experimental work of Louis Pasteur. Although initially interested in bacteria and their pathogenic properties, Pasteur became increasingly concerned with the prevention of infectious diseases and, thereby, became the first great experimental immunologist. Even though comparatively little was understood of the ways in which various bacterial pathogens caused disease, Pasteur realized that methods for immunization could be developed. These were initially based upon observations made with the chicken cholera bacillus. A level of immunity comparable to that elicited by the virulent organisms in surviving subjects could be stimulated by "attenuated" or modified strains. These strains were able to stimulate immunity without causing disease. This experimental analysis permitted the original success of Jenner's vaccination experiments to be understood. Pasteur, in honor of Jenner, called his treatment "vaccination". Vaccination is the method for stimulating immunity to an infectious disease by injection of the microorganism or its products.

It is easily understood, therefore, that immunology initially grew as a subdiscipline of bacteriology and was concerned primarily with the study of the development of immunity and specific defense mechanisms against infectious agents and their toxic products. The discovery of antibodies was the major accomplishment of this phase of immunological research. Roux and Yersin in 1888, at the Pasteur Institute, found the bacterial toxin of the diphtheria bacillus in the culture filtrates. Later immunity against the toxin was ascribed to the development of specific neutralizing substances or antitoxins in the blood of the immune animal, giving rise to the concept of antibodies. Such antitoxin could be passively transferred to a non-immune animal with immune serum. This result was first observed in the case of tetanus antitoxin by Von Boehring and Kitasato in 1890 at the Koch Institute in Berlin. The specific substances found in the serum of immune animals able to confer passive immunity were called antibodies and were the subject of intensive scrutiny. Antibodies were able to:

1. neutralize toxins

2. agglutinate bacteria

3. kill and lyse bacteria in the presence of normal serum. The components in normal serum required for lysis were found to be heat labile. Initially called alexine and later complement by Bordet, they are now known to include sixteen interacting serum proteins (Chapter 12).

4. opsonize bacteria for phagocytosis by macrophages or polymorphonuclear phagocytes

5. sensitize passively for anaphylactic (allergic) reactions.

All these phenomena displayed a high degree of specificity for the antigen that induced the antibody. They were generally protective for the patient who developed this immunity and constituted fundamental defense mechanisms against infectious agents. The immune sera which display these characteristic properties could confer passive immunity to normal, non-immune recipients. This form of immunotherapy, still in use today, is termed serotherapy.

The discovery that the antibody properties of antisera are attributable to specific protein molecules was made by Michael Heidelberger who showed that pneumococcal capsular polysaccharides precipitated specific serum proteins from rabbit anti-pneumococcal antisera. These antibodies or immunoglobulins are the molecules responsible for the precipitating, agglutinating, and complement-fixing properties of specific antisera. It was later established by A. Tiselius and E. Kabat that the bulk of antibodies in hyperimmune antisera had the electrophoretic properties of gamma globulins. The subsequent concern of immunologists was, for many decades, centered upon the properties of antibodies, their structure, the stimulation of their synthesis, and the nature of the complement system.

ANTIBODIES AND ANTIGENS

Antibodies are molecules synthesized upon stimulation by antigen and endowed with exquisite specificity for the antigen. Antigens are molecules which, when introduced to a subject, are able to stimulate the synthesis of specific antibodies capable of interacting with them. The structure of antibodies and the various classes to which they belong will be discussed in Chapter 3. At this time, we simply need to state that antibodies react with antigens by virtue of their antigen-combining sites and that each antibody molecule is made up of two identical half molecules, each containing a heavy and a light chain. Each molecule binds to one antigenic determinant at one of its ends where both heavy and light chains associate to create the combining site. The antigenic determinant is a small portion of the antigen, no more than a few amino acids long. Thus, antibody molecules bind two identical antigenic determinants. Interaction of antibody and antigen depends upon the steric configuration of both molecules, permitting a close fit between the antibody-combining sites and the corresponding determinant of the antigen.

The antibody molecules, besides binding to antigen, can interact with inflammatory cells and soluble molecules and thus can modulate important biological phenomena—such as cell lysis, phagocytosis, degranulation, and secretion of intracellular components from neutrophils, macrophages, and mast cells, etc. Antibody molecules are grouped into five major classes (IgG, IgM, IgD, IgA, and IgE) on the basis of structural differences in heavy chains. Each Ig class modulates specific biological effects, although each can bind to the same antigen with the same high degree of specificity. Thus, the antibody molecule is unique in that it is endowed with two distinct properties: the specific one of binding to unique antigens and the non-specific one of interacting with inflammatory cells and/or soluble serum components.

An important concept to bear in mind is that practically all natural antigens possess several antigenic determinants, each capable of eliciting antibodies. In addition to the heterogeneity in the antibody response to an antigen, resulting from numerous determinants on an antigen, the population of antibodies produced against a single determinant is also highly heterogeneous with respect not only to class of Ig but also to binding affinity, a reflection of the primary amino acid sequence of the combining site of the molecule (Chapter 3). The antibody register is, therefore, of enormous size and possesses a wide scope as well as marked specificity. Thus, we must consider antibodies produced against a given antigen as a population of antibodies with varying degrees of affinity for the various determinants of the antigen. As one would expect, therefore, antibodies produced against molecules with related structures will crossreact to a considerable extent, although a small population within these antibodies can be shown by absorption to be absolutely specific for the immunizing antigen. The degree of crossreactivity depends upon the structural similarities of the antigens. Thus, bovine serum albumin (BSA) and human serum albumin (HSA) stimulate the synthesis of rabbit antibodies which are extensively crossreactive, whereas anti-human serum albumin and anti-human gamma globulin (HGG) antibodies do not crossreact.

The study of the specificity of antibodies has depended very much upon the understanding of antigenic determinants. We owe to Karl Landsteiner the discovery that small, defined chemicals such as 2,4-dinitrofluorobenzene (DNFB) could be covalently bound to immunogenic molecules to form new antigens, the response to which is directed against the chemical group introduced. Such a chemical group which by itself is too small to stimulate a response but, nevertheless, reacts with the antibody, has been called a hapten. (The immunogenic protein to which the hapten is bound is termed the carrier.) Thus, antibodies against DNP-BSA will react with DNP-HGG. In solution, this interaction of soluble DNP-HGG with the antibody at an appropriate ratio results in the formation of a lattice of crosslinked molecules, which, as it grows, becomes insoluble and precipitates (Chapter 4). This reaction is inhibited by a monovalent hapten such as DNP bound to a small chain of lysines (Chapter 2).

What are the properties of antigens essential for immunogenicity? Chapter 2 analyzes this question. We can state now that the following classes of molecules are generally antigenic: 1) foreign proteins and polypeptides of size larger than eight amino acids; and 2) polysaccharides with repeated structural units. Generally speaking, small chemicals, lipids, and nucleic acids are weakly immunogenic. They can, when conjugated to an immunogenic protein carrier, behave as haptens and stimulate specific antibodies against these determinants.

The dissociation between antibody specificity and immunogenicity suggests the existence of separate recognition systems for the hapten and the carrier molecule at the cellular level in the induction of antibody responses (Chapter 8). The degree of immunogenicity of a molecule depends fundamentally on the extent to which such a molecule differs from homologous components of the host, since, generally speaking, autologous components which are strong antigens in a foreign species, are not immunogenic in the host of origin under normal conditions.

PRIMARY AND SECONDARY ANTIBODY RESPONSES

When a conventional antigen which an individual has never encountered is administered for the first time, one observes a latent period lasting several days during which antibodies are not detected in the serum nor antibody-producing cells in the lymphoid tissues. The more sensitive the method, the shorter is the latent period, but it is rarely less than three or four days. Following this period, the amount of antibodies in the serum increases exponentially to reach a peak level and then decreases. This is the primary response. It usually consists of IgM antibodies with sometimes a small IgG component appearing later, depending upon the antigen, the dose, and the route of immunization. If the animal is left to rest until the serum antibody concentration declines to low or undetected levels and then a similar or lower amount of the same antigen is administered, the second antibody response is much more rapid and stronger, the latent period is shorter, and the antibody produced is predominantly IgG in character. After reaching its peak, the secondary or anamnestic response decreases much more slowly. This is the phenomenon of immunological memory on which all prophylactic immunizations are based (Figure 1.1).

Another important feature of the antibody response is the increase of the average affinity of the antibody for the antigen with time of the immunization. This is generally referred to as maturation of the immune response. Increased antibody affinity with time has been observed both with conventional antigens such as diphtheria toxin,

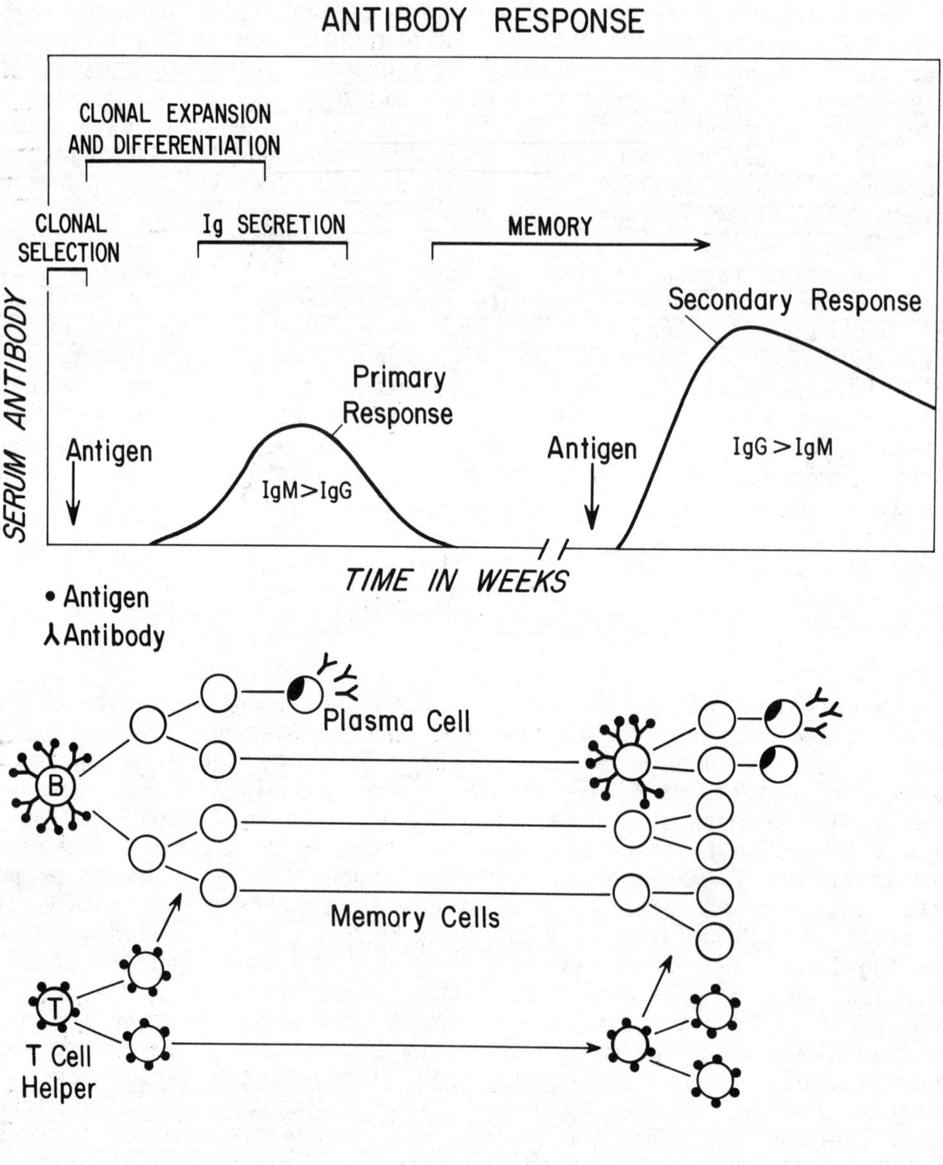

Figure 1.1. Antibody response in the serum against a conventional thymus-dependent antigen. The top panel depicts the serum levels of antibody after primary and secondary challenges. The bottom panel illustrates the cellular events in B cells, T cells, and plasma cells.

influenza virus, and hapten-protein conjugates. The studies with anti-hapten antibodies of Gregory Siskind and Herman Eisen have provided precise affinity measurement for this phenomenon. Thus, in the course of immunization, the affinity of late antibodies can increase by 10,000-fold over the affinity of early antibodies. In addition, this phenomenon is very much dependent upon the dose of antigen administered: the rate of maturation of antibody affinity increases with decreasing doses of antigen until a maximum is reached; if too little antigen is administered, antibody affinity no longer increases optimally.

The phenomenon of increase in antibody affinity with time of immunization is extremely important. The efficacy of humoral immunity depends as much, if not more, upon the affinity of the antibody for the antigen than upon the amount of antibody produced. Indeed, most defense phenomena involving antibody occur in body fluids at very low concentrations of antibodies and antigens.

THE CELLS OF THE IMMUNE RESPONSE

The events in the serum reflect the cellular dynamics of the immune response. The immune response results from the interaction of the antigen with lymphocytes bearing specific receptor proteins on the surface membranes. Lymphocytes are very heterogeneous cells that are grouped into two major classes, the T cells and the B cells. The T cells originate from the thymus gland where they mature and differentiate following interactions with the thymic stromal cells. The mature T cells then leave the thymus gland to continuously circulate from blood to lymph nodes and back to blood. T cells are represented by three major subsets: the T helper cells, the T suppressor cells, and the T cytolytic cells. T helper cells, as their name implies, regulate—help—other cells: B cells to secrete antibody, T cytolytic cells to become functional, and macrophages to become highly activated. Many of these functions are carried out by proteins elaborated by the T cell, called lymphokines or lymphocyte mediators (Chapter 7). The T suppressor cell functions to limit and terminate the immune response (Chapters 8 and 9). Immunity thus represents a fine balance between helper and suppressor functions. Shifts in this fine balance may result in abnormalities of immune function. T cytolytic cells are cells that attach to and kill tumor cells or virally infected cells (Chapters 7 and 11).

The B cells, or antibody-forming cells, derive from immature precursors found in abundance in bone marrow. When mature, the B cells are found in lymphoid organs in clusters called lymphoid follicles (Chapter 5). B cells interact with antigen by way of antibody molecules bound to their plasma membranes, acting as receptor proteins.

Following interaction with antigen and T cells, the B cells differentiate to antibody-forming cells called plasma cells. Plasma cells secrete antibody with the same specificity for antigen as that found in the receptor of the B cell from which it derived. This basic function of B cells, to have antibody as receptors and to secrete antibodies when stimulated, were hypothesized in 1902 by Paul Ehrlich at a time when there was no knowledge of lymphocytes nor of cell receptors. Ehrlich side chain theory stated that cells making anti-toxins had protoplasmic extrusions that would bind to the toxin and that this binding would induce more side chains that would then be shed to the outside, appearing as serum anti-toxins. Ehrlich's theory came too early in time to be understood, and no cellular work of significance was done until very recently.

By early 1950, theories explaining the great diversity in the specificity of antibodies fell into two groups: the instructive and the selective. The instructive theories postulated that antigen acted as a template over which antibody molecules folded and acquired their correct complementary configuration. The instructive theories were abandoned when it became evident that antibodies of different specificities had different amino acid sequences in their combining sites. The selective theories were first proposed by Niels Jerne and David Talmadge and postulated that antibodies of all specificities are produced prior to antigen administration, at low levels, and that the antibody molecule itself acts as the selective device to bind antigen and to permit specific antibody synthesis to be stimulated. Our understanding of immunologic phenomena was greatly fostered by the crucial contribution of Sir McFarlane Burnet, who envisaged selection at the level of the cell and proposed the "clonal selection theory of immunity". According to Burnet and the clonal selection theory:

1. Immunocompetent lymphocytes bear antibody receptors on their cell membrane. These receptors have identical specificity for antigen as the antibodies synthesized by their progeny when differentiated and activated.

2. Each immunocompetent lymphocyte bears antibody receptors of unique specificity (Figure 1.2).

We know now that each B cell reacts with a unique antigenic determinant, i.e., all the receptors on a B cell are monospecific. Thus, the immune system, as originally postulated by Burnet, functions by antigen binding to those lymphocytes with unique receptors of high affinity.

These selected lymphocytes are committed to bind antigen during their differentiation, prior to contact with antigen. The binding of antigen stimulates the selected B cells to divide, producing daughter cells of the same specificity. Clonal selection explains the progressive increase in antibody affinity with time. There is an

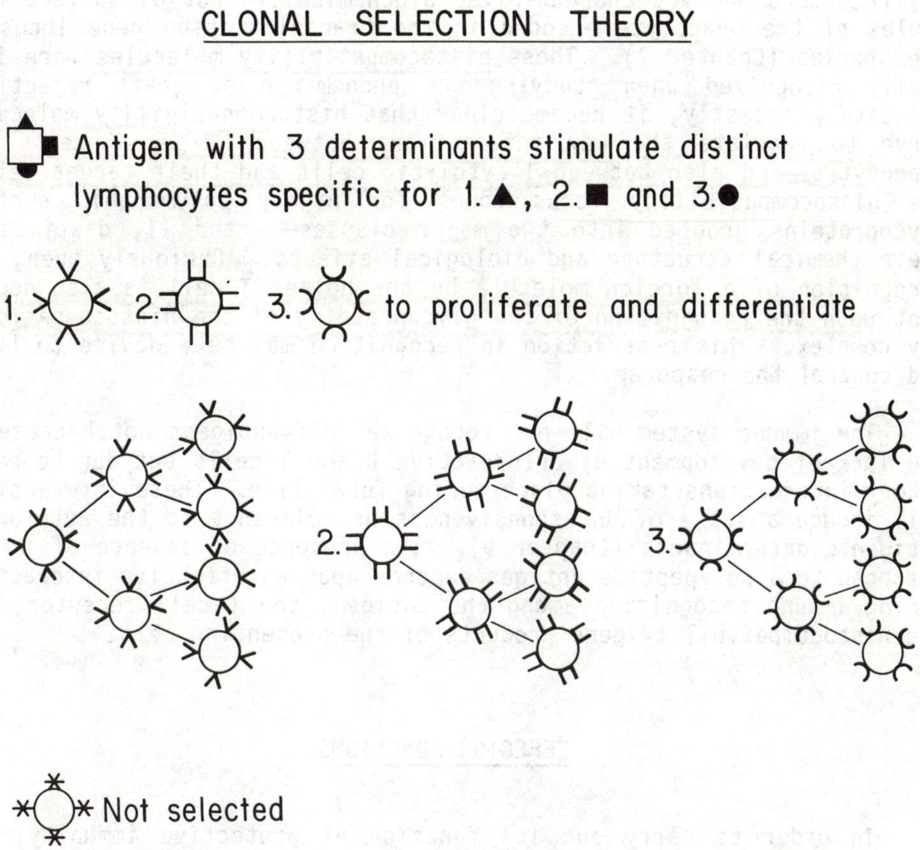

Figure 1.2. The figure depicts Burnet's Clonal Selection Theory. Different determinants on an antigen stimulate the response of different lymphocyte clones, each bearing antibody receptors for one of the determinants.

---

antigen-driven shift in favor of B cells producing antibodies of higher affinity. As antigen is metabolized and its concentration decreases, the high-affinity B cells will be preferentially stimulated to proliferate and differentiate.

The interaction of T helper cells with antigen, which is a fundamental step in the immune process, is highly complex, involving interaction with antigen-handling cells like the mononuclear phagocyte that serve as antigen-presenting cells (Chapters 5, 6, 7, and 8). This interaction involves the recognition by the T cell not only of antigen (by receptors not yet characterized biochemically) but of surface molecules of the phagocyte encoded in the transplantation gene locus of the species (Chapter 7). These histocompatibility molecules were initially recognized when studying the phenomenon of graft rejection. Relatively recently, it became clear that histocompatibility molecules serve to regulate the key interactions between helper T cells and phagocytes—and also between T cytolytic cells and their target cells. The histocompatibility locus codes for highly polymorphic surface glycoproteins grouped into two major classes—I and II, distinct in their chemical structure and biological effects. Curiously then, the recognition of a foreign molecule by the helper T cell is also dependent upon the recognition of the glycoproteins of the histocompatibility complex. This restriction in recognition may be a device to limit and control the response.

The immune system will not recognize self-antigens not because of the lack of development of autoreactive B and T cells but due to regulatory interactions taking place during fetal life. These interactions will induce a state of unresponsiveness or tolerance to the autologous antigenic determinants (Chapter 9). The presence or absence of immune response to a polypeptide antigen depends upon an effective interaction during immune recognition among the antigen, the T cell receptor, and the histocompatibility gene products of the presenting cell.

EFFECTOR FUNCTIONS

In order to carry out its function of protective immunity, the immunological system has developed a widespread number of effector reactions that result from the combination of antibodies with antigen and by the activation of T cells. As mentioned before, antibody molecules belong to five different subclasses. The IgM and IgG molecules are highly effective in fixing and activating complement thus generating a number of molecules that produce acute inflammation (Chapter 12). The IgG molecule, particularly when complexed to antibody and complement, binds avidly to surface structures of neutrophils and macrophages, enabling the complex to be phagocytized at a very high rate. IgG molecules cross the placenta and offer protective immunity to the fetus and the newborn. IgA molecules are found in secretion and serve in the elimination of some bacteria and viruses from mucosal surfaces. IgE molecules are found in trace amounts in blood but bind with very high affinity to mast cells. When antigen binds to the bound IgE, the mast cell degranulates, releasing its potent vasoactive amines that cause vasodilation and increase in permeability. IgE molecules were discovered for their harmful effect—the allergic response is a manifestation of an abnormal IgE antibody response (Chapter 14).

The effector mechanisms also include those mediated by T cells. T cells, by secretion of lymphokines, produce inflammatory reactions which activate macrophages (Chapter 7). These activated macrophages are essential for immunity to many intracellular bacteria and tumors.

In this brief survey, it is important to emphasize two major characteristics of the immune system. These two properties were needed in order for the individual to deal effectively with pathogens and thus for the species to survive and to be preserved. One, the system can recognize, and react to, a wide range of antigens encompassing not only all existing pathogens but, possibly, even those that have not been identified. Two, accompanying the wide library of receptor specificity, very selective effector systems developed, capable of coping with very diverse microbes and parasites. In order for the immune system to function, it, however, has to limit these two properties to foreign —non-self—molecules. Thus, complex cellular interactions and the restrictions imposed by the histocompatibility system developed as a way to critically control autoreactivity. Physiologically, the immune system should react only to non-self.

Finally, a brief mention of immunologically mediated diseases. Many pathological processes develop as a result of an abnormality in the immune process. These disorders range from abnormalities in the development of B or T lymphocytes or accessory cells, to lack of synthesis of complement proteins, to imbalances in regulatory interactions (Chapter 15). Autoimmunity diseases are caused by reactivity against autologous antigens (Chapter 13). The immune system is a network of carefully balanced, competing signals and responses. The immunopathologies are caused by an imbalance in the same mechanisms normally used to protect the individual—antibody, complement, activated macrophages, T cells, etc. (Chapters 13 and 14).

REFERENCES

Burnet, F. M. The Clonal Selection Theory of Acquired Immunity. Cambridge University Press, 1959.

Eisen, H. N. Immunology, Harper and Row, Hagerstown, 1980.

Humphrey, J. H., and White, R. G. Immunology for Students of Medicine, Third Edition. Blackwell Scientific, Great Britain, 1970.

Kabat, E. A., and Mayer, M. M. Experimental Immunochemistry, Second Edition. C. C. Thomas, Springfield, Illinois, 1961.

Klein, J. Immunology—The Science of Self-Nonself Discrimination. Wiley Interscience Publications, New York, 1982.

Landsteiner, K. The Specificity of Serological Reactions. Harvard University Press, Cambridge, Massachusetts, 1945.

Stites, D. P., Stobo, J. D. Fudenberg, H. H., and Wells, J. V. Basic and Clinical Immunology. Lange Medical Publishers, Los Altos, California, 1982.

CHAPTER 2

Antigens

Antigens are those chemical substances capable of inducing a specific immune response. Antigens, in general, do not have a characteristic or specific chemical composition that distinguishes them from analogous substances that are not antigenic; hence, the definition of an antigen is entirely an operational one depending on whether the substance in question stimulates an immune process. Usually, antigens induce the formation of antibody as well as cellular types of immune reactions, although there are instances in which one or the other type is preferentially stimulated. Antigenicity, or as some prefer to define it, immunogenicity, of a molecule depends to a great extent on the degree of foreignness of that molecule; that is, on the phylogenetical relationship betwen host and antigen. For example, rabbits will make an antibody response upon immunization with human albumin but not following immunization with rabbit albumin. The reverse is true; man responds immunologically to rabbit albumin but not to human albumin. Hence, for man, human albumin is not an immunogenic protein. Human and rabbit albumin have the same basic chemical composition except for relatively minor differences "recognized" by one or the other species.

For many years there has been extensive analysis of what makes a material antigenic and how a strong antigen differs from a weak one. The number of molecules that are antigenic for a given species is quite large, reflecting the extensive library of recognition structures available to the immune system. In essence, the antigenicity of a substance ultimately depends on a fine balance between the capacity of the antigen to stimulate the B lymphocyte, the cells destined to become antibody producers and, in most cases, the regulatory "helper" class of T lymphocyte, versus the effects of the same antigen in either not stimulating lymphocytes or in producing a state of tolerance or unresponsiveness (Chapter 9). Tolerance in some cases can result from the activation of the regulatory suppressor T lymphocyte. For a substance to follow one or the other pathway which will produce a positive (immunity) or a negative effect (tolerance and/or no response) depends on many variables, some of which will be considered below. First, a brief explanation of the methods used for studying antigens.

METHODS FOR STUDYING ANTIGENS

Antigens have been studied by various means. One procedure consists of isolating the foreign material, be it a protein, a carbohydrate, or a lipid, and introducing it into experimental animals, which are then assayed for the production of serum antibody or for cellular immune reactivity. Cellular immune reactions are conventionally assayed by skin testing—injecting a small amount into the skin and determining whether it provokes a delayed-type hypersensitivity reaction (Chapter 7). Other more simple and more quantitative tests are now available, consisting of measuring *in vitro* the activity of the T lymphocytes, the cells ultimately responsible for cellular immunity. These tests measure the proliferation of the T lymphocytes or their secretion of biologically active molecules.

Two very important developments in this study of antigenicity were the introduction of *haptens*, extensively studied in the pioneering experiments of Karl Landsteiner and associates, and the use of antigens synthesized in the laboratory.

Haptens. Landsteiner introduced the use of proteins to which small chemical groups (i.e., haptens) had been attached. He and his associates used a number of aromatic amines coupled at alkaline pH to tyrosine, histidine, or lysine side chains of immunogenic protein molecules by way of diazo linkages. The protein molecules were termed *carriers*. By conjugating known chemicals to protein molecules, it became possible to study the immune response directed to well-defined chemical groups. Figures 2.1 and 2.2 give examples of two of the most widely used haptens in immunology.

Immunization with a hapten-protein conjugate results in the production of a heterogeneous population of antibody molecules, the specificity of which can be analyzed *in vitro* using chemically related compounds. This can be done by testing either the same hapten used for immunization, but bound to different carrier proteins, or haptens that differ structurally from the immunizing one at some discrete position of the aromatic rings. Using this approach, Landsteiner and his associates were the first to analyze the fine specificity of antibodies and their capacity to discriminate among very fine chemical differences. This is seen in the example shown in Figure 2.3 taken from their now classical paper (Landsteiner and van der Scher, J. Exp. Med., 63:325, 1936).

The immunization with a hapten-protein conjugate may produce two major sets of antibodies: (1) those specific to the hapten and (2) those specific for the protein. (In some instances, there may be a minor set of antibodies directed to the region of attachment of the hapten to the carrier protein.)

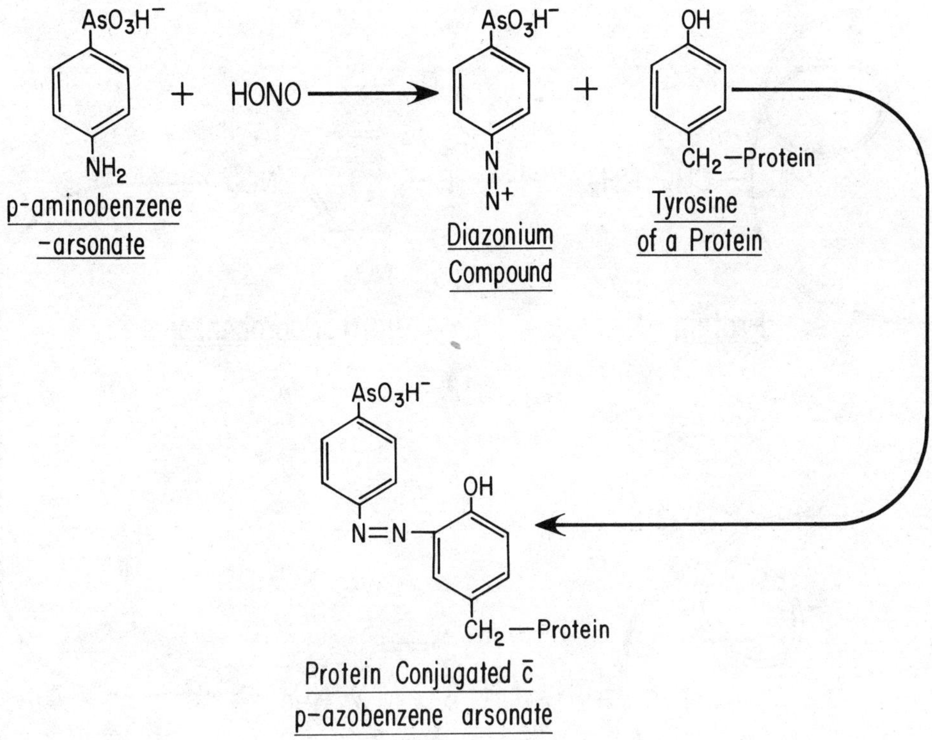

Figure 2.1. A compound like arsanilic acid can be diazotized and coupled to proteins. Conjugation usually takes place on tyrosines of the protein.

Let us consider the example of the dinitrophenyl (DNP) hapten (Figure 2.2). Rabbits immunized with guinea pig albumin containing a number of DNP groups (DNP-guinea pig albumin) make antisera that contains antibodies reactive with guinea pig albumin. (Normally, guinea pig albumin is immunogenic in the rabbit and will elicit antibodies regardless of whether it is chemically conjugated to DNP. These antibodies are produced unless the guinea pig albumin is very heavily conjugated with DNP; in this case, the heaviliy conjugated protein is partially denatured, or its native antigenic determinants are altered or masked.) Antibodies are also produced against the DNP hapten and can be readily identified by appropriate laboratory examinations. These antibodies bind to and precipitate DNP conjugates of carrier proteins unrelated to the one used for immunization, for example, DNP-ovalbumin. In the reaction between the anti-DNP antibodies and the

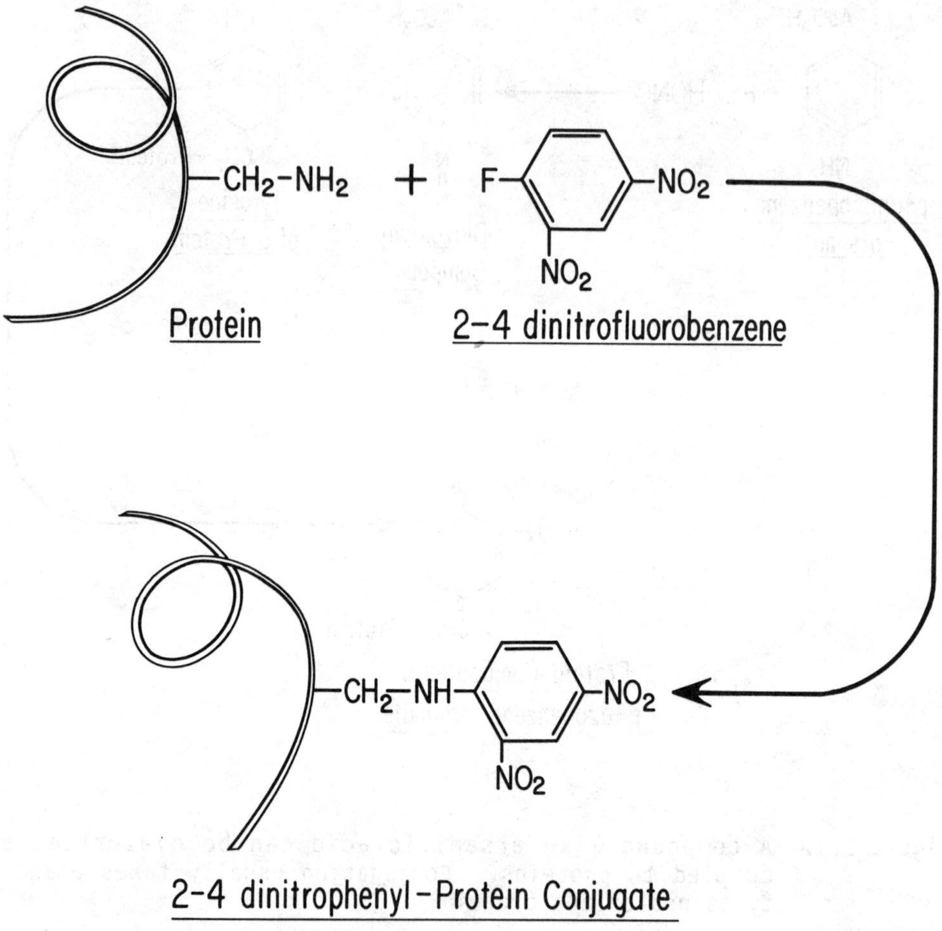

Figure 2.2. Dinitrophenyl groups can be readily conjugated to proteins. Conjugation usually takes place to the epsilon-amino groups of lysine.

DNP-ovalbumin, the addition to the mixture of an excess of unconjugated DNP hapten stops the precipitin reaction. The DNP hapten (DNP-OH) is monovalent (i.e., it binds to a single antibody-combining site). By binding to each of the combining sites of the antibody molecule, the haptens block the interaction with the multivalent DNP-carrier protein required for producing the lattice that leads to the precipitation. Table 2.1 illustrates these points.

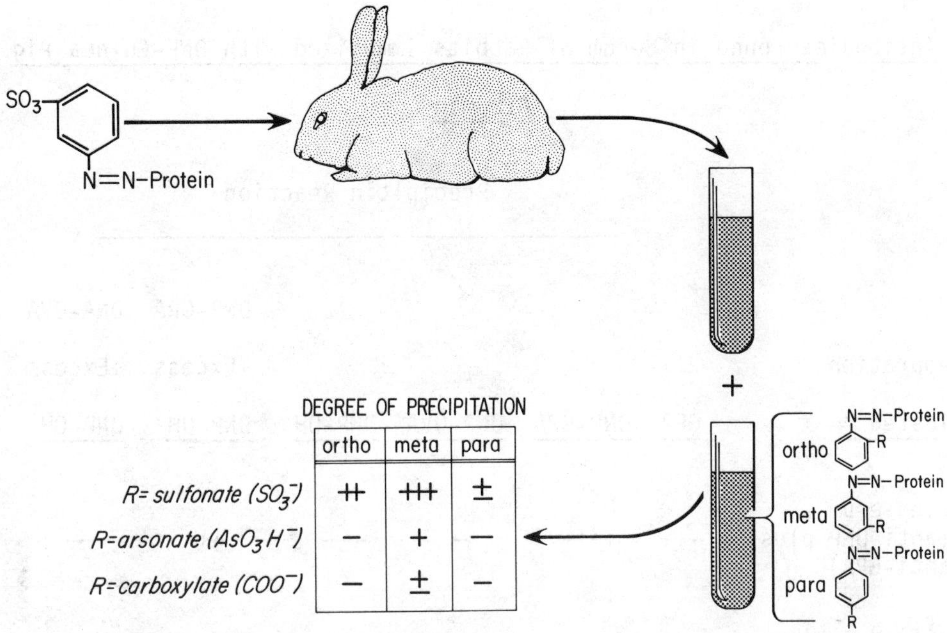

	ortho	meta	para
R= sulfonate (SO_3^-)	++	+++	±
R=arsonate (AsO_3H^-)	—	+	—
R=carboxylate (COO^-)	—	±	—

Figure 2.3. Immunization with meta-aminobenzene sulfonic acid conjugated to horse serum proteins resulted in antisera that, when analyzed in vitro, precipitated maximally with the immunizing antigen but less with aminobenzene arsenic acid and very little with aminobenzoic acid. Furthermore, the antisera were able to discriminate between the position of the acidic residue in the benzene ring; thus, ortho- and para-aminobenzene sulfonic acid precipitated less antibody than the meta derivative. These studies were later refined as more quantitative technology for measuring antibody-antigen reactions was developed.

A most important point to remember is that haptens in an unconjugated form, not bound to a carrier protein, will not produce an immune response. Thus, haptens are defined as those chemical determinants capable of combining with the antibody molecule but unable to stimulate an immune response unless they are chemically associated with an immunogenic carrier molecule. Haptens can be considered then as single antigenic determinants. Natural antigens, proteins, for example, contain different antigenic determinants and can be envisaged as bearing several "natural" haptens.

Table 2.1

Antibodies Found in Serum of Rabbits Immunized with DNP-Guinea Pig Albumin

Preparation Tested	Precipitin Reaction					
	GPA	DNP-GPA	DNP-OVA	DNP-OH	DNP-GPA +Excess DNP-OH	DNA-OVA +Excess DNP-OH
Whole serum (anti-DNP plus anti-GPA)	+++	++++	++	—	++	—
Purified anti-GPA	++	++	—	—	++	—
Purified anti-DNP	—	++	++	—	—	—

DNP-GPA = DNP-guinea pig albumin, the conjugate used for immunization
DNP-OVA = DNP-ovalbumin
DNP-OH = dinitrophenol, the free, unconjugated hapten
GPA = guinea pig albumin
+ = positive precipitation reaction; - no precipitation

The concept of haptens has led to important clinical applications. Antibodies can now be made against innumerable components that are normally not immunogenic because of their small size and/or because of a lack of host responsiveness (natural tolerance to the antigen, genetics, or simply poor immunogenicity). In clinical medicine, antibodies have now been made against most hormones, metabolites such as cyclic AMP and GMP, pharmacologically active peptides, and drugs. These antibodies are used in radioimmunoassay for measuring the amount of antigen (Chapter 4).

Finally, to be immunogenic, haptens need not be associated with a carrier by covalent interactions. There are several examples in which haptens bound to carriers by charge interaction are highly immunogenic. In this regard, DNA is an example of a large non-immunogenic molecule that can elicit a response when introduced bound non-covalently to an immunogenic carrier.

In Chapter 8 we analyze at length the basis of the hapten-carrier reaction in cellular terms which, in brief, represents an example of B-T cell collaboration. In most examples, the haptens are the determinants recognized by B cells under the experimental conditions of assay, while the carrier possesses additional determinants recognized by the T cells and largely responsible for the selective immunogenicity to thymus-dependent antigens.

Synthetic Polypeptides. Another approach to the study of immunogenicity involves the use of peptides made in the laboratory. Polypeptides can be formed of different amino acids linked by peptide bonds. These synthetic polypeptides can consist of homopolymers, polymers made up a of a single amino acid, or random copolymers, polymers made up of two or more amino acids in a random sequence, or block polymers in which small, known peptides are linked together. Any of these three kinds of peptides can be linked to a polypeptide backbone of known sequence to form a multichain copolymer.

The use of synthetic polypeptides has allowed the study of the effect of size, optical configuration, chemical complexity, and metabolism on immunogenicity. Also, and because these compounds have a limited structural heterogeneity—as opposed to many natural proteins made up of multiple determinants—they have been invaluable to study the genetic control of immune responses (Chapter 10).

A representation of one synthetic polypeptide, the (T,G)-A-L molecule is shown in Figure 2.4. This molecule has been used extensively to study the genetic control of immune responses.

FACTORS RESPONSIBLE FOR IMMUNOGENICITY

Several factors contribute to the immunogenicity of a molecule, many of which are interrelated and impossible to separate from one another.

Foreignness. A major requirement for immunogenicity concerns the phylogenetic relationship between host and antigens. Those molecules that are foreign to the host are the ones most capable of stimulating an immune response. In contrast, chemical compounds very close to, or

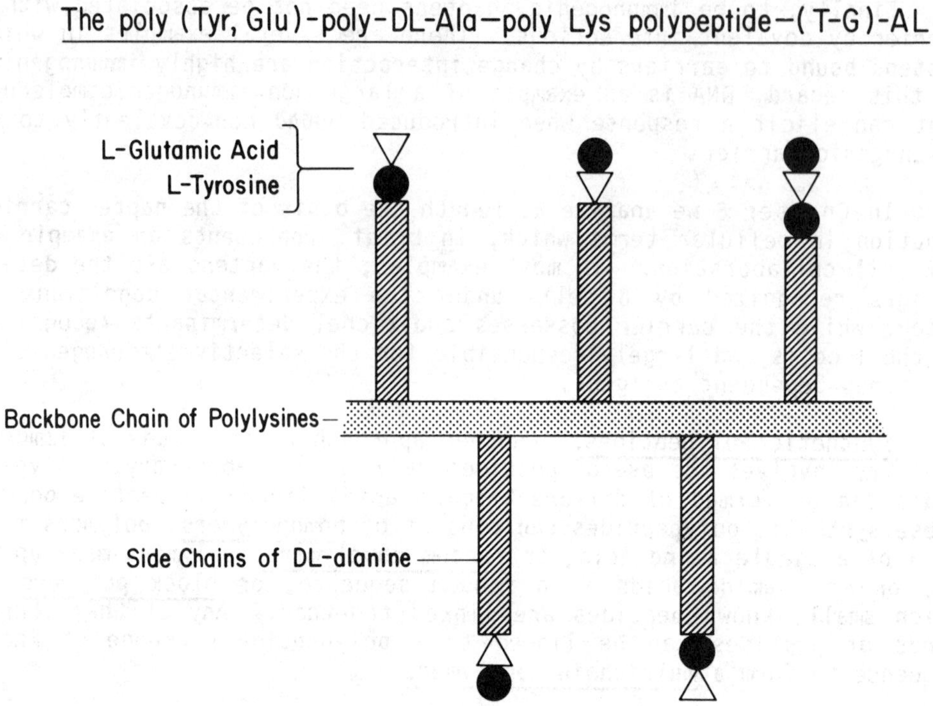

Figure 2.4. The molecule consists of a backbone of L-polylysines to which side chains of DL-alanine are attached. L-tyrosine and L-glutamic acid are placed at the ends of the alanine side chains. Most of the the antibody response is directed to these end groups.

---

identical with, the individual will not stimulate immunity. In general, to elicit antibody responses, the more foreign the antigen in relation to the host, the stronger the antibody responses. This is probably because the host recognizes a larger number of distinct antigenic determinants in the antigen. Thus, for example, the antibody responses that a goat makes against turkey albumin is of greater magnitude than against bovine or sheep albumin. It should be noted, however, that antibody responses can be produced to protein antigens within members of the same species if these differ from each other by subtle chemical differences (isozymes, for example, or Ig allotypes). To obtain such responses, however, one requires strong immunization procedures. In contrast to antibody responses, cellular immunity reactions of lymphocytes against cells and tissue antigens, such as the histocompatibility antigens, are very strong within members of the same species (Chapter 6).

Immunity against self—autoimmunity—can be generated by appropriate immunization, involving chemical changes in the antigen or its association with immunogenic carriers and/or the use of strong adjuvants (Chapter 13 considers these points). The fact that autoimmunity can indeed be produced has led immunologists to postulate that the individual, at least during some stage in its development, does contain specific lymphocytes bearing the recognition structures for self-antigens —as well as those lymphocyte-bearing receptors for foreign ones. The difference between immunity and self-tolerance depends, therefore, on the regulatory interactions that tip the balance toward a positive or negative response.

Chemical Composition of the Antigen. Immune responses can be produced against a wide range of molecules differing in their chemical composition. The most extensively studied antigens are proteins and polysaccharides, which can be strongly immunogenic when administered either in soluble form or as part of a more complex structure, like, for example, a bacterial cell wall. Lipids, steroids, and nucleic acids are either weakly immunogenic, or not at at all, unless they are associated with an immunogenic carrier (the hapten concept discussed above). As a general rule, the more complex the antigen, in terms of both size and chemical composition, the more apt it is to produce a strong immune response. Particulate antigens—bacteria, viruses, foreign red cells—are all very strongly immunogenic materials. Large foreign proteins, for example, hemocyanins, are powerful antigens. In these examples, both size and chemical complexity play a fundamental role.

There is no fixed general rule concerning the size that an antigen must have to be immunogenic, nor is there a good relationship between strength of an antigen and size. Very small natural proteins, the classical example being glucagon of 2,600 daltons, are immunogenic. In general, the larger the antigen, the more the chance of chemical complexity and of the presence of different antigenic determinants within the molecule, which is one of the factors responsible for strong immunogenicity. Some reasons for the increased immunogenicity associated with complex antigens are known. Indeed, the cellular studies of recent years have indicated that: 1) the cooperation between determinants recognized by T cells and those recognized by B cells and 2) the uptake of antigen by the macrophages, are two interrelated and very critical factors in establishing the immunogenicity of an antigen.

One major factor in immunogenicity, then, is the availability and number of determinants in the antigen recognized by helper T cells. This finding has now been analyzed extensively with hapten-carrier conjugates and extended also to natural proteins, such as the glucagon molecule in which one part of the molecule is recognized by T cells and helps in the development of immunity to another part recognized by the B cells (Chapter 8). Genetic studies with synthetic polypeptides carried out in inbred strains of mice have shown that T cell recognition is under a precise genetic control. Different strains differ in their capacity to develop positive immunity to different synthetic polypeptides with limited structural heterogeneity. As an antigen increases in chemical complexity, there will be more opportunity for the individual to possess the cooperating lymphocytes recognizing some or all of the different determinants. In contrast, as the chemical complexity is reduced and the different number of antigenic determinants becomes limiting, then the changes of lacking helper T cells will be higher. Using synthetic polypeptides, it has been found that homopolymers made of L-amino acids are poorly immunogenic. In contrast, polymers of two or more amino acids, depending on the species, are able to induce responses. In many cases, the presence of aromatic acids, in particular tyrosines, becomes an important factor. For example, addition of small peptides containing tyrosine to gelatin will make this poor antigen immunogenic. The general consensus, then, is that diversity in composition is a necessary factor in immunogenicity. Finally, the second reason why large, complex antigens are immunogenic is because they are readily taken up by macrophages. Antigens that bypass uptake by macrophages, because of very small size, are usually poorly immunogenic.

Other important chemical features for immunogenicity have been analyzed, mainly with the use of hapten attached to carrier protein or with synthetic antigens. The shape of the molecule is not a critical factor in immunogenicity. However, the structure of the carrier molecule does play a modulating role in the overall immunogenicity of an antigenic determinant. In this respect, the charge of the molecule and the optical configuration of the antigen are important. Immunization with a hapten bound to carrier proteins that are either negatively or positively charged will elicit anti-hapten antibodies, the average electrical charge of which varies inversely with that of the carrier. Thus, the charge of the carrier plays some role in the selection of the appropriate lymphocyte. However, charge is not an essential factor in that completely uncharged natural molecules such as dextran or, for that matter, synthetic polymers can be immunogenic. The optical configuration determines the extent of metabolism of the antigen. Thus, synthetic polypeptides made up of D-amino acids, which are poorly degraded because of their resistance to proteases, are very poorly immunogenic. Of interest is the fact that D-polypeptides are immunogenic if bound to natural metabolizable proteins (in this case, the D-polypeptide behaves operationally as a hapten). Hence, the overall handling of the molecule and not that of the particular antigenic determinant, plays the critical role.

Route of Immunization and Dose of Antigens. Other important factors in determining immunogenicity are the route of immunization, dose of antigen, immunization schedule, and use of adjuvants. Most particulate antigens—bacteria, red cells, viruses, or large polymers—elicit antibodies after inoculation by intracutaneous or intravenous routes, at a broad range of doses. In contrast, many of the soluble proteins and carbohydrates require more critical immunization schedules, sometimes involving several inoculations. With these antigens, the amounts used for immunization may be critical, and the addition of adjuvants may be necessary to boost the response. In these cases, conditions that usually lead to increased uptake of the antigen by the phagocytes or to an inflammatory reaction, enhance immunogenicity.

Adjuvants refers to a number of materials that are used to augment an immune response. Many of the adjuvants are bacteria or their products such as killed *Bordetella pertussis* or endotoxins from Gram-negative organisms. Killed mycobacteria are particularly powerful adjuvants; for example, inoculated together with known protein antigens, they increase the response by severalfold. The use of dead tubercle bacillus incorporated in water-in-oil emulsions (Freund's adjuvant) is a popular way to augment responses to proteins in experimental work. The mode of action of adjuvants is complex. Most adjuvants act by increasing macrophage and T cell helper function.

Genetics. This is a critical factor that is analyzed in Chapter 10.

Cellular Interactions. Many antigens interact with T lymphocytes and stimulate their various functional responses. These include most proteins, either in soluble form or as part of the structure of a microorganism or a cell surface. Carbohydrates, in contrast, stimulate T lymphocytes to a very limited extent, if at all. With regard to B cell stimulation, antigens are customarily grouped into two sets, depending on whether there is a requirement for T lymphocytes to cooperate for the production of antibody. *Thymic-dependent antigens are those that require the interaction of B cells with antigen in the presence of specific T helper cells. These include most protein antigens. Thymic-independent antigens stimulate B cells with a very limited participation, or in the apparent absence, of T lymphocytes.* Usually, it follows that thymic-independent antigens interact poorly with T lymphocytes. Thymic-independent antigens include the lipopolysaccharides of Gram-negative bacteria (LPS) and many carbohydrates in which the antigenic determinant is repeated in the molecule several times. The response to many but not all thymic-independent antigens is restricted to IgM antibodies and shows poor immunological memory. Many, but not all, thymic-independent antigens stimulate large numbers of B cells to multiply and differentiate to antibody secretion—these are considered to be *polyclonal* activators and are not restricted to stimulating those B cells having specific receptors for the antigenic determinants. The best example is LPS. LPS at high doses interacts with many sets of B cells and stimulates their proliferation and differentiation to antibody-secreting cells. The antibody-secreting cells make the antibody to which they were genetically committed regardless of the nature of the stimuli. At limiting doses, however, the LPS binds *preferentially* to the B cell clones having specific receptors to LPS; and the antibody will be mostly anti-LPS antibodies.

SOME BIOLOGICAL CONSIDERATIONS

What is the structure of the antigenic determinants of an antigen molecule recognized by B cells and antibodies? A complex protein or a polysaccharide antigen contains various antigen determinants, some of which are more powerful than others in stimulating antibody responses; hence, there will be particularly immunodominant groups in a molecule. A particular factor in immunodominance is the accessibility of the determinant. Those antigenic groups that are hydrophilic and exposed to the aqueous environment are apt to be immunodominant in contrast to those that are hidden and folded within the molecule. Immunodominant groups are strongly represented by the end of amino acid chains or sugar side chains. In the example of the (TG)A-L polypeptide shown in Figure 2.4, the antibodies are mostly directed to the tyrosyl-glutamyl (TG) part of the antigen and not to the alanyl (A) side chain. If the sequence of side chains is reversed so that the TG is attached directly to the polylysyl backbone and the alanyl chains are now at the end, then the antibodies are directed mostly to the alanyl groups and not to the TG.

What is the actual size of the antigen determinant? It is small and represented by a structure that has complementarity to the antibody-combining site—of about 35 x 10 Å. The size of the antigen determinant has been estimated for proteins or sugars by determining the minimal size of a particular polypeptide chain or sugar side chain required to inhibit antigen-antibody precipitin reaction. Using the dextran system, the pioneering studies of E. Kabat and associates estimated the site to fit about a hexasaccharide; with protein, the antibody-combining site can accommodate four to eight amino acids. This point is also considered in Chapter 3.

FATE OF THE ANTIGEN

Usually, the bulk of the antigen introduced into an individual is degraded and eliminated as amino acids and/or small peptides. The exception to this are the peptides formed of D-amino acids that bypass catabolism. As mentioned before, these are very weak antigens.

What do the different kinds of lymphocytes recognize when an antigen is introduced? The native antigen? The antigen degraded extensively? The primary amino acid composition or part of the antigen? A new structure, the antigen somehow associated with a tissue structure? These questions are at the heart of a crucial and difficult area of immunology, to which we have only partial answers.

There is variation in the fate of antigens, depending to a great extent upon their chemical composition. Several situations, which are not mutually exclusive, have been observed:

1. Antigen is recognized before extensive degradation. It appears that for globular proteins the B lymphocytes recognize the protein before it suffers extensive degradation by the normal catabolic processes. The B lymphocyte recognizes antigen by way of a membrane-bound Ig, then differentiates following complex steps, to a cell that secretes antibody **having the same property of combining with antigen as the receptor Ig** (Chapter 5). Thus, sampling the serum antibody and studying whether it combines with antigen in its native state or in a denatured form indicates whether the antigen was recognized prior to, or after, biochemical changes took place. The answer is that the antibody is directed mostly to the protein in its native state, to conformational determinants. What happens if you immunize with a denatured, unfolded protein? Will the individual make antibodies to it? Yes. Globular proteins, if denatured and then injected into animals, will give rise to antibodies that bind part of the primary amino acid sequence of the protein and not the protein in its native state. These are antibodies to sequential determinants. It is obvious, then, that sets of B cells are found in an individual with receptors capable of recognizing conformational or sequential determinants. Yet, when one immunizes with a globular protein, the B cells that are usually selected by antigen are those having the receptors for conformational determinants. Hence, the conclusion is that the protein antigens must be recognized by the B cells, to a great extent, **before there is extensive alteration by the normal catabolic processes**.

2. Recognition after some degradation. **In contrast to the recognition globular proteins by B cells, T cells recognize many globular proteins following their partial denaturation (T cells usually interact with antigen in association with a macrophage)**. For example, immunization with ribonuclease results in antibodies that are directed mostly to conformational determinants, while the T cell reactivity (in the form of delayed skin reactions) is directed to sequential determinants of the ribonuclease. **It should be emphasized now that the recognition** of antigen by T lymphocytes is regulated by the major histocompatibility gene complex of the species (Chapters 8 and 10).

With some bacteria, antibodies are produced to some antigenic determinants that are produced only after enzymatic digestion. For example, infection with Group A streptococci gives rise to antibodies that react with A carbohydrate but also to some antibodies that react with an A "variant". The normal antibodies to A carbohydrate recognize mainly n-acetylglucosamine; those of the A variant recognize rhamnose, which is accessible only following hydrolysis of n-acetylglucosamine by enzymes.

3. Recognition after biochemical changes in the host. The most extensive example are those of small compounds that undergo metabolism and become incorporated into proteins, being, in fact, transformed into hapten-carriers that are immunogenic. For example, penicillin is immunogenic after extensive chemical changes resulting in a highly reactive material that conjugates to proteins producing a new immunogen. Penicillin is degraded to penicillenic acid, which is highly reactive, eventually leading to the formation of penicilloyl-protein conjugates. Another important example is the skin sensitivity to small chemicals. The chemicals conjugate to skin proteins, forming immunogenic compounds. The most frequent conjugates involve some plant products like the urushiol of poison ivy, or heavy metals like nickel (Chapter 6).

BLOOD GROUPS

Knowledge of blood group antigens is essential since blood transfusions are used extensively in medicine. Early attempts to transfer blood from one person to another frequently had disastrous results. This was the case even when the intended recipient had never previously received blood. The existence of "naturally occurring" antibodies to certain highly immunogenic antigens on red cells was the cause of this problem. The blood group systems include the ABO, Rh, Lewis, MN, P, Kell, Duffy, and Kidd. The ABO and Rh are the most important and will be the only ones discussed here.

The ABO System. The ABO system includes four different blood groups: A, B, AB, and O. This designation of each blood group is that of the antigen present on the red cell surface. Thus, Type A individuals have A antigen; Type B have B antigens; AB have both; and O have neither. Since there is generally tolerance to self-antigens, we can predict that no individual will have antibodies against an antigen on their own red cells. The unexpected fact is that we all have easily detectable levels of antibodies against whichever antigen we lack. Thus, a Type A individual has anti-B; a Type B has anti-A, Type O has both anti-A and anti-B; and Type AB has neither. Most of the naturally occurring anti-A and anti-B antibodies are of the IgM class (Chapter 3). These arise presumably as a result of immunity to similar or cross-reacting antigens found in the bacteria of intestinal tract.

The antigens of the ABO system are complex oligosaccharides located on the red cell surface. Similar saccharides are quite common in the animal and plant world. Figure 2.5 shows the structure of the terminal end of the molecules that make up the ABO system. Each of the sugars is added sequentially by enzymes that are under genetic control.

The ABO system is under the control of a genetic locus with three major alleles--A, B, and O--with A and B dominant over O. Table 2.2

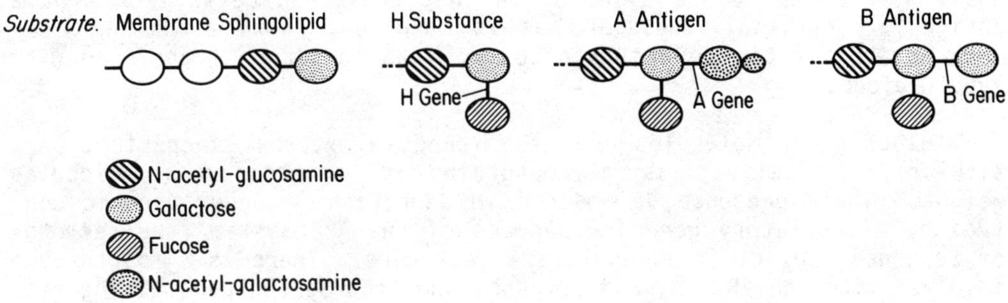

Figure 2.5. Structure of molecules in the ABO system. The genes responsible for the production of the A and B red blood cell antigens are glycosyltransferases. These enzymes add terminal carbohydrates to the H substance which serves as backbone for the two antigens. The A gene is responsible for the addition of N-acetylgalactosamine, while the B gene adds galactose, forming, respectively, the A and B antigens. The H substances is created when a fucosyl transferase adds fucose to the terminal galactose.

---

shows the possible genotypes, the corresponding red cell phenotypes, and the serum antibodies found in each case.

The blood group molecules on the red cells are formed by a single large polysaccharide attached to sphingolipids. To the polysaccharide are added the various sugars that form the A or B antigens. The addition of fucose by a fucosyl transferase creates the H substance which is not an antigen in normal individuals (all individuals have the H substance and, therefore, are immunologically unresponsive to it). The H substance is an obligatory precursor for the expression of the A or B genes. The fucosyl transferase required for production of the H substance is under control of genes (H gene) different from the ABO genes. The addition of n-acetyl galactosamine to the terminal galactose of the H substance creates the A antigen. The A gene codes for the enzyme responsible for this addition. (Individuals not having the A gene, and therefore not having the A antigen in their red cells, will be able to make antibodies to it; in fact, all such persons have naturally acquired antibodies thought to come about by exposure to environmental A substance.) In individuals having the B gene, there is addition of galactose to the terminal galactose of the H substance creating the B antigen.

There are rare individuals who lack the fucosyl transferase needed to add fucose and create the H substance. These rare individuals will appear to be Group O (in that their red cells lack A or B antigen). The individuals with this mutation, known as Bombay, can make antibodies to the H substance and thus cannot be transfused with Type O blood.

Blood group molecules are also found in external secretion, particularly in saliva, as glycoproteins of heterogeneous molecular weight. Their presence or absence in secretion is under genetic control by a regulatory gene independent of the ABO system (the secretor or Se gene); 80% of individuals are secretors. There is a fourth gene involved with the ABO, H, and Se gene, and that is the gene giving rise to the Lewis blood group antigen. Lewis represents a system of soluble antigen found in saliva and plasma. The red cells do not produce the Lewis antigens but instead acquire it from plasma. The expression of the main two Lewis specificities depends on an interaction between the H and Se gene. The Lewis gene codes for a fucosyl transferase that attaches fucose to the core polysaccharide at the next to the last sugar moiety.

In blood banks, red cells are typed by mixing them with antisera containing a high titer of antibody against one of the antigens, resulting in agglutination of the red cells. These sera are usually obtained from individuals who have been accidently mistransfused or from women who have borne children of another blood type.

It is clear that there are two ways to obtain a transfusion mismatch. In one case the recipient may have antibodies against the transfused red cells. This is avoided by giving the proper blood group. If this were the only consideration, it would be perfectly safe

Table 2.2

Genotype	Red Cell Phenotype	Serum Antibodies
A/A	A	anti-B
A/O	A	anti-B
B/B	B	anti-A
B/O	B	anti-A
O/O	O	anti-A and anti-B
A/B	AB	none

to give any blood to an AB individual and Type O blood to anyone. (Indeed, it is fairly safe; and in war or other emergency, Type O blood is valued as a universal donor.) However, the transfused blood, although relatively small in volume, does contain plasma and hence antibodies. In usual medical practices, only precisely matched blood is given; after typing with conventional antisera, a cross-match and a back-cross are done by mixing the recipient's serum with the prospective donor's red cells and vice versa to check for the presence of any incompatibility due to antigens other than ABO (of which there are many, but most are weakly immunogenic and less often a problem).

The Rh System—Erythroblastosis Fetalis. This is another system of red cell antigens that is less well understood and has not been chemically characterized but has assumed great importance and has led to one of the greatest therapeutic triumphs for immunology. Rh stands for Rhesus. The system was first discovered by Landsteiner and Weiner (1940), who serendipitously found that rabbit antibodies to Rhesus monkey red cells agglutinated the red cells of 80% of normal humans. The antigen in human red cells was called Rh. At about the same time (1939), Levine and Stetson found antibodies in the serum of a woman who had delivered a stillborn. The antibodies were later found to be anti-Rh antibodies made by the mother against Rh antigens of the fetus.

There are a very large number of antigens detected in the Rh system, many of which cross-react and are difficult to sort out—most of them are weakly immunogenic and seldom cause trouble, with the exception of one antigen, known variously as D or Rho. Perhaps the easiest way to understand the Rh system is to think of three antigenic sites, each of which has two alternative antigens. One of these is D, which may be either present or absent—thus defining what is usually called Rh positive or Rh negative. In addition, there are C, c, E, and e—for each pair only one alternative is present. Possible combinations include Dce, DCe, DcE, DCE, ce Ce, cE, and CE. Each of these combinations is coded for by a single gene. A little thought reveals that there are thirty-two possible genotypes.

Typing in the Rh system can be very complex, and its complexity is increased because the antigens are weak, and antisera to them do not cause as strong agglutination as the ABO antisera do. Special techniques are used to detect Rh determinants such as doing the agglutination in solutions of albumin or other charged molecules. Such molecules decrease the surface charge of the red cells and hence their mutual repulsion—this makes agglutination easier. There are two reasons why some red cell antigens are difficult to detect; one is that the antibodies to them are primarily of the IgG class. IgG is less good at agglutinating because it has only two binding sites compared to ten for IgM. The other reason is that some antigens such as Rh are quite sparsely distributed on the red cell surface, decreasing the probability of cross-linking the red cells.

Another technique used to detect the presence of weak antigens or antibodies is the indirect Coombs test. In this test, a serum, either that of a prospective transfusion recipient or a typing serum, is mixed with red cells, and the unbound antibody is washed away. Then a Coombs reagent which is an anti-immunoglobulin antibody (for example, a rabbit anti-human globulin) is added. The second antibody creates much greater agglutination because it amplifies the cross-linking effect of the first antibody.

When the D antigen is present on red cells, the person is said to be Rh positive regardless of the status of the other antigens of the Rh system. There are no detectable natural antibodies to D either in Rh-negative or Rh-positive individuals. The only way to develop such antibodies is for an Rh-negative individual to receive Rh-positive red cells. This may obviously occur as the result of a mismatched transfusion that will cause no trouble for the recipient because of the absence of natural antibodies. (However, subsequent transfusion with Rh-positive blood can cause hemolysis.) Another important route by which an Rh-negative person may receive Rh-positive cells is for an Rh-negative mother to give birth to an Rh-positive child. Since D is dominant, such a child must have been fathered by an Rh-positive man. It is very common for maternal and child blood to mix at the time of delivery due to disruption of the highly vascular placenta. The first occurrence of such a transfusion of the child's blood into the mother causes no problem; however, the mother will be immunized and will proceed to make antibody directed to D over the following several weeks. With a subsequent pregnancy, the mother's anti-D response will be boosted by small amounts of Rh-positive red cells from the fetus. She will make large amounts of IgG antibodies directed against D that will cross the placenta and induce hemolysis in the fetus. Such a fetus is in serious trouble for two reasons. First, it is going to be anemic in utero and may develop heart failure (hydrops) with edema and even death in utero. Second, it will have a very large load of hemoglobulin free in the circulation that will be converted to bilirubin. The fetal liver is unable to excrete much bilirubin until after birth so that high levels accumulate and cause tissue damage, especially in the brain (kernicterus).

This condition, known as erythroblastosis fetalis, can be diagnosed by: 1) the history of a previous Rh-positive child born to an Rh-negative woman; and 2) the presence of Rh-positive cells and/or a high level of bilirubin found in the fetus by amniocentesis (the draining of amniotic fluid or fetal blood by a long needle in the uterus). It is usually treated by exchange transfusion of Rh-negative red cells into the fetus in utero and by inducing early birth with intensive exchange transfusion and measures to reduce bilirubin levels immediately after birth. The treatment is difficult, and death or brain damage sometimes occur. The same disease process called isoimmune hemolytic disease of the newborn can occur due to incompatibilities other than Rh, but the others are much less common.

Erythroblastosis fetalis shows promise of being almost totally eliminated by a very clever application of immunotherapy. It was noted that the presence of an ABO incompatibility prevented maternal immunization. For example, an O, Rh-negative mother would give birth to an A-positive child but would not become immunized against D. The precise explanation for this was not clear, but the observation led to the concept of giving the mother a high titer of anti-D antibodies around the time of delivery in the hope of preventing Rh sensitization. This procedure has been dramatically successful and prevents sensitization with a very high reliability. Since it has been widely applied, the incidence of erythroblatosis has dropped dramatically. It is now standard practice in every hospital to give any Rh-negative woman an injection of concentrated gamma globulin from a donor with a high titer of anti-D within twenty-four hours of delivery of an Rh-positive, ABO-compatible child or at the time of suspected miscarriage if there was any possibility of an Rh incompatibility. Administration of anti-D, however, is not very helpful for women who are already sensitized.

The mechanism by which the administration of antibody prevents the immune response is not known for certain. Likely possibilities include: 1) the antibody binds to fetal red cells as they enter the maternal circulation and covers the antigen; or 2) causes the red cells to be phagocytized before they can stimulate an immune response; or 3) the presence of the antibody complexed to the antigen might induce a transient state of tolerance to the antigen—this phenomenon has been demonstrated in experimental systems.

Regardless of the mechanism, the ability to prevent an immune response is a powerful tool that may see application to other diseases. The prerequisites for such therapy to be successful are that we know exactly the offending antigens and that exposure to the antigen is transient or self-limiting.

REFERENCES

Goodman, J. W. Antigenic determinants and antibody combining sites. In: The Antigens, M. Sela, ed. Academic Press, Inc., New York, 3: 127, 1975.

Landsteiner, K. The Specificity of Serological Reactions. Harvard University Press, Cambridge, Massachusetts, second edition, 1945.

Race, R. R., and Sanger, R. Blood Groups in Man. Blackwell, Oxford, England, sixth edition, 1976.

Reichlin, M. Amino acid substitution and the antigenicity of globular proteins. Adv. Immunol., 3:71, 1975.

Zmijewski, C. M. Immunohematology. Appleton, Century, Crofts, New York, third edition, 1978.

CHAPTER 3

Antibodies and Their Functions

Protein molecules that combine specifically with antigens are termed antibodies; collectively, proteins with antibody activity are referred to as immunoglobulins. Alternative designations that have, in the past, been applied to these proteins include the term gamma globulins which arose from the observation that the bulk of serum antibody molecules migrated electrophoretically in the gamma region (see Chapter 4). All immunoglobulin molecules have a common structure consisting of four polypeptide chains, two large and two small, arranged as shown in Figure 3.1. The large polypeptide chain is termed the heavy or H chain; the smaller one is termed the light or L chain. Human immunoglobulins have been assigned to five classes based on primary structure of their respective heavy chains; these classes are IgG, IgA, IgM, IgD, and IgE; the respective heavy chains are gamma, alpha, mu, delta, and epsilon. There are two types of light chains, kappa and lambda. In human serum, approximately 65% of IgG molecules have two gamma heavy chains and two kappa light chains, while 35% have two gamma heavy chains and two lambda light chains. The same distribution applies for circulating IgA and IgM molecules; the kappa/lambda ratio for IgD and IgE molecules has not yet been established (Figure 3.2). This chapter describes in detail human immunoglobulin which, together with mouse and rabbit immunoglobulin, are the most thoroughly studied. The conclusions drawn from studies in humans are readily applicable to all species.

IMMUNOGLOBULIN G

Since much of our knowledge of immunoglobulin structure was derived from studies performed with IgG molecules, these experiments will be reviewed briefly. R. Porter, in 1959, demonstrated that treatment of rabbit IgG antibody molecules with the enzyme papain, in the presence of cysteine, separated the molecule into two major fragments.

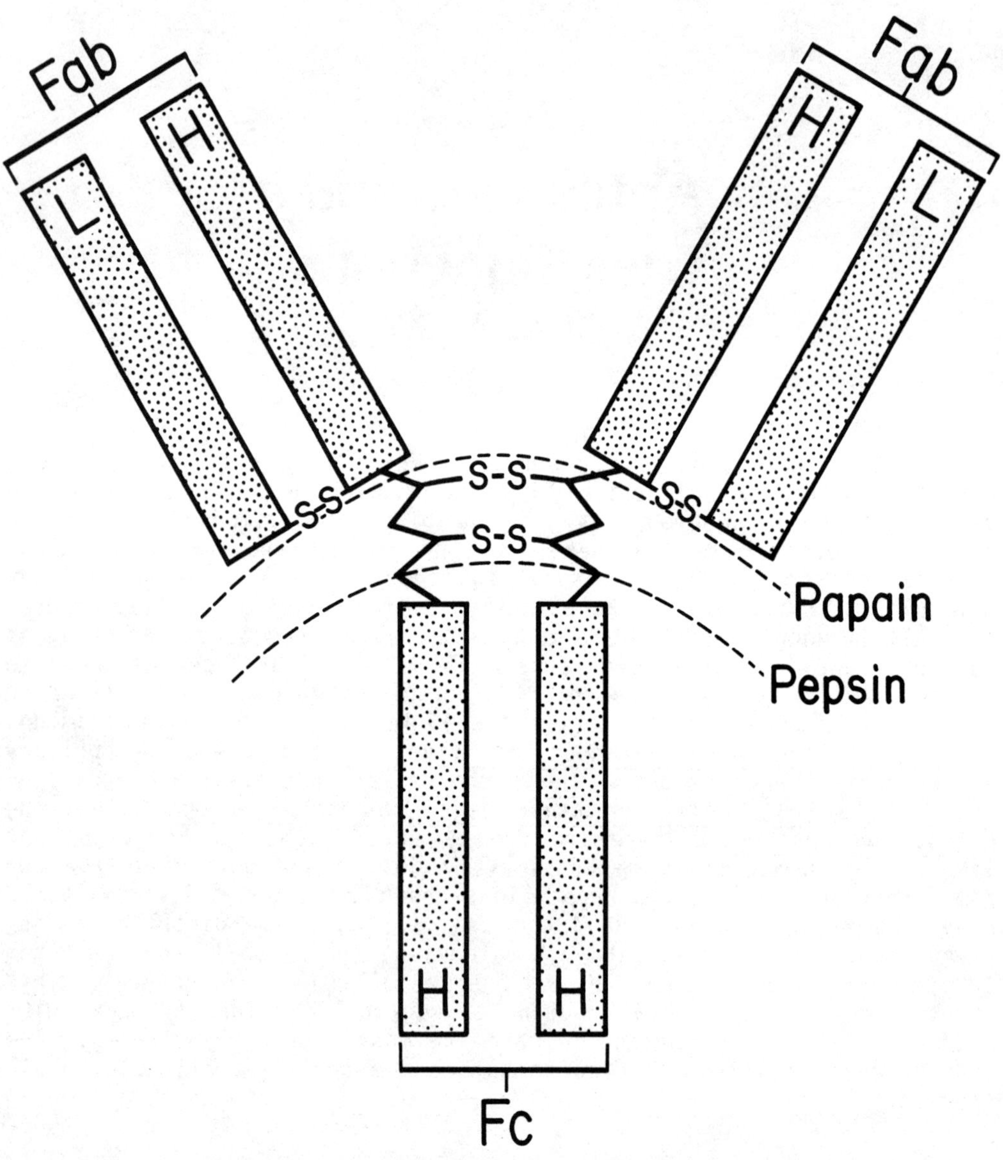

Figure 3.1. Schematic representation of an IgG antibody molecule. A pocket or cleft capable of binding the same unique determinant is present in each Fab fragment; certain biological properties of IgG antibody molecules reside in sites or configurations present on the Fc fragment. The approximate sites of cleavage by the enzymes papain and pepsin are shown.

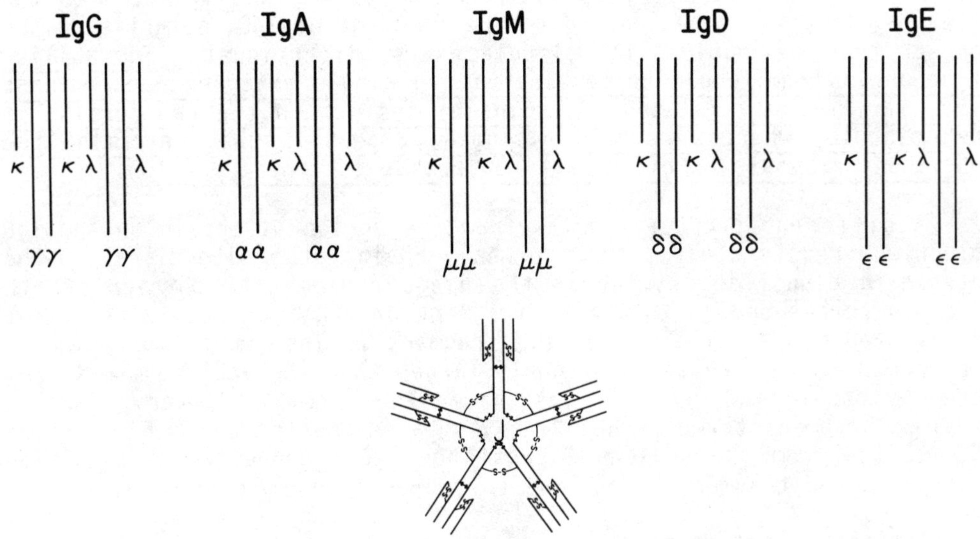

Figure 3.2 Schematic representation of the five classes of human immunoglobulins. Differences among the classes reside in the primary structure of their heavy chains; two kappa or two lambda light chains are found on a certain percentage of the monomers in each class. Circulating IgM antibody molecules consist of five IgM monomers combined into a pentameric structure which also contains the J or joining chain. (The S-S bonds between light and heavy chains as well as those between heavy chains are not shown in the stick diagrams in the upper portion of the figure.)

One of these fragments retained the antigen-binding capacity of the intact molecule and hence was termed Fab fragment (ab refers to antigen binding). The other fragment did not combine with antigen but was readily crystallizable and hence was called Fc fragment (c refers to crystallizable). Each fragment had a molecular weight of approximately 50,000 daltons; Fab fragments accounted for approximately two-thirds and the Fc fragments for one-third of the papain-digested IgG. It is now known that papain cleaves immunoglobulin G approximately in the middle of the heavy chain in a segment called the hinge region. Cysteine appears to have had a dual function: activation of the enzyme papain and reduction of some disulfide links between the heavy chains.

The subsequent discovery that certain biologic properties of antibody molecules, such as transport across the maternal-fetal membranes, interaction with the classical complement system, and fixation to the heterologous tissues resided in the Fc fragment of IgG, established the concept that immunoglobulin molecules were bifunctional. The ability of an antibody molecule to combine with a single antigenic determinant (or a very closely related determinant) resides in the Fab portion of the molecule, whereas certain biologic properties that determine the subsequent disposition of the antigen reside in the Fc portion.

A different product results from the action of pepsin on the IgG molecule. Pepsin cleaves the IgG heavy chains at a site distal to the interchain disulfide bridges in the hinge region; the portion of the molecule corresponding to the Fc fragment produced by papain treatment is digested by pepsin into peptide fragments. The two antigen-binding fragments, each of which is slightly larger than the Fab fragments produced by papain and hence is designated Fab', remain linked. Thus, a bivalent fragment termed F(ab')2, having a sedimentation coefficient of 5S, results from the action of pepsin on IgG. Reduction of disulfide bond(s) in the fragment gives rise to two antigen-binding fragments.

Additional information on the structure of IgG was provided by G. Edelman, who treated these molecules with reducing agents in the presence of urea. This treatment led to a decrease in molecular weight, suggesting that the IgG molecule consisted of disulfide-linked peptide chains. Less drastic reduction (resulting in the splitting of only a few disulfide bridges), followed by treatment with propionic acid, permitted the separation by gel filtration of two components with molecular weight of 50,000 and 25,000 daltons. The function of propionic or other organic acids in these experiments was to overcome noncovalent hydrophobic bonds between the peptide chains and to impose positive charges upon the chains leading to their mutual repulsion. Based on the molecular weight of the original IgG molecule (150,000) and the porportion of high and low molecular weight components, it was concluded that such molecules consisted of two heavy and two light polypeptide chains.

Subsequently, reduction and alkylation of the Fab fragment followed by gel filtration in urea and propionic acid led to the recovery of one light chain and the amino terminal one-half of a heavy chain designated the Fd fragment. The relationship between fragments and chains was clarified and the model of immunoglobulin structure shown in Figure 3.1 was adopted. It should be emphasized that, in addition to the disulfide bridges between the peptide chains, there are a number of other intermolecular forces contributing to the stability of the four-chain structure.

Properties of IgG: IgG molecules have a molecular weight of 150,000 and a sedimentation coefficient of 7S. Each molecule consists of two kappa or two lambda light chains and two gamma heavy chains.

Table 3.1

Characteristics of Human Immunoglobulins: Classes and Subclasses

	IgG	IgA	IgM	IgD	IgE
Heavy chain	Gamma	Alpha	Mu	Delta	Epsilon
Subclasses	Gamma 1,2,3,4	Alpha 1,2	Mu 1,2	—	—
Light chain	Kappa or Lambda	Kappa or Lambda	Kappa or Lambda	Kappa or Lambda	Kappa or Lambda
J chain	—	±	+	—	—

Four subclasses of IgG have been identified on the basis of antigenic and structural differences residing in the heavy chains designated gamma-1, gamma-2, gamma-3, and gamma-4. The relative distribution of these four subclasses among serum IgG molecules is 65 to 70%, 23 to 28%, 4 to 7%, and 3 to 4% for IgG1, IgG2, IgG3, and IgG4, respectively. Some differences among the subclasses include the anodal migration on electrophoresis of IgG2 and IgG4 and the cathodal migration of IgG1 and IgG3, as well as the greater molecular weight of the gamma-3 heavy chain 60,000 daltons, compared to 52,000 for gamma-1 and gamma-2. Tryptic peptide maps of Fc fragments indicated that seventeen to twenty-two of the twenty-four peptides were shared between the four subclasses. Differences in tryptic peptides ranged from four between gamma-1 and gamma-2 to eighteen between gamma-3 and gamma-4. There appears to be no difference in the carbohydrate content of the subclass proteins. Treatment with pepsin, papain, and trypsin has shown considerable variation in susceptibility to enzymatic digestion of the different subclasses of IgG. Limited information is available on their metabolism; IgG3 appears to have the shortest plasma half-life, lowest synthetic and highest catabolic rate of the four subclasses. IgG3 molecules are also characterized by an unusually large number of inter-heavy chain disulfide bonds.

The antibody response to some antigens is characterized by a proportional representation of IgG antibodies of all four subclasses, but there is a tendency for certain antibodies to be associated primarily with one of the subclasses. Spontaneously occurring antibodies to clotting factors in patients tend to be IgG4 proteins. Antibodies to certain carbohydrates such as dextran tend to be IgG2 proteins. Subclass restriction has been observed among anti-nuclear antibodies; for example, anti-DNA antibodies are found primarily in the IgG1 and IgG3 subclasses.

Table 3.2

Characteristics of Human Immunoglobulins

	IgG	IgA	IgM	IgD	IgE
Molecular weight	150,000	150,000-350,000	900,000	180,000	190,000
Sedimentation coefficient ($S_{20}w$)	7	7(9-15)	19	7	8
Carbohydrate (approximate percent)	3	7	12	12	12
Biological survival (plasma T-1/2 days)	21	6	5	3	2
Placental transfer	+	—	—	—	—
Activation of classical complement system	+	—	+	—	—
Serum concentration (mg per 100 ml)	1,100	250	100	3	.01

IMMUNOGLOBULIN M

IgM has a molecular weight of about 900,000 daltons. Each molecule consists of five identical subunits of about 180,000 daltons, consisting of two kappa or lambda light chains and two mu heavy chains. The latter have a molecular weight of about 70,000. Five monomeric units are formed in a circle via disulfide bonds between heavy chains of the subunits to form a pentamer. In addition, the IgM molecule contains an additional chain, the J or joining chain. Based on the presence of ten Fab units, it would be expected that IgM antibody molecules would have an antigen-binding valence of ten. While this value is found experimentally for some IgM antibody molecules, it has not been found in all instances, a valence of five being observed in some cases. This disparity in valence is as yet unexplained. Most, but not all IgM antibodies appear to be capable of interacting with the classical complement sequence in the presence of antigen. The complement binding site is present on the heavy chain of the antibody molecule in the Cmu4 domain (see discussion of domain concept below).

Two types of oligosaccharide units are present in IgM; "simple" consisting of mannose and N-acetylglucosamine and "complex" consisting of mannose, N-acetylglucosamine, fucose, galactose and sialic acid. These carbohydrate units are attached to the Cmu3 domain.

The J chain is a component only of polymeric immunoglobulins of many species such as IgM, and IgA. Based on electrophoretic mobility, antigenic cross-reactivity and equable content of amino acids, few differences exist among the J chains of diverse species. J chain was first recognized when polymeric immunoglobulins were subjected to cleavage of disulfide bonds and subsequent analysis by electrophoretic procedures. J chain appeared as a band of protein migrating anodally faster than L chains of immunoglobulins. Subsequently this fraction was isolated and antisera to J chain were prepared. Studies conducted with these antisera disclosed that J chain antigenic determinants are rarely accessible in intact polymeric immunoglobulins; J chain antigenic determinants are revealed after denaturation.

The J chain consists of approximately 118-125 amino acid and 7 to 8 carbohydrate residues for a molecular weight of about 15,000 daltons. An unusual aspect of the amino acid composition is the presence of six cysteine residues. According to one model, two cysteine residues are involved in linking J chain to two of the five subunits of IgM; the remainder presumably being utilized for the formation of intrachain disulfide bridges. Possibly intracellular J chain initiates polymerization by binding to one IgM subunit through a disulfide bridge. This process may bring about polymerization among other subunits. After the fifth subunit has been added the circle may be completed by the union of a sulfhydryl group on the mu chain with another sulfhydryl group on the same J chain (Figure 3.2).

Based on immunofluorescence and biosynthetic studies, it appears that J chain is synthesized by plasma cells engaged in the production of IgM (and IgA) immunoglobulins. J chain may constitute the rate-limiting factor in synthesis of these proteins.

IMMUNOGLOBULIN E

IgE molecules consist of two epsilon heavy chains and two kappa or lambda light chains. Each IgE molecule appears to have one interheavy-light and two interheavy-heavy chain disulfide links. The molecular weight of IgE is 190,000 and the sedimentation coefficient is 8S. The carbohydrate content is approximately 12%; carbohydrate is associated only with the heavy chain. IgE is present in normal human serum in very low concentration; the mean value is about 10 ug per 100 ml of serum. It has the shortest survival, highest fractional catabolic rate and lowest synthetic rate of all the immunoglobulin classes. The half-life in serum is approximately two to three days. These characteristics have required the study of IgE myeloma proteins for much of our information of this class of immunoglobulins, but meticulous immunochemical studies of normal serum IgE proteins were important in the discovery of this class.

IgE is susceptible to denaturation by treatment with heat and reducing agents under conditions that have little effect on other immunoglobulins with the exception of IgD. Heating of IgE at 56°C for thirty minutes results in irreversible conformational changes in the carboxy-terminal portion of the heavy chain.

IMMUNOGLOBULIN A

Monomeric IgA molecules have a molecular weight of 150,000 daltons; polymers range in weight up to 350,000 daltons. Each molecule consists of two kappa or two lambda light chains and two alpha heavy chains. Polymer forms of IgA contain the J or joining chain; polymers consisting of two or three IgA monomers may be found in normal serum and constitute a small fraction of serum IgA.

Two subclasses of IgA have been identified on the basis of differences in structure of the heavy alpha chain, IgA1 and IgA2. IgA2 molecules may be further classified into two categories based on the presence of the genetic markers A2m(1) and A2m(2). (For further discussion of genetic markers on immunoglobulin molecules, see below). IgA2 molecules bearing the A2m(1) marker lack disulfide links between the heavy and light chain; these bonds are present in the A2m(2) variant (and in all IgA1 molecules). Both the IgA1 and IgA2 subclasses have two inter-heavy chain disulfide bonds.

Secretory IgA. The predominance of IgG which is characteristic of serum is also found in other internal secretions such as the aqueous fluid of the eye, cerebrospinal, amniotic, synovial, pleural and peritoneal fluids. The immunoglobulin pattern of external secretions, however, is characterized by a predominance of a different immunoglobulin, secretory IgA (SIgA). The pattern characterizes saliva, tears, nasal, tracheobronchial, intestinal and cervical fluids, as well as bile and urine. It should be stressed that other immunoglobulins, including IgG, IgM and IgE are also present in external secretions in amounts greater than can be accounted for by transudation from serum. To a considerable degree, these immunoglobulins as well as secretory IgA are the product of diverse plasma cells present in the lamina propria of the respiratory and gastrointestinal tracts.

The majority of IgA molecules in external secretions exist as dimers composed of two 7S IgA monomers plus two other non-immunoglobulin proteins, J chain and secretory component (SC). The IgA monomer consists of two alpha heavy chains and two kappa or two lambda light chains. In an IgA dimer, both monomers have the same type of light chains. The J chain associated with polymeric IgA is similar, if not identical, to that associated with IgM (see IgM section). Secretory component is a protein with a molecular weight of 71,000 daltons. One model of the structure of SIgA is shown in Figure 3.3.

Two IgA monomers are linked end-to-end via their carboxy termini; the J chain is shown to be disulfide-bonded in a concealed and central position between the Fc ends of the IgA monomers. The SC polypeptide chain is shown coiled about the double Fc cylinders. The molecular weight of SIgA is 390,000 daltons, and its sedimentation coefficient is 11S.

The site and sequence of assembly of SIgA have been determined from immunofluorescence and biosynthetic studies. Plasma cells containing IgA predominate in the lamina propria of the respiratory and

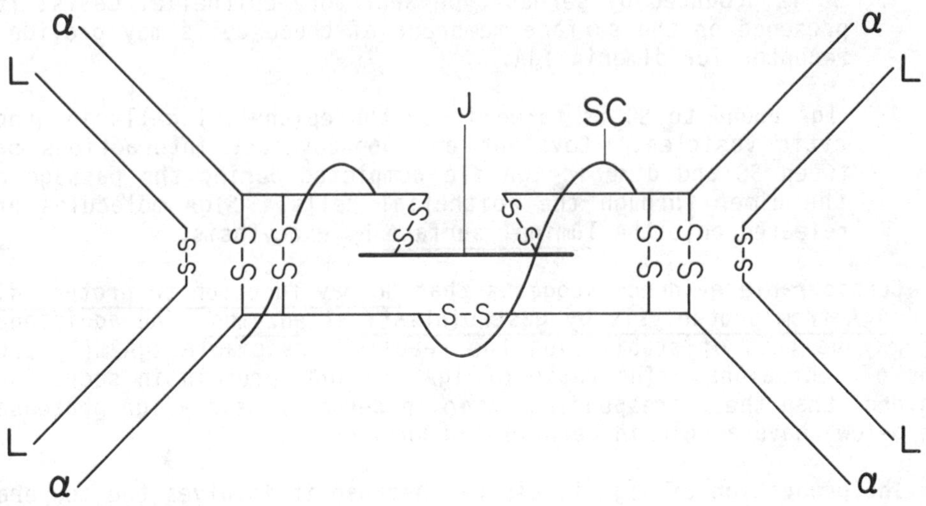

Figure 3.3. SIgA consists of two IgA monomers linked via disulfide bridges between the heavy chains of the monomers plus two additional proteins (J chain and secretory component SC). J chain is shown in an internal location between the carboxy terminal ends of the two sets of chains; SC is shown coiled about the Fc ends of the two IgA monomers. The IgA monomers shown belong to the IgA2m(1) category lacking disulfide links between the heavy and light chains.

gastrointestinal tract; the density of IgM- and IgG-containing plasma cells in the gastrointestinal tract is approximately one-tenth to one-twentieth of that of IgA-containing cells. Secretory component has been localized in mucosal epithelium, in intracellular spaces of the mucosa and on the surface of the epithelial cells lining the lumen of secretory glands; SC is not found in plasma cells. J chain has been localized to plasma cells of the lamina propria. Based on these studies as well as immunohistologic techniques that permitted differentiation between free and bound SC, the following sequence was proposed:

1. The IgA dimer with J chain is formed intracellularly in plasma cells of the lamina propria and is secreted into the interstitial fluid.

2. Although apparently free to move into either the intestinal lumen or the lymphatic channels and thus eventually into the systemic circulation, most of the dimeric IgA moves toward the lumen. In doing so, it must pass through the basement membrane beneath the epithelial cells of the mucous membranes and between and through the epithelial cells.

3. SC is produced by serous-type secretory epithelial cells; its presence on the surface membrane of these cells may provide a receptor for dimeric IgA.

4. IgA bound to SC is taken in by the epithelial cells in endocytic vesicles. Covalent and non-covalent interactions between SC and dimeric IgA are completed during the passage of the dimer through the epithelial cells. SIgA molecules are released onto the luminal surface by exocytosis.

Considerable evidence suggests that SC may function to protect dimeric IgA from proteolysis by gastrointestinal enzymes. An additional role may be that of stabilizing the readily dissociable IgA2m(1) proteins of secretions. The ratio of IgA2 to IgA1 protein in secretions is higher than the corresponding ratio in serum; possibly IgA proteases (see below) have a role in determining this ratio.

The production of SIgA is unusual because it involves the cooperative interaction of two different cells, plasma cells and serous epithelial cells. In addition to its presence in SIgA, secretory component also occurs in an unbound form in secretions, its synthesis appears to be independent of immunoglobulin production. Patients who are unable to produce immunoglobulin molecules may nevertheless have secretory components in their external secretions.

IgA protease. Several bacterial species, including some normally residing in the intestinal tract, secrete a proteolytic enzyme with substrate specificity for IgA. This enzyme cleaves a bond in the hinge region of IgA1. This bond is absent in IgA2 which is not cleaved by the enzyme.

IMMUNOGLOBULIN D

The immunoglobulin D class was discovered as a result of studies of an unusual human myeloma protein (see below for discussion of myeloma proteins) and much of our knowledge of IgD is based on the study of such proteins. Normal human IgD is difficult to investigate because of the low concentration of this protein in serum, average of 30 ug per ml, and because of the tendency of IgD to aggregate and fragment during isolation. IgD molecules are susceptible to proteolysis by the enzyme plasmin, formed during the clotting of blood. IgD, as well as IgE, is susceptible to denaturation by heat and acid treatment under conditions that do not affect IgG, IgA or IgM.

IgD molecules consist of two delta heavy chains and two kappa or two lambda light chains linked by three interchain disulfide bonds, two interheavy-light chains and one interheavy-heavy chain. The sedimentation coefficient of IgD is 7S and the molecular weight 170,000 to 200,000 daltons. IgD is a glycoprotein; carbohydrate is distributed among at least three glycopeptides attached to the delta heavy chain.

IgD is a minor component of serum immunoglobulins. However, there is an unusual distribution of IgD concentration among normal individuals. Approximately 70% of the normal population has about 20 to 50 ug IgD per ml of serum, 15% have less than 3 ug per ml and the third group has 100 to 400 ug or more per ml. The biologic basis of this unusual distribution is uncertain. The rate of synthesis of IgD is 100 times lower than that of IgG. IgD has a fast catabolic rate. The serum half-life is about three days.

Little is known of the biologic function of serum IgD. Serum levels of IgD are increased during chronic infection but an increase in IgD has not been associated with any specific infection. Antibody activity has been identified in the IgD class by indirect techniques; antibodies identified have been anti-nuclear, anti-thyroid, anti-insulin, anti-penicillin and anti-diphtheria toxin specificity. IgD in its native or aggregated form does not interact with the classical complement system nor does it prepare guinea pig tissue for passive cutaneous anaphylactic reactions. In a large proportion of human B lymphocytes, both IgD and monomeric IgM are present in the cell membrane.

CELLS OF ORIGIN AND PATTERNS OF IMMUNOGLOBULIN SYNTHESIS

Immunoglobulin molecules are synthesized by lymphocytes of the B cell series and by their progeny, the plasma cells (Chapter 5). B lymphocytes constitute a small percentage of the circulating lymphocytes but constitute the majority of cells in the follicles of lymph nodes and spleen. Plasma cells are normally absent from the circulation but are found in lymph nodes, spleen, bone marrow and diffusely distributed in the lamina propria of the respiratory and gastrointestinal tracts. In B cells, immunoglobulin molecules are synthesized, and incorporated into the plasma membrane; in plasma cells, immunoglobulin molecules are synthesized and secreted into the external environment of the cell. The majority of circulating human B lymphocytes bear either monomeric IgM or monomeric IgM and IgD molecules in their plasma membranes. The minority of circulating B lymphocytes bear IgA, IgG, IgD or IgE in their plasma membranes. There is considerable evidence for the sequential development of IgG- or IgA-bearing B lymphocytes from IgM- or IgM-plus IgD-bearing precursors (Chapter 5). B cells interact with antigen via the antibody molecules present on the cell surface. Generally, a plasma cell synthesizes and secretes antibody molecules made up of one class of heavy chain and one type of light chain.

In some instances, immunization with a single antigen leads to the appearance of plasma cells producing the corresponding IgM, IgA, IgG, IgD, and IgE antibodies. In other instances, the antibody response is less heterogeneous. The precise mechanism governing the appearance of plasma cells producing antibody molecules with identical antigen-binding specificity but with different heavy chains, remains to be delineated.

Within individual plasma cells, light and heavy chains of immunoglobulin molecules are synthesized on small and large polyribosomes. Light chains are released into an intracellular pool and may have a role in releasing heavy chains from their sites of assembly. Possibly one L and H chain first combine to form a half molecule and two half molecules unite to form the four chain moiety. Under normal circumstances, there appears to be synthesized a slight excess of L and H chains. Whether some plasma cells show a completely balanced pattern of synthesis (i.e., one in which equal numbers of light and heavy chains are produced) and others show a somewhat unbalanced pattern, or whether all plasma cells show a slightly unbalanced pattern of synthesis is not established. Neoplastic plasma cells may show either of these patterns of synthesis and, in addition, may show a markedly unbalanced pattern of synthesis with production of only L or H chains (see below).

Myeloma and Bence Jones proteins. Multiple myeloma is a neoplastic disease of plasma cells. At the time of clinical presentation, patients with this disease may have multiple tumor masses totalling in weight one half to one kilogram. According to one concept, these tumor masses represent the progeny of a single normal plasma cell that, many years earlier, was transformed into a neoplastic plasma cell by some, as yet unidentified, agent. (Recent studies suggest that the transforming event affects a pre-B cell or possibly, a stem cell. If so, the transformed cell appears to be capable of differentiating to the plasma cell stage). The transforming event permits the plasma cell to escape from the normal constraints on cell proliferation; however, in most instances it does not alter the protein synthetic and secretory capabilities of the plasma cell. Since each cell in the tumor mass is identical with every other cell and since each cell produces and secretes an identical product, the serum of patients with myeloma constitutes a source of large amounts of intact homogeneous immunoglobulin protein.

In some instances it has been possible to identify the antigen-binding specificity of the myeloma protein. Antibody activity directed against bacterial antigens has been observed with considerable frequency. It seems likely that if a very large number of antigens were used as probes, then more such proteins would be found to combine with specific antigens. In the majority of cases, the neoplastic plasma cells also produce an excess of light chain protein which, like its normal counterpart, is secreted into the interstitial fluid, reaches the circulation and is transported to the kidney. In the kidney, some of the light chain protein is catabolized and some excreted intact. The urine of patients with multiple myeloma thus becomes a second source of homogeneous immunoglobulin protein, in this instance, homogeneous light chain protein.

The presence of homogeneous light chain protein confers unusual solubility properties on the urine of patients with multiple myeloma. After adjustment of the urine with buffer of an appropriate pH and ionic strength, heating to $56^{\circ}C$ for 15 minutes leads to the appearance of a precipitate. This precipitate, which consists of the homogeneous light chain protein, dissolves upon further heating to $100^{\circ}C$ for three minutes. This unusual phenomenon was first observed by Bence Jones and the term Bence Jones protein was applied to the substance which is now recognized to be homogeneous light chain protein.

In some instances, the neoplastic plasma cells of patients with multiple myeloma appear to have lost the ability to synthesize heavy chains while maintaining light chain production. This variant of multiple myeloma is termed "light chain disease" and it is characterized by the presence of Bence Jones protein in serum and urine. In a different neoplastic disease, malignant lymphoma, a subset of patients is characterized by the presence of neoplastic lymphocytes or plasma cells which produce only the heavy chains of the immunoglobulins. Three variants of "heavy chain disease" are recognized at present: gamma, alpha and mu. In heavy chain disease, the heavy chain product of the neoplastic cells tends to be abnormal; synthesis of the heavy chain begins appropriately at the amino terminus and ends with an appropriate carboxy terminal sequence, but deletions of variable lengths occur near the amino terminal end.

PRIMARY STRUCTURE OF IMMUNOGLOBULINS: REGIONS WITH VARIABLE AND CONSTANT AMINO ACID COMPOSITION

Availability of homogeneous light chains and intact immunoglobulin molecules permitted the elucidation of the primary structure of these proteins. Detailed studies of a limited number of antibody molecules have also been carried out. The amino acid sequence of approximately one hundred light chain proteins has been determined. Light chain proteins of the kappa type were found to consist of 214 amino acids. All kappa chains were found to have the same sequence in the carboxy terminal half of the molecules, except that certain kappa chains had the amino acid leucine at position 191, while others had valine in this position. None of the kappa chains examined had the same amino acid sequence composition in the amino-terminal half of the chain. The two portions of the kappa light chain have been designated V kappa and C kappa representing the segments of variable and constant amino acid sequence. A similar pattern is found among lambda light chains.

Heavy chains have also been found to consist of segments of variable and constant amino acid sequence composition; the VH segment of IgG consists of approximately 115 amino acids and the CH segment of approximately 330. The CH segment in turn consists of three regions or domains of approximately 110 amino acids termed CH1, CH2, and CH3 which show extensive homology with each other (Figure 3.4).

Further examination of the VL or VH segments discloses that variation is constrained: certain residues do not change from one protein to another, only a limited number of different amino acids occur at certain other positions; however, some positions of the variable region show great variability in sequence composition (hypervariable regions). The less variable residues in between the hypervariable regions are termed framework residues (for example, the light chain proteins of either kappa or lambda type have the amino acid threonine at position 5, glutamine at position 6 and glycine at position 16. All kappa light chains have isoleucine at position 2 and leucine at position 11; all lambda light chains have proline at position 7 and glutamine at position 17). Variation in amino acid composition at certain positions, 9 and 13 in the kappa chain, permit the assignment of kappa variable regions to three subgroups V-kappa I, V-kappa II and V-kappa III, which are always associated with the C-kappa segment. Similarly, five subgroups of V-lambda segments have been identified and found to be regularly associated with the C-lambda segment. Three regions of the VL segment show extreme sequence variability; these are located at positions 24 through 34, 50 through 56 and 89 through 97.

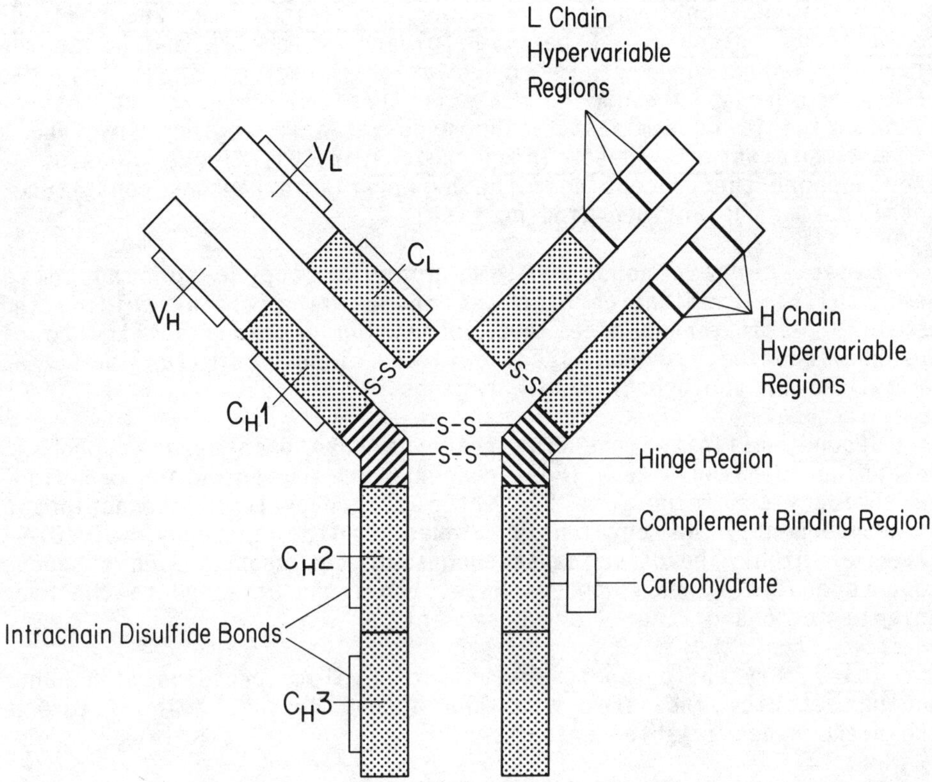

Figure 3.4. Schematic representation of an IgG antibody molecule showing additional details of its structure.

The variable segment of the heavy chain also has certain residues which appear invariant, for example valine at position 2, leucine at 4, glutamine at 6 among others. In addition, certain residues permit the assignment of VH segments to four subgroups. These four V_H subgroups are not restricted to one class or subclass of heavy chains but may be found in association with the CH regions of the gamma, alpha, mu, delta or epsilon heavy chains. <u>Four regions in the VH region show marked variability in amino acid sequence composition and constitute the hypervariable regions of heavy chains</u>; these regions are located at positions 31 through 37, 51 through 68, 86 through 91 and 101 through 109. While the extensive sequence variations in these regions has been stressed, a second major source of variation in structure arises from minor additions or deletions of amino acids in the hypervariable regions.

According to current concepts, the VH and VL regions contribute to the formation of antigen-binding pocket or cleft in the Fab portion of the antibody molecule. Extensive folding of the VH and VL segments serves to bring three of the hypervariable regions of VL into close spatial proximity so as to form a structure complementary to that of a given antigenic determinant. The hypervariable regions involved are termed complementarity determining regions or CDR. Three lines of evidence support the concept that the hypervariable regions constitute or contribute to the antigen-binding site:

First, certain mouse myeloma proteins appear to bind antigen specifically. Examination of a set of myeloma proteins arising independently in different mice, but possessing a common ability to bind phosphorylcholine, showed identical or closely similar amino acid composition in the hypervariable regions.

Second, affinity labelling reagents have been used as probes of the antigen-binding site. These reagents are haptens which can bind to the antibody-combining site by virtue of noncovalent interactions and may subsequently be covalently linked to the antibody molecule by virtue of highly reactive constituents of the hapten. On subsequent sequence analysis, such haptens have been found attached to the hypervariable regions of the VH or VL segments.

Third, crystallographic analysis of myeloma proteins with hapten-binding activity indicated that the actual contact amino acids were within the hypervariable regions.

The remaining residues of the VH and VL segments are now viewed as maintaining the hypervariable regions in appropriate alignment in the antigen-binding site. Hence, these residues constitute the framework of the combining site. It should again be stressed that amino acid substitutions, additions or deletions in the complementarity-determining regions make it possible to generate the large number of unique antigen-binding sites required to cope with the vast diversity of antigens.

The size of the antigen-binding pocket or cleft in anti-polysaccharide and anti-protein antibodies has been estimated. The binding site of the former accommodated an oligosaccharide of six or seven residues, while the latter accommodated a peptide of approximately four to seven residues. The strength of the bond between an antigen-binding pocket and its corresponding antigenic determinant depends on geometric complementarity and several other noncovalent interactions. The degree of complementarity between site and determinant influences the number of bonds that develop. These interactions include hydrogen bonds, bonds between anionic and cationic groups and electronic van der Waals forces.

IMMUNOGLOBULIN DOMAINS

In Figure 3.4, the presence of intrachain disulfide bonds is indicated in the VL and CL segments of the light chain and the VH, CH1, CH_2, and CH3 segments of the heavy chain. Thus, in each segment, the intrachain disulfide bond establishes a loop involving approximately 60 amino acids (Figure 3.5). Each segment appears to be folded into a compact globular domain; the links between adjacent domains appear to be less tightly folded and hence more accessible to enzymatic attack. Thus, it has been possible to cleave the junction between VL and CL and VH and CH1 and to thereby produce an Fv fragment composed of VL and VH. This fragment had a molecular weight of approximately 25,000 and consisted of two polypeptide chains of approximately 110 amino acids held together only by noncovalent bonds. The Fv fragment had all of the antigen-binding specificity of the intact antibody molecule from which it was obtained.

The region in the heavy chain which was previously cited as being particularly vulnerable to attack by papain and pepsin is termed the hinge region. This region consists of about 15 amino acid residues and includes the cysteines that form the inter-heavy chain disulfide bridges. There is no sequence homology between the hinge region and other segments of the immunoglobulin light or heavy chains, and the amino acid sequence of the hinge region is characteristic of each class and subclass of heavy chain.

ANTIGENIC MARKERS ON IMMUNOGLOBULINS

Immunoglobulin molecules are proteins and hence are immunogenic upon administration to animals of unrelated species or individuals of different genetic background in the same species. Several different types of antigenic determinants may be recognized on immunoglobulin molecules. First, there are antigenic determinants which characterize all gamma, alpha, mu, delta, or epsilon heavy chains and all kappa or lambda light chains. These antigenic determinants are termed isotypic determinants. A rabbit antiserum directed against the isotypic determinants on the gamma heavy chain, for example, will "recognize" the IgG molecules present in all normal human sera.

Second, there are antigenic determinants present on the gamma heavy chain and kappa light chains of some but not all normal individuals. For example, the previously mentioned substitution of a single amino acid, either leucine or valine, at position 191 in the C kappa segment of kappa light chains produces a sufficient change in the protein so as to constitute a unique antigenic determinant recognizable by appropriate antisera. These antigenic determinants are called

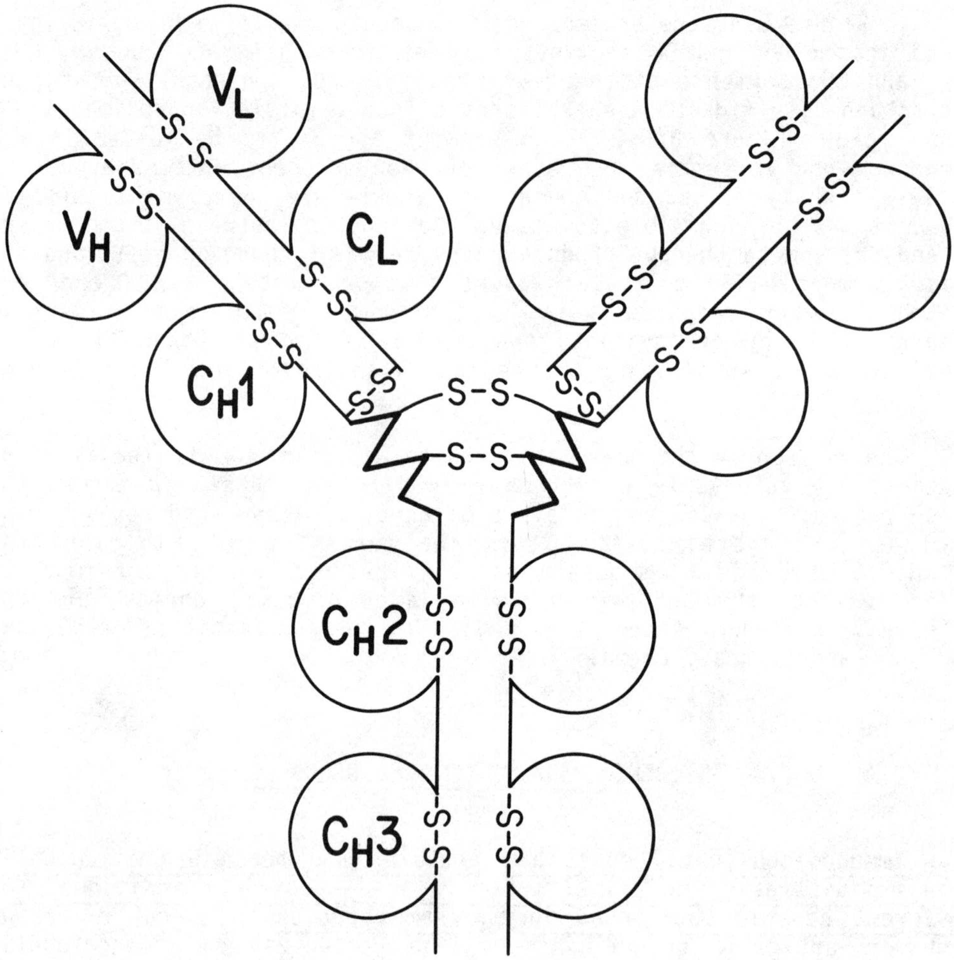

Figure 3.5. Schematic representation of an IgG antibody molecule, taking into account the approximately 60 amino acid loops generated by intrachain disulfide bonds in the various segments of the molecule. Each segment is folded into a compact globular domain stabilized by disulfide bonds. Globular domains are linked via segments of less tightly folded peptide chains.

allotypic determinants. Kappa chains with leucine at position 191 bear the InV(1,2) allotypic determinants; those with valine in this position bear the InV(3) allotype. Approximately twenty allotypic determinants have been recognized on gamma heavy chains; these are termed Gm markers and are found chiefly on the Fc, and to a lesser extent on the Fd segment of the gamma chains. Each subclass of IgG has its own allotypic markers which are under genetic control by codominant alleles. The inheritance of allotypes follows mendelian rules. A homozygous individual has a certain allotypic determinant on all IgG molecules of a subclass, while a heterozygous individual may have this marker on approximately one half of the IgG molecules. In a heterozygous person, individual plasma cells show evidence of allelic exclusion by producing gamma heavy chains with either one or the other allotypic marker. This observation underscores the severe restriction in expression of the genetic potential of a mature plasma cell. The plasma cell can produce only one type of light chain constant region and only one class of heavy chain constant region, as well as only one VH and one VL sequence. The inheritance of allotypes is detailed in Chapter 10.

A third type of marker is the idiotypic antigenic determinant. This antigenic determinant arises from the unique configuration of amino acids constituting the combining site of an antibody molecule. Generally, idiotypic determinants are dependent on the arrangement of both light and heavy chain hypervariable regions. The presence of hapten or antigen in the combining site of an antibody molecule would be expected to interfere with the reaction of anti-idiotypic antibody with the antibody against which it is directed.

BIOLOGIC FUNCTIONS OF ANTIBODY MOLECULES

Certain biologic functions associated with antibodies of the five different classes are summarized in Table 3.3. This table also introduces the concept that the capacity to produce antibodies may be either beneficial or injurious to the host depending upon special circumstances. The injurious consequences of antibody-antigen interaction are the subjects of Chapters 13 and 14.

Antibody molecules of several classes have the ability to neutralize the soluble exotoxins produced by bacteria. Antibody molecules may interfere with the action of toxins by combining with antigenic determinants in or near the active site of the toxin thereby blocking the reaction with substrate. Alternatively, antibody molecules may combine with determinants remote from the active site of the toxin; such combination may alter the configuration and hence the activity of the site.

Table 3.3

Biologic Activities of the Five Classes of Human Antibodies

Class of Antibody	Beneficial Activities	Injurious Activities
IgG	Toxin neutralizing Agglutinating Opsonizing Bacteriolytic (with aid of complement system)	Antigen-IgG antibody complexes are capable of mediating tissue injury; examples: Arthus reaction, serum sickness
IgM	Toxin neutralizing Agglutinating Bacteriolytic (with aid of complement system) Antigen receptor on B lymphocytes	Same as above
IgA	Toxin neutralizing Agglutinating ? Opsonizing	?
IgD	Antigen receptor on B lymphocytes	?
IgE	Mediate changes in vascular permeability	Local and systemic immediate permeability, hypersensitivity, or anaphylactic reactions

Antibody molecules of several classes have the ability to agglutinate or clump bacteria, viruses, fungi, yeasts and other potential parasites. Clumping facilitates the task of phagocytic cells by interfering with the movement of the parasite and by permitting the phagocyte to deal with clusters of organisms rather than having to deal singly with each parasite.

The term "opsonizing" refers to the role of antibodies in preparing bacteria and other parasites for phagocytosis (Chapter 5). Adherence of bacteria to the plasma membrane of the phagocytic cell is a necessary step in engulfment. Although some uncoated bacteria adhere to the surface of phagocytes such as polymorphonuclear leukocytes and monocytes, others, including many virulent organisms, show little adherence. Addition of IgG antibodies to such organisms leads to adherence of the organisms to the phagocytes via specific cell surface receptors for the Fc end of the antibody molecules. Addition of complement to the antibody-coated parasite further enhances adherence and phagocytosis. This enhancement of phagocytosis is mediated via additional cell-surface receptors for the complement component C3b (Chapter 12).

Antibodies capable of activating the complement sequence, such as most IgG and some IgM antibodies, are capable of damaging certain strains of gram-negative bacteria. These antibodies are termed "bacteriolytic" although the lytic action is provided by the complement system acting in concert with the enzyme lysozyme.

Biologic properties of IgG subclasses. Antibody molecules of the four IgG subclasses differ in certain biologic properties. The ability to initiate the classical complement sequence is a property of IgG1, IgG2, and IgG3; IgG4 molecules fail to react with Clq, a subcomponent of the first component of complement. IgG1, IgG3 and IgG4 molecules possess a site or configuration permitting their interaction with mast cells of an unrelated species, the guinea pig; IgG2 molecules lack this ability. All four subclass proteins can bind to the Fc receptors of neutrophils, but only IgG1 and IgG3 antibodies can bind to receptors on monocytes. The monocyte binding site has been localized to the CH3 domain. (A peptide containing ten amino acids derived from the CH3 domain, bound to monocytes and inhibited their interaction with intact IgG1 and IgG3 antibody-coated erythrocytes). Immunoglobulins of all four subclasses are transported across maternal-fetal membranes; whether any subclass of IgG is over- or under-represented in the fetal compared to the maternal circulation remains to be firmly established (Table 3.4).

The Special Biologic Properties of Secretory IgA Antibodies. Secretory IgA antibodies are capable of neutralizing toxins and of neutralizing the infectivity of viruses. The mechanism of virus neutralization has not been established. In addition, SIgA antibodies are capable of agglutinating bacteria and other parasites. There continues to be controversy over the ability of SIgA antibodies to interact with the classical complement system and over the existence of receptors for SIgA on macrophages. An accepted role for SIgA antibodies is that of interfering with the adherence of bacteria to mucosal surfaces. Adherence is a prime requisite for colonization of mucosal surfaces; bacteria that do not adhere are unable to establish themselves on the mucosal surfaces.

An additional role for SIgA antibodies in the gastrointestinal tract may be that of excluding intact soluble proteins from the systemic circulation. Experiments in normal animals suggest that a small fraction of ingested proteins may be taken up intact by the epithelial cells and transported from the mucosal surface into the lymphatic and venous circulation. Immunization with protein antigens leads to inhibition of their uptake. The process of "immune exclusion" probably

Table 3.4

Biologic Properties of Subclasses of Human IgG

	IgG1	IgG2	IgG3	IgG4
Complement fixation (at C1 step)	+	+	+	—
Passive cutaneous anaphylaxis*	+	—	+	+
Binding to Fc receptors on neutrophils	+	+	+	+
Binding to Fc receptors on monocytes	+	—	+	—
Placental transfer	+	+	+	+
Percentage distribution in normal serum	65-70	23-28	4-8	3-4

*In guinea pigs (Chapter 14)

involves the formation of antigen-secretory antibody complexes in the mucous coat of the intestine followed by degradation of the complexes by surface-associated enzymes.

IgE Antibodies as "Gatekeepers". The biologic potency of IgE antibodies arises from their unique ability to combine via configurations in the CH3 and CH4 domains with specific receptors on the surface of host mast cells and basophils (Chapter 14). This interaction leaves the antigen-binding end of the IgE molecule available for combination with antigen. Bridging by antigen of adjacent IgE antibodies triggers the release of pharmacologic mediators, such as histamine, from the mast cell or basophil. Histamine alters the permeability of adjacent small blood vessels, thereby permitting intravascular antibodies of diverse classes and phagocytic cells to leave the vascular channels and to accumulate at the local site. Thus, by altering vascular permeability, the IgE antibody-mast-cell-mediator system exerts a gate keeper function at the sites where this system is disposed. These sites include the skin and mucosal surfaces in contact with the external environment.

REFERENCES

Capra, J. D. and Kehoe, J. M. Hypervariable regions, idiotypy and antibody-combining sites. Adv. Immunol. 20:1, 1975.

Davies, D. R., and Metgzer, H. Structural basis of antibody function. Ann. Rev. Immunol., 1:87, 1983.

Haber, E., and Krause, R. M. (eds.) Antibodies in Human Diagnosis and Therapy, Raven Press, New York, 1977.

Moller, G. Immunoglobulin E. Immunol. Rev., 41: 1978 (contains twelve chapters dealing with various aspects of IgE structure and function).

Natvig, J. B. and Kunkel, H. G. Human immunoglobulins: classes, subclasses, genetic variants and idiotypes, Adv. Immunol., 16:1, 1973.

Nisonoff, A., Hopper, J. R. and Spring, S. B. The Antibody Molecule, Academic Press, New York, San Francisco, London, 1975.

McNabb, P.C. and Tomasi, T.B., Jr. Host defense mechanism at mucosal surfaces, Ann. Rev. Microbiol. 35:477, 1981.

CHAPTER 4

Methods of the Immunologist

PRECIPITIN REACTIONS IN LIQUID MEDIA

Antigens and their corresponding antibodies interact with one another through reversible, non-covalent forces to form antigen-antibody complexes. These interactions are influenced primarily by the ionic strength and pH of the medium and by the concentration of the reactants. The reversibility of the reaction is dependent on the affinity of the antibody for the antigen; the higher the affinity, the less reversible the reaction becomes (i.e., Ag + Ab <---> AgAb). The interaction of soluble antibody with soluble antigen is termed the precipitin reaction. M. Heidelberger and his associates employed the precipitin reaction as a quantitative method for determining the amount of the antibody present in an antiserum. Varying amounts of antigen, in their case a capsular polysaccharide from *Streptococcus pneumoniae*, were mixed with a constant amount of antiserum and incubated. After incubation, the supernate and precipitate were retained. The precipitate was washed free of contaminants and analyzed for total nitrogen by means of the Kjeldahl method. Since the antigen used contained no nitrogen, any nitrogen detected in the precipitate must have been of antibody origin. The amount of nitrogen or the total amount of precipitate could then be plotted as a function of the amount of antigen added and represented as shown in Figure 4.1. The supernates were divided and to each half of the solution was added either additional antigen or antibody. Supernates obtained from tubes to which small amounts of antigen had initially been added, showed additional precipitate upon the addition of antigen. Hence such supernates contained excess antibody and the region of the precipitin curve from which such supernates were obtained was called the zone of antibody excess. Addition of antibody (or antiserum) to supernates obtained from tubes to which large amounts of antigen had initially been added, led to the formation of a precipitate. Hence, such supernates contained excess antigen and the region of the precipitin curve from which these supernates were obtained was called the zone of antigen excess. Supernates obtained from tubes intermediate between the other two, failed to form additional precipitate upon addition of either antigen or antibody. The region of the precipitin curve from which these supernates were

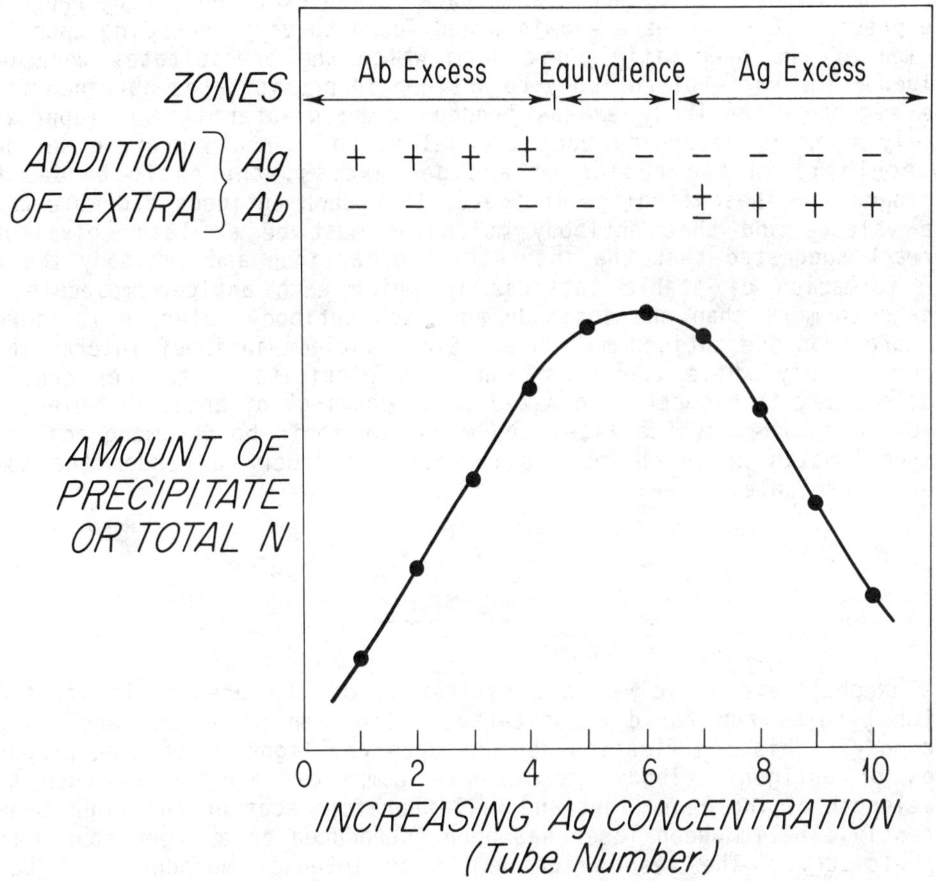

Figure 4.1. Precipitin curve resulting from the addition of increasing amounts of antigen to a constant amount of antiserum in a series of tubes. The regions of antibody excess, equivalence, and antigen excess are indicated.

---

obtained was called the zone of equivalence implying that the initial mixture of the antigen and antiserum was appropriate for the complete precipitation of antigen and antibody. From the amount of protein present in the precipitate at equivalence it was possible to calculate the amount of antibody present in the anti-pneumococcal polysaccharide antiserum. This method of analysis is also applicable to protein antigens because at equivalence all of the antigen added is present in the precipitate. By subtracting this amount of protein from the total protein in the precipitate, it is possible to estimate the anti-protein antibody content of an antiserum.

The composition of the precipitate formed over the entire range of the precipitin curve were examined and found to vary depending upon the region of the precipitin curve from which the precipitates were obtained. The ratio of antibody to antigen in precipitates obtained from the region of antibody excess tended to be greater than 1 (approximately 4 or 5, depending upon the valency of certain protein antigen molecules); in the region of antigen excess, the ratio tended to approach 1. These findings indicated that such antigens had more than one valence and that antibody molecules must be at least bivalent. Marrack suggested that the interaction of antigen and antibody led to the formation of stable lattices in which each antigen molecule is linked to more than one antibody and each antibody molecule is linked to more than one antigen molecule. Since antigen-antibody interactions occur rapidly while the formation of a precipitate requires considerable time, it has been suggested that "packing" of antibody molecules involved in the lattice (i.e., by means of ionic bonds among adjacent immunoglobulin heavy chains) is required in order to render the complexes insoluble.

NEPHELOMETRY

Nephelometry involves a modification of the precipitin reaction which permits the rapid quantitative estimation of either antigen or antibody. This modification depends upon the light scattering properties of antigen-antibody complexes. Complexes are larger than the wavelength of incident light and will therefore scatter the light beam. Recently a helium-neon laser has been introduced as a light source for nephelometry. The laser light emits an intense, monochromatic beam that is claimed to enhance the sensitivity of the procedure. In contrast to the classical precipitin reaction which measures the concentration of antigen or antibody at equivalence, nephelometry determines the concentration of either reactant in the antibody excess region of the precipitin curve (i.e., at a point where antigen-antibody complexes are still small). For the nephelometric titration of antigen, antigen is incubated with a constant amount of antibody in a special tube or cuvette. After an incubation interval varying from several minutes to an hour, a beam of light is passed through the cuvette and the degree of scatter of the light beam is measured by an electronic detector. The concentration of antigen is determined from a standard curve constructed by measuring the light scattering of antigen solutions of known concentration. The rapidity with which the concentration of protein antigens can be measured by nephelometry makes it likely that many clinical laboratory tests such as the determination of immunoglobulin or complement component concentration will be performed with this instrument.

PRECIPITATION REACTIONS IN GELS

Precipitation reactions may be carried out in various semisolid media. Two types of reactions in gels will be described: double immunodiffusion and radial immunodiffusion. The double immunodiffusion technique was developed by Ouchterlony. In this technique, a series of wells are cut in a layer of agar in a Petri dish or on a glass slide. Solutions of antigen and antibody are placed in adjacent wells and allowed to diffuse towards each other. During the incubation period, both reactants diffuse radially into the agar establishing a concentration gradient which diminishes progressively with increasing distance from the well. An opaque precipitation forms in the gel at the interface of the diffusion fronts of antigen and antiserum. The location of the precipitin band depends upon the concentration of antigen and antibody initially placed in the wells. If the concentration of antigen is dilute with respect to that of the antiserum, then the antibodies contained therein must diffuse further from the well in order to reach equivalence with antigen. If the antiserum is relatively dilute in comparison to the antigen solution, then the precipitin band tends to form closer to the antiserum well. It can be readily appreciated that an inappropriate concentration of either the antigen or the antiserum may lead to a failure of the reactants to form a precipitate. The molecular size of the antigen or antibody also influences the location of the precipitin band. High molecular weight components, such as IgM molecules, tend to diffuse slowly in agar hence their precipitin bands will form close to the source of these components.

Double diffusion in agar provides a powerful tool for studying the relationships among antigens in solution. In Figure 4.2 three types of precipitin reactions are shown.

<u>In panel A,</u> antigen solution (A) was placed in two wells opposite a <u>single well</u> containing antiserum to (A); precipitin bands formed between the antigen and antiserum wells and the bands fused in a <u>pattern of identity</u>.

<u>In panel B,</u> two solutions containing unrelated antigens, (A) and (B) <u>were placed</u> in peripheral wells and antiserum containing antibodies to both (A) and (B) was placed in the central well. Following diffusion, two intersecting precipitin bands were seen. This pattern of precipitation is one of <u>non-identity</u>.

<u>In panel C</u>, two solutions of antigen were placed in the peripheral wells. One contained molecules of antigen (A); the second contained solutions of molecules bearing two antigenic determinants (A) and (a). The antiserum well contained antibodies directed against (A) and (a). Antibodies to (A) diffused into the gel until they encountered antigen molecules bearing the (A) determinant, whereupon precipitation occurred. Antibodies to (a) diffused into the gel until they encountered antigen molecules bearing the (a) determinant. Since there are no such

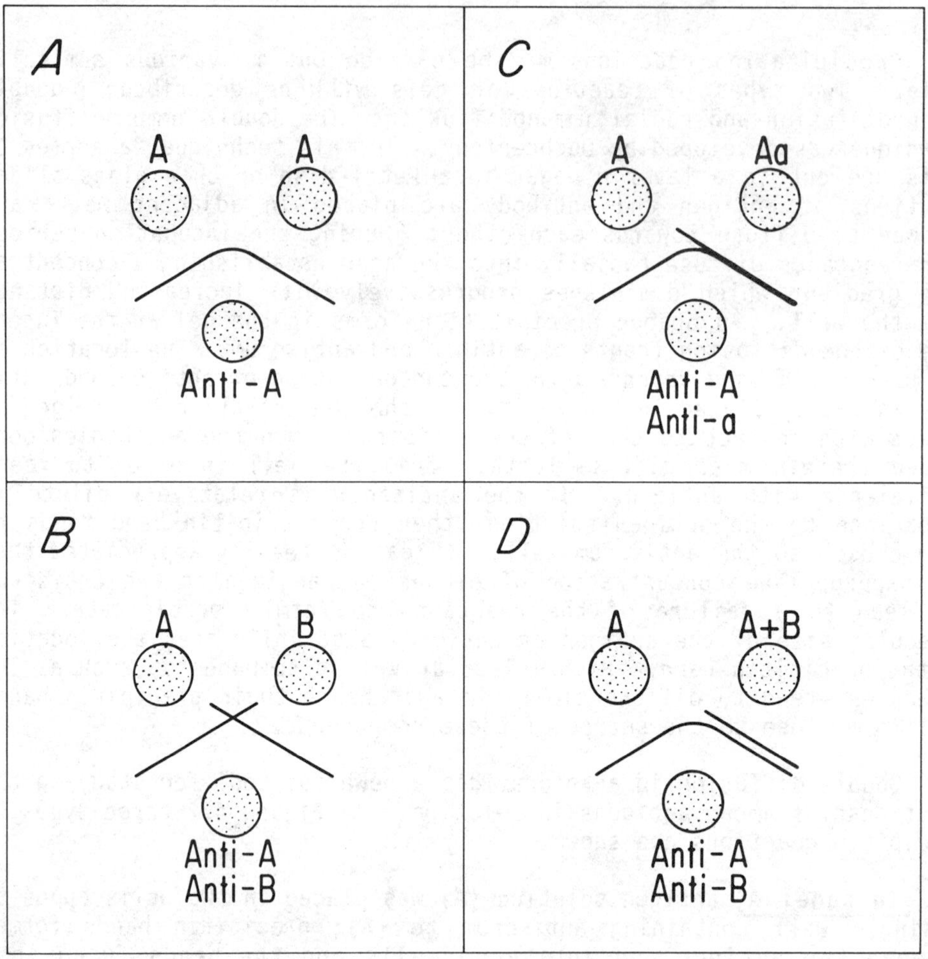

Figure 4.2. Double diffusion in agar showing the precipitin patterns characteristic of the reaction of identity (panel A), reaction of non-identity (panel B), and partial identity (panel C). A complex pattern is shown in panel D.

---

determinants on molecules diffusing from the well containing antigen (A), these antibodies diffused through the first precipitin band until they encountered (a) on (Aa) molecules diffusing from the second antigen well. Precipitation occurred and resulted in the <u>spur</u> of the precipitin band. It should be noted that the initial precipitin band between antiserum and (Aa) antigen was formed by antibodies to (A), as well as antibodies to (a) reacting with the corresponding determinants on the same antigen molecule and that the spur was formed only by antibodies to (a) and the (a) antigen on the (Aa) molecule. For this reason, the spur tends to be a weaker precipitin band. This pattern of precipitation is termed a reaction of partial identity.

In Panel D, a solution of antigen (A) and a solution of antigen (A) plus (B) were placed in peripheral wells (in this example, antigenic determinants (A) and (B) were on separate molecules); antiserum containing antibodies to A and B was placed in the central well. Antibodies to (A) and antigen (A) formed precipitin bands that fuse in a pattern of identity. Antibodies to B were unaffected by the initial precipitin band and diffused through it until equilibrium conditions were reached with antigen (B), whereupon a second precipitin band was formed.

Radial Immunodiffusion. A variation of double immunodiffusion, single, or radial immunodiffusion (RID), permits the accurate determination of the concentration of either antigen or antibody by means of a relatively simple method. In this procedure, a certain dilution of monospecific antiserum is mixed with molten agar. The mixture is poured into a mold and allowed to gel. A series of wells are cut in the agar and filled with solutions of antigen. Antigen diffuses into the agar forming a precipitate with the antibodies contained in the agar. Consequently, an opaque circle forms around the antigen well. In time, additional antigen diffuses from the well and dissolves the antigen-antibody precipitates initially formed. The opaque circle expands until equivalence between antigen and antibody is reached. At this time, a permanent ring is formed. By observing the growth of the precipitin ring, it was determined that a linear relationship existed between the square of the diameter of the ring and the concentration of antigen in the well.

Application of RID in the clinical laboratory include its use in determining the concentration of immunoglobulin or complement components in the serum of patients. In Figure 4.3, three standard solutions of different antigen concentrations and a sample of unknown concentration were placed in the wells of an RID plate. After incubation for a sufficient interval to permit equilibrium to be reached, the diameters of the rings were measured. The square of the diameter of the standard rings was plotted on the x axis and the concentration of the antigen in the standard solution was plotted on the y axis in order to generate a standard curve. The concentration of antigen in the test sample was determined from the standard curve by finding the concentration of antigen corresponding to the square of the diameter of the ring formed by the test sample.

The RID method is popular because of its ease of performance, versatility and low cost. It requires no special equipment and can be used with virtually any combination of soluble antigen and precipitating antibody.

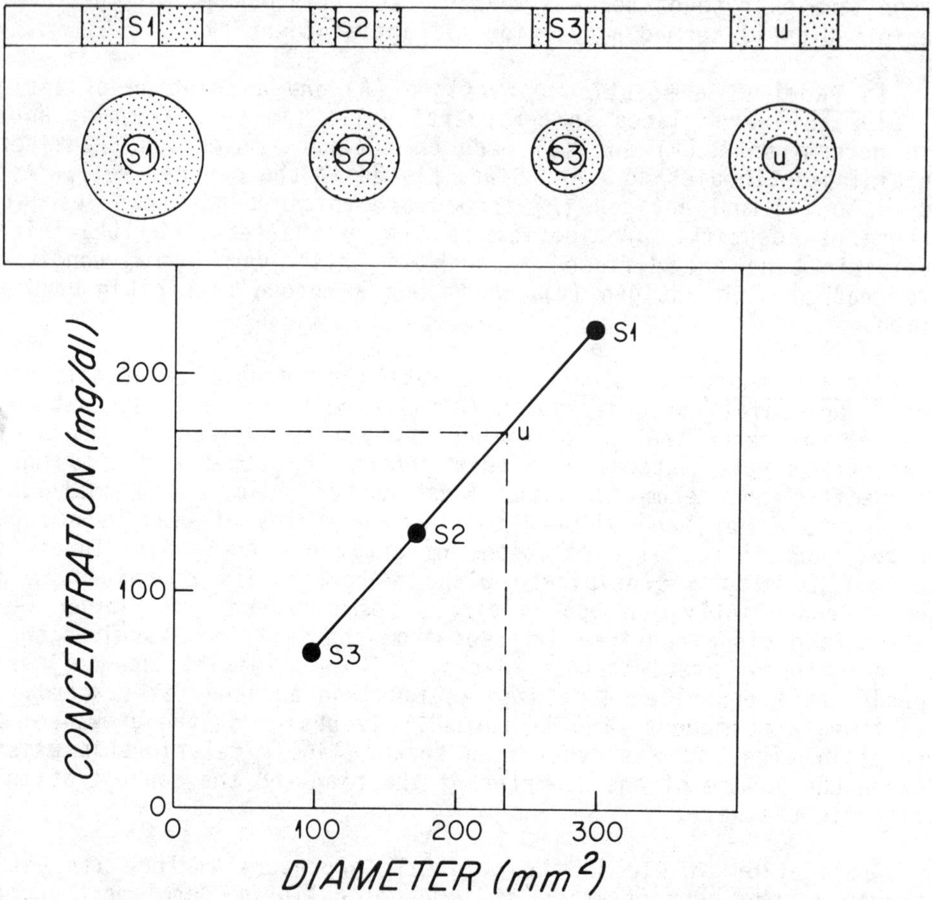

Figure 4.3. The graph shown illustrates the relationship between antigen concentration and the diameter of the precipitin rings.

AGGLUTINATION REACTIONS

A major difference between agglutination and precipitin reactions is that the antigen in the former is insoluble. The insoluble antigen may be an intrinsic antigenic determinant of the cell membrane of an erythrocyte or the cell wall of a bacterium. Addition of antiserum will, under appropriate conditions, cross-link the antigenic determinants on separate particles causing the particles to come together or clump. Agglutination involving antigenic determinants which are an intrinsic constituent of the particle is termed active agglutination or in the case of erythrocytes, hemagglutination. A normally soluble antigen may be combined with a variety of insoluble particles such as erythrocytes, bentonite (clay) particles or polystyrene latex beads, and may thereby be rendered insoluble. Agglutination involving antigenic determinants which are not an intrinsic constituent of the particle is termed passive agglutination.

The agglutination reaction is widely used to detect the presence of antibody and to estimate the relative amount of antibody in an antiserum. Although the procedure cannot be used to establish the actual amount, by weight, of antibody, it can be used to compare the relative potency of different antisera. The agglutination reaction is also popular because of its versatility. Particles to be used in passive agglutination can be prepared by methods ranging from simple adsorption of antigen to covalent linkage of antigen and particles. For example, lipopolysaccharide (LPS), a soluble component of the cell wall of gram-negative bacteria, can be rendered insoluble by mixing the purified LPS with a suspension of normal erythrocytes. A soluble protein such as IgG can be rendered insoluble by covalent linkage to erythrocytes; a cross-linking agent such as glutaraldehyde may be used for this purpose. Alternatively, erythrocytes may be treated with tannic acid solutions so as to alter their surface properties. Following treatment with tannic acid, various proteins or hapten-protein conjugates will bind firmly to the surface of the altered erythrocyte.

The agglutination reaction is performed by adding a constant volume of a suspension of particles bearing intrinsic or extrinsic antigenic determinants, to a constant volume of serially diluted antiserum. The reactants are thoroughly mixed and incubated. During the period of incubation, the particles settle out of suspension to the bottom of the test tube or microtiter plate. The presence of antibodies leads to clumping of the particles which may be scored according to various schemes. Generally, in the absence of the corresponding antibody, the particles settle out in a uniform layer (0 agglutination). In the presence of large amounts of antibody, strong agglutination occurs and clumps of particles settle out (4+ agglutination). Lesser amounts of antibody produce patterns of agglutination intermediate between the former patterns (3+ to 1+). In the agglutination reaction, the antibody content of an antiserum is expressed as the titer which represents the reciprocal of the final dilution of antiserum capable of yielding visible agglutination.

The agglutination reaction proceeds in two stages. The first stage involves the rapid interaction of antigen and antibody on the surface of the particle. During this stage a bivalent antibody molecule may bind to two antigenic determinants on the same or adjacent particles. The second stage involves the cross-linking of adjacent particles or small agglutinates, into large, easily visible aggregates

(Figure 4.4). Several factors may prevent the agglutination of particles by the appropriate antiserum; these include electrostatic forces, an excess of antibody and the sparsity or inaccessibility to antibody of antigenic determinates on the surface of the particle. Agglutination of particles may be prevented by the presence of electrostatic forces which are generated by charged groups on the surface of particles such as erythrocytes. Sialic acid residues on the surface of erythrocytes impart a negative charge to the surface. The negative charge on all erythrocytes in a suspension leads to their mutual repulsion. This effect must be overcome before antibody molecules can bridge adjacent particles. The repulsive force may be overcome by changing the ionic strength of the test medium; the presence of certain ions in sufficient concentration will negate the effect of surface charges on the particle and allow the particles to approach closely enough for antibody molecules to cross-link and thus agglutinate the particles.

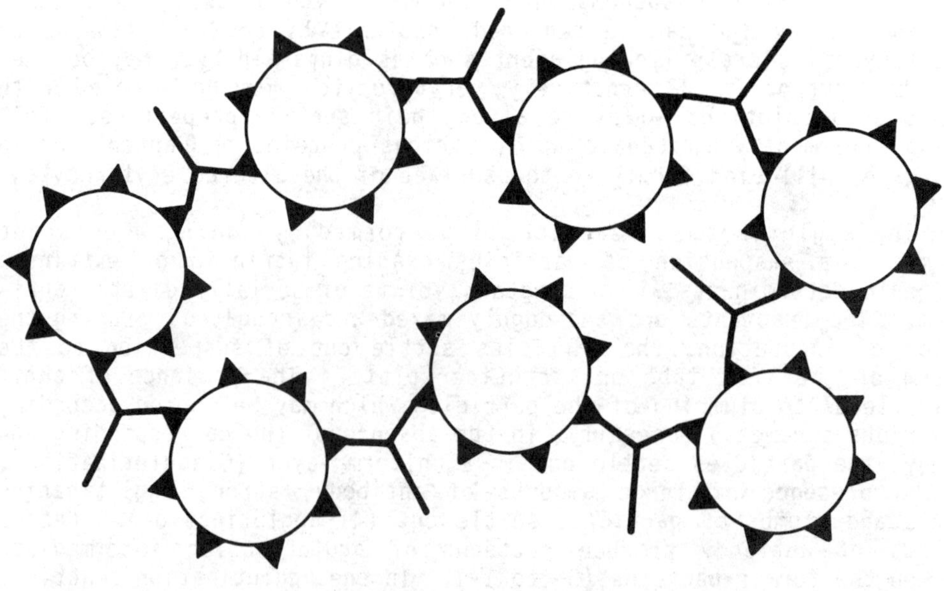

Figure 4.4. Schematic representation of the agglutination of erythrocytes by bivalent antibody molecules. The intrinsic antigenic determinants are represented by triangles. Although a limited number of antibody molecules are shown in the figure, multiple IgG, but fewer IgM, antibody molecules are required to link the cells.

In the precipitin reaction, the region of antibody excess is characterized by the presence of small, insoluble complexes. In the agglutination reaction, antibody excess does not lead to the formation of partial agglutination but instead may be responsible for the failure of agglutination. The zone in which no agglutination is observed despite evidence that the particles are coated with antibody, is termed the prozone. The prozone phenomenon occurs most frequently with very high titered antiserums at low dilutions; a negative agglutination test is seen until the antiserum is sufficiently diluted. The prozone phenomenon probably results from the extensive coating of antigenic determinants on a particle by antibody molecules; this coating prevents cross-linking by covering all or most available determinants.

The sparsity of antigenic determinants or the inaccessibility to antibody of antigenic determinants on the surface of the cell or other particles can also interfere with agglutination. If the number of antigenic determinants are few or they are widely scattered over the surface of the particles, then the cross-linking forces exerted by antibody molecules may be insufficient to overcome the repulsive forces between particles. Similarly, if antigenic determinents are present in the depths of the erythrocyte membrane, an IgG antibody molecule might be able to combine with one such determinant but be unable to reach (because of its limited size) a similar determinant in the membrane of an adjacent cell.

The presence of anti-erythrocyte antibodies which are incapable of agglutinating the cells may be revealed by the addition of a second antiserum termed an antiglobulin or Coombs' reagent. This reagent is an antiserum directed against the immunoglobulin present in the primary, non-agglutinating, system. The addition of anti-immunoglobulin serves to agglutinate the erythrocytes not by virtue of intrinsic surface antigenic determinants but by binding to the immunoglobulin molecules attached to these determinants. The appropriate Coombs' reagent may be used to detect the presence of non-agglutinating antibody on a cell or other particles, as well as to determine the immunoglobulin class of the antibody and to reveal the presence of complement components.

The agglutination reaction is also affected by the class of antibody involved; IgM antibody molecules are more effective in agglutinating particles than are IgG antibody molecules.

COMPLEMENT MEDIATED HEMOLYSIS

The complement proteins to be described in Chapter 12 comprise a group of plasma proteins that interact with each other following an antigen-antibody reaction. The end result of the activation of complement--or the "fixation of complement"--is the production of a lesion in the membrane of the cell bearing the antigen, and to which antibody is bound. For example, antibodies to red cells in the absence of complement will induce their agglutination, depending on the dose of antibody. The addition of fresh serum results in the lysis of the antibody-coated red cells. The degree of hemolysis can be measured in the spectrophotometer.

Complement dependent hemolysis has been used extensively in both clinical and experimental work. The assay can be used to: 1) titrate hemolytic complement in the serum; a serum is diluted severalfold and added to a constant number of red cells coated with a standard amount of antibody; depending on the amount of complement, different degrees of hemolysis can be measured; 2) study, or titrate, individual complement proteins; this is done as above but adding excess of all the complement proteins except the one to be titrated and 3) measure antibodies; this is similar to the hemagglutination test described above; after incubation of cells with antibody, complement is added and hemolysis is measured. The reciprocal of the highest dilution of antiserum capable of producing lysis is taken as the hemolytic titer. As with hemagglutination, IgM antibodies are about one-thousandfold more active on a molar basis than are IgG antibodies.

ELECTROPHORESIS METHODS

The observation that charged particles migrate in an electrical field led to the development of several important tools for characterizing complex mixtures of proteins. Tiselius, in 1937, performed electrophoresis of serum in a liquid medium; serum was separated under the influence of an electrical field into four components: albumin, alpha, beta and gamma-globulins. Following separation, it was possible, for the first time, to associate antibody activity with proteins migrating in the gamma-globulin fraction. Subsequent modifications have replaced the liquid medium by various supporting media including paper wicks, cellulose acetate strips and layers of agar or agarose. These supports are all hydrated, porous materials which provide mechanical rigidity, eliminate convection and vibration disturbances, but do not interact with the migrating proteins. Electrophoresis is performed in the presence of a buffer selected so that all of the proteins in a mixture are on the same (either positive or negative) side of their respective isoelectric points. Separation of serum proteins for example is conducted with buffers at or close to pH 8.6. At this pH, most serum proteins have a net negative charge. Serum albumin has the highest net negative charge per molecule and hence migrates closest to the anode; gamma-globulins have a small net negative charge at this pH and hence tend to remain near the origin. Electrophoretic separation is continued until the major protein constituents of the mixture have separated into discrete zones, hence the term zone electrophoresis. In addition to the variables already considered, the location of these zones is influenced by an additional force termed electroendosmosis. For simplicity, this force may be viewed as a flow of buffer passing through the supporting medium in a direction opposite to that of the electrical field. All of the proteins applied to the supporting medium would be carried towards the cathode, were it not for their ability to resist this flow in proportion to their charge density. Electroendosmosis accounts for the distribution of gamma-globulin on the cathodal side of the origin in most supporting media.

An example of the electrophoresis of serum in an agarose gel is shown in Figure 4.5. Serum was applied to the slit cut in the agarose gel. Electrophoresis was continued for one hour. Thereafter, the agarose plate was placed in a mixture of glacial acetic acid, ethanol and water in order to "fix" the proteins in place. The plate was then washed, dried and stained with Amido black dye. The stained bands indicate that this procedure is capable of resolving serum proteins into seven discrete zones.

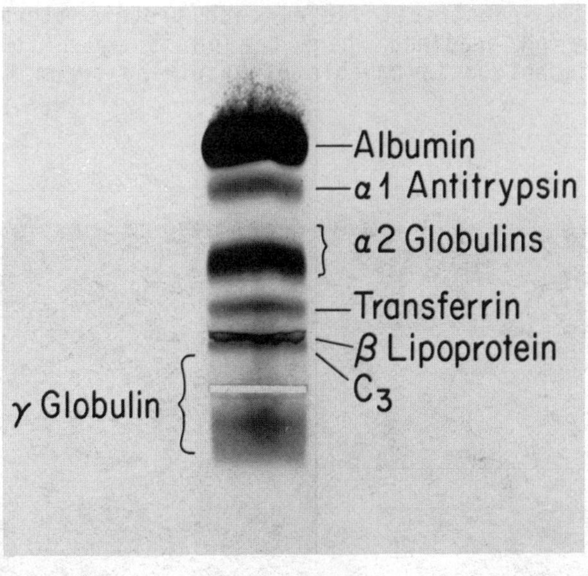

Figure 4.5. Separation of the components of normal human serum by electrophoresis in agarose gel. The migration of albumin is in the direction of the anode.

<u>Immunoelectrophoresis.</u> Immunoelectrophoresis (IEP) combines zone electrophoresis with double immunodiffusion in a method developed by Grabar and Williams. This technique permits the identification of single components in complex mixtures, provides a means for monitoring

purification schemes and finally serves as one criterion of purity of the isolated product. In the clinical laboratory, IEP is widely used to estimate the amount of IgG, IgA and IgM as well as to identify M-components (homogeneous immunoglobulin molecules or their fragments). Immunoelectrophoresis is performed in a thin layer of agar or other supporting medium on a glass slide. In the example shown in Figure 4.6, normal human serum was applied to wells cut in the agar and subjected to an electrical field. Following electrophoretic separation of the protein components, troughs were cut in the agar parallel to the direction of the electrical field. Monospecific antisera directed against the gamma, alpha and mu chain of immunoglobulins were applied to the troughs. Antibodies diffused from the trough until they encountered the corresponding antigens initially distributed into the gel under the influence of the electrical field. Precipitin bands formed in the gel revealing the location of IgG, IgA and IgM proteins.

Isoelectric focusing. Another powerful electrophoretic method is isoelectric focusing invented by H. Svensson. In this procedure, a mixture of proteins is subjected to an electrical field in a gel support in which a pH gradient has initially been generated. Under the influence of the electrical field, each protein migrates toward that portion of the pH gradient where the pH is equal to its isoelectric point. This technique is capable of resolving serum into a minimum of

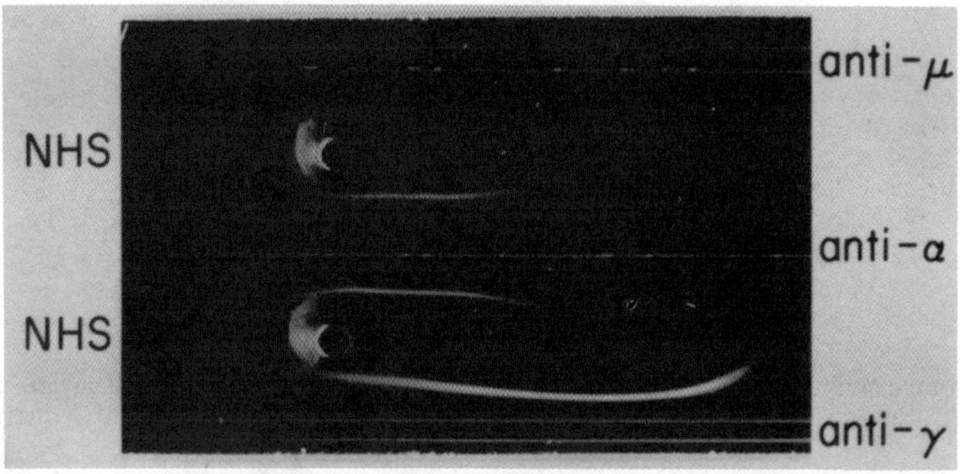

Figure 4.6. Immunoelectrophoresis of normal human serum. The location in the agar of the proteins was revealed by the precipitin bands developed by anti-mu, anti-alpha, or anti-gamma antisera placed in the troughs. (Anode is to the left.)

forty discrete bands. Isoelectric focusing, like other electrophoretic procedures described above, can be converted from an analytical to a preparative procedure.

RADIOIMMUNOASSAY

Radioimmunoassay is based upon the exquisite specificity of antibody molecules and the sensitivity of detectors for small amounts of radioactivity. The radioimmunoassay was developed by Berson and Yalow to measure insulin molecules in human plasma. The concentration of insulin normally present is far below the limits of detection by conventional chemical assay procedures. The principle of one type of radioimmunoassay, the competitive binding assay, is illustrated in Figure 4.7. A constant amount of antibody of high affinity for antigen is added to a series of tubes. To each tube is added a small amount of radiolabeled antigen, as well as increasing amounts of unlabeled antigen (sequence in row 1). Following a period of incubation, antibody-bound labeled and unlabeled antigen must be separated from unbound or free antigen. Several different methods are available; some methods remove antibody (together with bound antigen) from the mixture, while others remove free antigen. An example of the former method involves the use of 50% saturated ammonium sulfate. Most antibody molecules are insoluble in 50% saturated ammonium sulfate, whereas many antigens are soluble at this concentration. Another example involves the use of a second antibody directed against the antibody employed in the first stage of the assay. Rabbit anti-insulin antibody together with bound insulin may be removed from a mixture with free antigen by precipitation with a goat anti-rabbit immunoglobulin antiserum. Free antigen may be removed from a mixture of antibody-bound and free antigen by adsorption to activated charcoal. In all of the examples, the radioactivity associated with antibody and that remaining free is determined.

The sequence in row 2, Figure 4.7, illustrates that, at equilibrium, the combining sites of the antibody molecule contain only radioactive antigen. The ratio of bound to free antigen is 1. In the second panel, one combining site contains a labeled and one an unlabeled antigen molecule. The ratio of bound to free labeled antigen in this illustration is 0.33. In the third panel, a large number of unlabeled antigen molecules compete with a small number of labeled antigen molecules for a limited number of antibody binding sites. At equilibrium, it is quite likely that all the sites will be occupied by unlabeled antigen. Hence, the ratio of bound to free antigen will approach zero. The relationship of the amount of unlabeled antigen added, to the bound over free (B:F) ratio is illustrated in the bottom panel of the figure. This is an example of a standard curve constructed with known amounts of unlabeled antigen; the antigen concentration of an unknown sample can be derived from the standard curve and the B:F

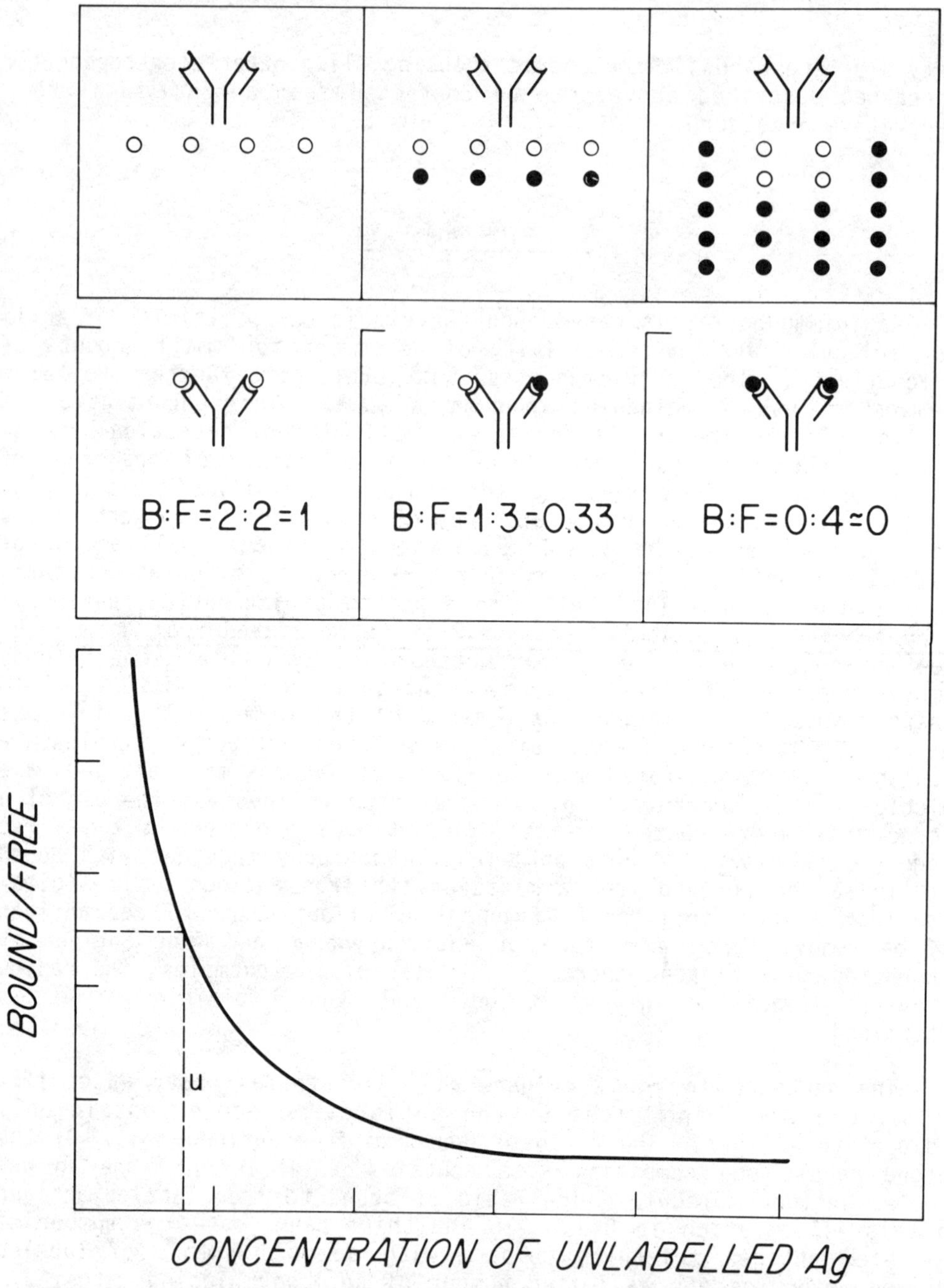

Figure 4.7. Principles of the competitive binding radioimmunoassay. Explanation is in the text. Open circles equal radioactive antigen; dark circles equal non-radioactive antigen.

ratio obtained upon the addition of the unknown sample to a standard mixture of antibody and labeled antigen.

Requirements for the successful application of the radioimmunoassay include: highly specific antibody, a high degree of purity of antigen used for the induction of antibody and for standardizing the assay, limited damage to the antigen as a result of the process employed in radiolabeling, the absence of nonspecific or cross-reactive interfering substances in the test material, and the ability of the test to detect antigen at concentrations that are physiologically active. A large number of advances in modern endocrinology were made possible by the development of radioimmunoassays capable of measuring the nanogram or picogram amounts of hormones in biologic fluids.

(A recent modification of the radioimmunoassay is the Enzyme-Linked Immunosorbent Antibody or ELISA. The test consists of linking the antibody used in the detection assay to an enzyme—such as alkaline phosphatase—after which the enzyme substrate is added. The amount of substrate degraded by the enzyme-linked antibody is then read spectrophotometrically.)

RADIOALLERGOSORBENT TEST

The radioallergosorbent or RAST represents a special application of the radioimmunoassay for the detection of IgE antibodies directed against inhaled or ingested allergens (Figure 4.8) (Chapter 14). In this procedure, allergen is covalently linked to an activated particle such as cellulose beads or paper disks. Test serum containing putative IgE anti-allergen antibody, as well as other classes of anti-allergen antibody, is added and the reactants incubated. During the incubation period, anti-allergen antibodies combine with the solid phase immunoadsorbents. After washing away extraneous proteins, radiolabeled monospecific anti-IgE antibody is added. After a second incubation, the particles are again washed and the particle-associated radioactivity is measured. The amount of radiolabeled anti-IgE antibody bound is directly related to the amount of specific IgE anti-allergen antibody present in the test sample. The IgE antibody content of the test sample is expressed in arbitrary units of 0 to 4+. The RAST procedure has been modified to provide a numerical estimate of the amount of IgE anti-allergen antibody. This is done either by determining the amount of IgE protein present in a sample before and after exposure to solid-phase allergen or by measuring the amount of IgE protein eluted from allergen-coated absorbents. Both methods are relatively cumbersome and require the availability of a reliable radioimmunoassay for IgE protein. Both modifications of the RAST procedure have revealed that a surprisingly large fraction of the circulating IgE protein in serum of allergic patients consists of IgE antibodies directed against a single allergen.

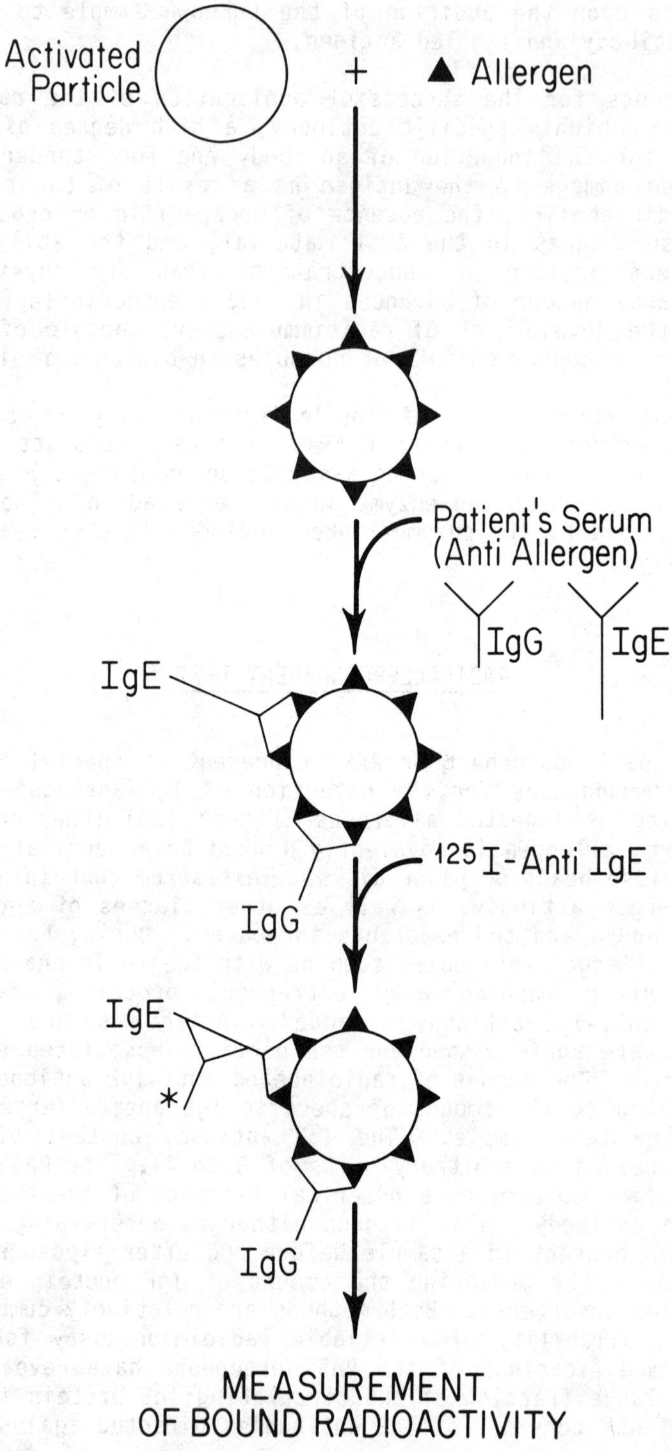
Activated Particle
+
Allergen
Patient's Serum (Anti Allergen)
IgG
IgE
IgE
^{125}I-Anti IgE
IgG
IgE
*
IgG
MEASUREMENT OF BOUND RADIOACTIVITY

Figure 4.8.

In experimental work, quantitation of specific antibodies in serum and of their isotype can be made by a similar procedure as described above: antigen is bound to a particle, which is then reacted with test serum. The amount of antibody bound is titrated by labeled antibody to the antibody. For example, N. Klinman has developed a highly sensitive method to measure mouse anti-DNP antibodies secreted by cells in culture, by mixing antiserum with DNP bound to an immunoabsorbent and then using radioiodinated antibodies to mouse IgG or IgM.

IMMUNOFLUORESCENCE

Certain molecules have the ability to be excited to a higher energy state by a particular wavelength of light. Upon the return of the excited electrons to their normal energy state, the excess energy is released in the form of light. The wavelength of the emitted light is generally longer than the wavelength used to excite the molecules. This excitation-emission process is termed fluorescence when it occurs over a very short period of time (on the order of 10^{-9} to 10^{-8} sec). In 1941, A.H. Coons developed a technique for covalently linking fluorescent dyes to antibody molecules. Thus, it became possible, under appropriate conditions, to visualize antibody molecules; the method by which this process is accomplished is termed <u>immunofluorescence</u>. The immunofluorescence method permits the localization of antigen or antibody on the surface of live cells in suspension or in the cytoplasm or nuclei of cells in frozen sections of tissue. For example, this method is widely used to identify B lymphocytes on the basis of the reaction between their surface immunoglobulin molecules and fluorescein-conjugated anti-immunoglobulin antiserum (Chapter 5). In the ultraviolet microscope, B lymphocytes are recognized by a peripheral linear or beaded rim of fluorescence.

The two fluorescein dyes most commonly used by the immunologist are fluorescein isothiocyanate (fluorescein or FITC) and tetramethylrhodamine isothiocyanate (rhodamine or TRITC). These molecules have characteristic excitation and emission wavelengths. FITC has an excitation maximum of 490-495 nm and an emission maximum of 517 nm; FITC emits with an apple-green color. TRITC is maximally excited at 550 nm and emits its red-orange color at 580 nm.

A special fluorescence microscope, a modification of a light microscope, is used to detect FITC- or TRITC-labeled molecules. A beam of light from a mercury arc or quartz lamp passes through a series of glass or gelatin exciter filters located between the lamp and the microscope stage; these filters restrict the wavelength of the transmitted light to the desired excitation wavelength (490 nm for FITC or 550 nm for TRITC). The excitation beam impinges on the material on the microscope stage causing the dye to fluoresce. Another filter, the barrier filter, located between the stage and the ocular, allows only the emitted wavelength (517 nm for FITC and 580 nm for TRITC) to pass.

Two "staining" procedures are commonly used in immunofluorescence: direct and indirect. In the direct or one-step staining procedure, fluorescein or rhodamine is linked to the isolated IgG fraction of an antiserum containing antibodies directed against a specific component of cells or tissue. Alternatively, the fluor may be linked to antigen for use in localizing specific antibody being synthesized in cells or tissue sections. The material under study is incubated with the labeled antibody or antigen for thirty to sixty minutes. Thereafter, the specimen is washed and examined by fluorescence microscopy. The identification of B lymphocytes cited above is an example of the direct immunofluorescence method. The indirect method involves a two-step procedure (Figure 4.9). An example of this procedure is the widely used assay to detect anti-nuclear antibodies in serum of certain patients. In this procedure, serum is applied to cryostat-sectioned

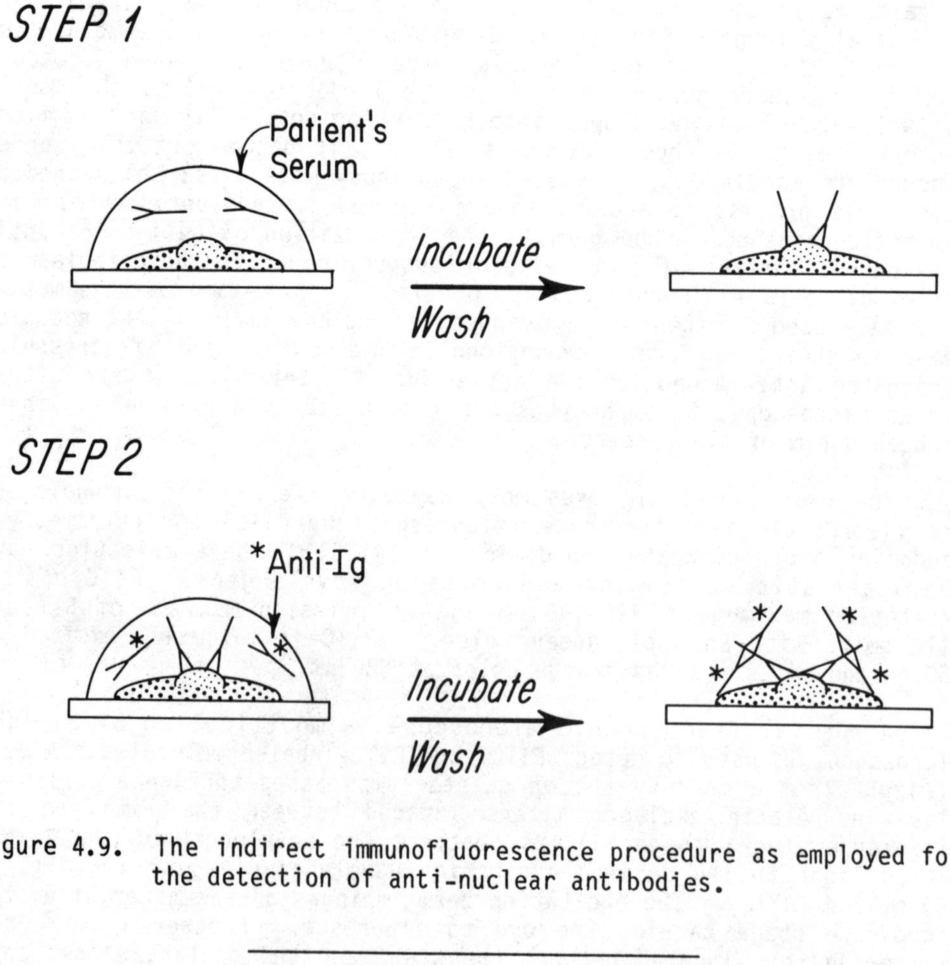

Figure 4.9. The indirect immunofluorescence procedure as employed for the detection of anti-nuclear antibodies.

and acetone-fixed slices of rat or mouse liver on a glass slide. Any anti-nuclear antibodies present in the test serum bind to the corresponding nuclear antigen in the section of liver. After incubation, the slide is washed and then overlaid with a drop of fluorescein-conjugated, anti-human immunoglobulin antiserum. During a second incubation, antibodies to human immunoglobulin bind to the anti-nuclear antibodies initially deposited on the substrate nuclei. After a second washing, the slide is examined by fluorescence microscopy. The presence of anti-nuclear antibodies is indicated by fluorescence of the substrate nuclei.

The indirect staining method has obvious advantages over the direct staining procedure. The expense of conjugating to fluorescein the gamma-globulin fraction of each patient's sera in order to test for the presence of anti-nuclear antibodies by the direct procedure, would make the detection of these antibodies extremely expensive as well as laborious. Furthermore, the indirect procedure leads to greater intensity of fluorescence because several fluoresceinated anti-human immunoglobulin antibodies can attach to a single molecule of anti-nuclear antibody.

The indirect immunofluorescence procedure can also be used to detect antibody in the cytoplasm of plasma cells, the antibody secreting cells (Chapter 5). Following fixation with acetone, plasma cells on a glass slide are overlaid with unlabeled antigen. After incubation, the slide is washed, overlaid with fluorescein-conjugated antiserum and reincubated. After a second washing, cells are examined by fluorescence microscopy. Fluorescence of the cytoplasm of certain plasma cells indicates that these cells contained antibody capable of binding the specific antigen applied in the first step of the procedure.

PLAQUE ASSAY FOR DETECTING INDIVIDUAL ANTIBODY-SECRETING CELLS

Single cells secreting antibody molecules can be identified by a hemolytic technique termed the Jerne plaque assay after its developer. In this procedure, lymphoid cells from an animal immunized with sheep or other erythrocytes, are mixed with a suspension of the corresponding erythrocytes. The mixture of lymphoid cells and erythrocytes is combined with molten agar, poured into a mold and allowed to gel. During a subsequent incubation at 37°C, anti-erythrocyte antibodies produced by lymphoid cells are secreted into the agar, diffuse, and combine with erythrocytes. After the initial incubation, the surface of the agar is flooded with a source of complement, usually fresh guinea pig serum. After a second incubation, the agar is examined for circular clear zones or plaques, representing regions in the gel where complement-mediated lysis of antibody-coated erythrocytes has occurred.

The direct plaque assay described reflects the presence of lymphoid cells secreting antibodies of high hemolytic efficiency. These antibodies are usually of the IgM class. Lymphoid cells secreting IgG anti-erythrocyte antibodies are generally not detected by the direct plaque assay; to demonstrate the presence of such cells requires an indirect procedure. In the indirect plaque assay, lymphoid cells and erythrocytes are incubated for one hour. Thereafter, the surface of the agar is flooded with anti-IgG antibodies and incubation is continued. After the second incubation, the anti-IgG antibodies are decanted and the complement source added. The total number of plaques formed is determined and the number of indirect plaques is obtained by subtracting from the total, the number of direct plaques counted on a duplicate plate. The indirect plaque assay permits the identification of the specific class of antibody-producing cells.

The plaque assay can be further modified to detect cells producing antibodies to non-erythrocyte antigens such as haptens or soluble proteins. For this purpose, erythrocytes can be coated passively with antigen or antigen can be linked to their surfaces by methods cited above.

IMMUNOCYTOADHERENCE

Immunocytoadherence refers to the attachment of certain cells or particles to specific receptors on the membrane of lymphoid cells. It is a technique with wide application. For example, it can be used to detect antibody forming cells. The antigen must be particulate, bacteria or red cells, or may be a soluble protein attached to an indicator particle such as a red cell. The antibody forming cells are mixed with the antigen, usually at 37°C and then examined under the microscope. The particulate antigen is bound all over the surface of the antibody-secreting cells.

Immunocytoadherence can be used to detect receptors on the membranes of lymphocytes such as the Fc receptor (Chapter 5), the C3 receptor (Chapters 5 and 12) and the receptor for sheep red cells in human T cells (Chapter 5).

LYMPHOCYTE TRANSFORMATION

A widely used _in vitro_ assay of cellular immune function involves the measurement of lymphocyte transformation following stimulation by antigens or mitogens. Unstimulated lymphocytes are characterized by a large acentric nucleus surrounded by a thin rim of cytoplasm; these cells show a relatively low rate of synthesis of protein, RNA and DNA. Following stimulation with antigen, certain lymphocytes obtained from previous immunized animals undergo dramatic alterations detailed in Chapters 5 and 8. The cells enlarge and develop a prominent cytoplasmic component filled with rough endoplasmic reticulum (a characteristic feature of cells engaged in active protein systhesis). The synthesis of RNA and DNA is also increased. The stimulated lymphocytes assume the appearance of lymphoblasts (hence the term blast cell transformation) and may undergo mitotic division. Blast cell transformation can be scored morphologically by counting the number of such cells among the population of lymphocytes or by measuring the incorporation of radiolabeled precursors into newly synthesized protein or DNA.

Blast cell transformation may be induced in a lymphocyte population by stimulation with specific antigens or mitogens _in vitro_. Among the commonly used mitogens are the plant lectins, phytohemagglutinin, Concanavalin A and pokeweed mitogen and the bacterial cell wall component, lipopolysaccharide. Cultures of lymphocytes, usually those obtained from peripheral blood, are incubated with either an antigen or mitogen. The cultures are maintained at 37 degrees C for several days in an atmosphere of 5% CO-2. Optimum stimulation with mitogen is usually achieved in about three days; optimum stimulation with antigen usually requires about seven days. During the final hours in culture, tritiated thymidine is added to the culture medium. The labeled thymidine added is incorporated into newly synthesized DNA. The experiment is terminated by depositing the cells onto a glass-fiber filter, washing the cells and disrupting them with trichloracetic acid which also serves to precipitate DNA into the interstices of the filter. After additional washing to remove unincorporated labeled thymidine the filter is dried, and its content of radioactivity determined by liquid scintillation spectroscopy. Thus, the number of counts per minute (cpm) incorporated into DNA is determined. Blast transformation is expressed as the stimulation index which reflects the ratio of cpm incorporated into DNA in the stimulated culture to the cpm incorporated by the unstimulated control lymphocytes. Although a biochemical evaluation of lymphocyte transformation has many advantages including the ease with which multiple samples can be tested, only morphologic evaluation of cells at the end of the period in culture permits an estimation of the fraction of the lymphocyte population that is reacting to the stimulus.

Among the lymphocytes obtained from actively immunized animals, only a small proportion are capable of responding to antigen _in vitro_. Mitogens, however, are capable of non-specifically stimulating a very large fraction of the lymphocyte population. The _in vitro_ responses of lymphocytes to antigens and mitogens provide _important_ information about the functional capabilities of these cells _in vivo_ (Chapter 5).

CELL-MEDIATED LYSIS

Cell-mediated lysis is an important assay to measure the activity of three types of cells: cytolytic T cells (Chapter 7), Killer or Natural Killer (NK) cells (Chapter 5), and activated macrophages (Chapter 7). The assay consists of measuring the release from the target cell of radiolabeled Cr bound to cytosol proteins. Radioactive chromium in the form of sodium chromate penetrates the cells and in the cytosol is reduced to chromic ion which binds tightly to a variety of proteins. (A very small amount is slowly released with time and is taken as a background value in each assay.) If the cell is damaged, the cytosol proteins are released in a soluble form. The amounts released, usually measured after eighteen hours, correlates with the degree of cell death. For the cytolytic T cell assay, graded numbers of lympocytes are incubated with a standard number of target cells and the values expressed as percent specific cytolysis at various T cell-to-target ratios. The targets for the cytolytic T cells are tumor cells or virally infected cells. A similar procedure is followed for measuring NK cell activity, except that the choice of targets is of great importance. Only some—like the line YAC-1—are sensitive to killing by NK cells. The killing of targets by macrophages is detailed below. A related assay for cytolysis consists of using target cells coated with specific antibody. Activated macrophages, neutrophils, or NK cells which bear receptors for IgG can bind to such cells and lyse them (antibody-dependent cellular cytotoxicity or ADCC).

LYMPHOKINES AND GROWTH FACTORS

Lymphokines are protein molecules secreted by T cells upon activation by antigen or lectins (Chapter 7). The amounts of lymphokines released by the T cells can be taken as a measure of their degree of activation. All lymphokines are assayed in biological tests examining their effects on different cell types. Included among the lymphokines is a protein termed interleukin-2 (IL-2) or T cell growth factor. IL-2 stimulates the growth of T helper or cytolytic cells after their initial stimulation by antigen. IL-2 is assayed by adding the culture supernatant to a standard T cell line dependent for its growth exclusively on IL-2. The T cell lines can be generated in culture in a number of ways, by repeated stimulation of T cells with antigen on macrophages or with alloantigens on foreign lymphoid cells. After the initial growth, these T cells are then maintained on IL-2. Eventually, clones of cells propagate, their growth depending entirely on the amounts of IL-2 in the medium. The assay developed by S. Gillis and K. Smith uses a cytolytic T cell line that grows only in the presence of IL-2: the supernatants to be tested are added at graded dilutions, and the degree of proliferation is measured twenty hours later by the incorporation into the DNA of the growing T cells of tritiated labeled thymidine pulsed for a four-hour period. The reciprocal of the dilution of supernatant inducing 50% of a maximal response is taken as a unit value and compared to a standard IL-2 preparation.

A number of lymphokines are measured by their effects on macrophages. These include factors discussed in Chapter 7 that inhibit macrophages from migrating (Migration Inhibitory Factor), that activate macrophages to kill tumors or microbes (macrophage-activating factor) or that induce macrophages to synthesize Ia antigens. In the macrophage inhibitory factor assay, the suspension of macrophages is placed in a capillary tube mixed with graded dilutions of the test supernatant. The tube is then placed in a culture dish. After a few hours, the macrophages migrate out, and the area of migration is estimated. The degree of inhibition of migration correlates with the amounts of the factor. There are several tests for measuring macrophage cytocidal activity. The most popular consists of mixing macrophages in culture with a target tumor cell labeled with radioactive Cr (see "Cell-Mediated Lysis"), the culture supernatant, and a small amount of bacterial endotoxin. After eighteen hours, the culture fluid is harvested, and the amounts of the Cr released by the cell are measured in a radioactive counter. The tumor cells must be selected for their sensitivity to the macrophage cytocidal effect.

For testing lymphokines that induce Ia, the macrophages are cultured from three to six days with the test supernatant. By this time of culture, all untreated macrophages have lost their membrane Ia antigens. The lymphokines stimulate Ia expression in a dose-dependent manner. Ia is estimated with monoclonal antibodies using a cell radioimmunoassay or counting, by immunofluorescence, the number of Ia-bearing macrophages.

Interferons are proteins that induce an anti-viral effect on cells (Chapter 7). A standard cell line, usually L cells, are incubated with the test material for twenty-four hours, after which a cytolytic virus is added (usually Vesicular Stomatitis Virus) for about twenty hours. The virus will lyse the L cells unless these have been incubated with interferon. The interferon-treated L cells will inhibit viral replication. The test supernatants are diluted, titred, and compared to known standards of interferon.

Interleukin-1 (IL-1) is another important mediator secreted not by lymphocytes, as are the lymphokines, but by macrophages (Chapter 5). IL-1 is assayed by estimating its effects on the growth of thymocytes in culture. Freshly harvested thymocytes are in DNA cycle and incorporate tritiated thymidine. However, their multiplication ceases after twenty-four hours of culture. Thymocytes cultured in IL-1, however, maintain their growth. The IL-1 assay consists of culturing thymocytes with different concentrations of the test supernatant for seventy-two hours, after which the cells are given tritium-labeled thymidine and later examined for the incorporation of the label into DNA.

MONOCLONAL ANTIBODIES PRODUCED BY HYBRID CELL LINES

A widely applicable method for producing highly specific antibodies has been recently developed by G. Kohler and C. Milstein. Antibody-forming cells can be fused with malignant plasma cells to form hybrid cells. Fusion is usually produced by the addition of the chemical polyethylene glycol. The method makes use of malignant plasma cells that are poor producers of immunoglobulin and are unable to survive in selected culture media because of certain genetic abnormalities. After fusion, the cell hybrids that survive and secrete antibody are selected as permanent culture lines. These cell hybrids have the growth potential of the tumor line and the genes for immunoglobulin synthesis derived from the parental antibody forming cells. The hybrids secrete antibodies of a single specificity (a monoclonal antibody). These highly purified antibodies are valuable reagents for immunochemical assays, particularly for distinguishing cell surface antigens, such as tissue specific and differentiation antigens. Moreover, the cell fusion technic has confirmed the clonal selection hypothesis, inasmuch as each "hybridoma" secretes a unique homogeneous antibody.

USE OF THE FLUORESCENCE ACTIVATED CELL SORTER

Quantitative cytofluorimetry using a fluorescence activated cell sorter is a new method for measuring cell surface bound ligands and separating subclasses of lymphocytes.

Cells are first labeled with a fluorescein tagged antibody, then washed to remove unbound ligand and passed through the cell sorter. The sorter consists of a flow system in which the cells pass through a small orifice. They emerge "single file" in a liquid stream which then passes through a focused laser beam. This scattered light is detected by the machine and creates a signal which is a measure of the size of the cell. At the same time, if the cell has bound fluorescent antibody, the laser beam excites the fluorescence and this also creates a signal proportional to the amount of antibody on the cell. These size and fluorescence signals are digitalized and analyzed. The sorter gives precise definition of numerous subclasses of cells due to the extreme flexibility offered by the use of fluorescent antibody. It also permits the immunologists to identify cells on the basis of their surface markers.

In addition, the fluorescence activated cell sorter can physically separate—sort out—the positive from the negative cells. This sorting, therefore, permits the collection and examination of specifically tagged cells. The developments of this machine, which was pioneered by Dr. Leonard Herzenberg and associates, at Stanford University, and at Los Alamos Scientific Laboratories, has proved to be extremely useful in biomedical research.

REFERENCES

Adams, D. O., Edelson, P. J., and Koren, H. (eds). Methods for Studying Mononuclear Phagocytes. Adademic Press, New York, 1981.

Bloom, B., and David, J., (eds.) In Vitro Methods in Cell-Mediated and Tumor Immunity, Academic Press, New York, 1976.

Garvey, J. S., Cremer, N. E., and Sussdorf, D. H. Methods in Immunology, third edition, W. A. Benjamin, Inc., Reading Mass., 1977.

Kohler, G., and Milstein, C. Derivation of specific antibody-producing tissue culture and tumor lines by cell fusion, Eur. J. Immunol., 6, 511, 1976.

Mishell, B. B., and Shiigi, S. M. (eds). Selected Methods in Cellular Immunology. W. H. Freeman and Company, San Francisco, 1980.

Rose, N. R. and Freidman, H., (eds.) Manual of Clinical Immunology, American Society for Microbiology, Washington, D. C., 1976.

Weir, D. M. (ed.). Handbook of Experimental Immunology, Third Edition. Blackwell Scientific Publications, London, England, 1978.

Williams, C. A. and Chase M. W. (eds.), Methods in Immunology and Immunochemistry, Academic Press, New York, Vol. I (1967); Vol. II (1968); Vol. III (1970); Vol. IV (1977); Vol. V (1970).

CHAPTER 5

The Cellular Basis of Immunity

Various types of cells participate in an immune response. The principal cells of the lymphoid tissues are the lymphocytes. Lymphocytes have receptor molecules on the membranes that enable them to recognize and interact with antigen molecules. Under appropriate interactions with antigen, the lymphocytes are activated and carry out various effector functions.

Lymphocytes are divided into two major categories, the B and the T lymphocytes. (The B refers to the bursa of Fabricius of birds or to the bone marrow in mammals; the T refers to the thymus.) B lymphocytes, the progenitors of antibody-forming cells, derive from the bone marrow stem cells through a process of antigen-independent maturation that takes place in birds in the bursa of Fabricius, a lymphoepithelial organ found in the posterior wall of the cloacae. No primary lymphoid organ for B cell differentiation has been identified in mammals, although part of the process takes place in the bone marrow. The T lymphocytes, responsible for important regulatory functions and for cellular immunity, derive from the thymus, a primary lymphoid organ located, in most species, in the anterior superior mediastinum. B and T lymphocytes are not homogeneous and include various subsets. There is a third category of lymphocyte that does not show the classical characteristics of T and B cells. These have received the ill-defined name of null cells. Null cells may include stem cells and certain types of cytolytic cells like the natural killer cells (Chapter 11). Their definite identification as a third lymphocyte population has not been established.

Other cells make essential contributions to the immune response by carrying out crucial effector functions. The mononuclear phagocytes act as accessory cells by taking up antigen for lymphocyte stimulation. They also participate as effector cells by ingesting and/or killing bacteria, tumor cells, and foreign substances as well as by releasing a number of inflammatory molecules. Polymorphonuclear neutrophils, eosinophils and basophils, and mast cells participate in the inflammatory response mediated by antibodies.

This chapter considers the properties of lymphoid organs and of the main cells involved in immunity, as well as some of the functional events taking place in response to antigen. It also includes an analysis of various techniques used for the study of immune cells and their interactions. Details of the cellular interactions that result in an immune response are considered in later chapters. We will describe first the histology of primary and secondary lymphoid organs, the recirculation of lymphocytes, and the changes in lymph nodes in response to antigen. We then will describe B cells, T cells, NK cells, and macrophages in detail, considering their surface properties, functions, their pathways of differentiation, and the ways in which to identify them.

CELLULAR ORGANIZATION

The lymphocytes are in a highly dynamic state. A large number of them (about half) recirculate as individual cells in blood and lymph fluids. The lymphocytes are the main cells of the lymphoid tissues--thymus, lymph nodes, and spleen--and an important constituent of some organs like the respiratory and gastrointestinal tract.

Two major types of lymphoid organs can be distinguished: The primary and secondary lymphoid organs. A primary lymphoid organ is one where antigen-independent differentiation of lymphocytes takes place; that is to say, mature T and B cells are generated from stem cells. (Stem cells are early cells with the capacities for self-renewal as well as for generating cells with differentiated properties.) The only primary lymphoid organ identified in mammals is the thymus. The secondary lymphoid organs are the lymph nodes and spleen formed by mature B and T cells as well as by antigen-trapping cells such as the phagocytes. It is in the secondary lymphoid organs where antigen is concentrated and where the specific immune reactions are generated.

Thymus Gland. The thymus is a bilobed organ that derives from the endoderm of the third and fourth branchial pouches. It is a lymphoepithelial organ containing lymphocytes (named thymocytes) and epithelial cells. The thymus is the first lymphoid organ to develop during ontogeny. It increases progressively in size during fetal and neonatal life, reaching its full dimension in early puberty, after which there is a steady involution. By late life, the thymus is markedly atrophied.

The thymus is organized into two main compartments, the cortex and the medulla. The cortex, the more prominent of the two, contains numerous thymocytes, many epithelial cells, and a few macrophages, all closely packed together, leaving little free extracellular spaces. The thymocytes in the cortex are of small and medium sizes with a few large cells found predominantly at the periphery of the cortex, where mitoses are frequent. The epithelial cells have a stellate shape, adhering to the thymocytes and establishing contact with other epithelial cells by small desmosomes. The macrophages in most species tend to concentrate near the corticomedullary areas. The cortex is the area where thymic differentiation takes place. The cortical thymocytes are immature and progressively differentiate to T cells which eventually migrate to the medulla where they then exit to the blood.

The medulla of the thymus contains small thymocytes loosely arranged and not as tightly packed as in the cortex. Many of the thymocytes of the medulla are mature T cells in the process of leaving the gland. The medulla also contains epithelial cells of varying sizes and shapes, many of which organize into Hassall's corpuscles, concentric layers of flat, squamous-type epithelial cells with abundant cytoplasm. An interesting difference between cortex and medulla is their degree of permeability to plasma proteins. The vessels of the cortex are highly impermeable to proteins, thus isolating the maturing thymocytes from contact with circulating proteins; in contrast, the medullary area is highly permeable. The functional significance of this anatomical difference is not known.

The maturation of T cells within the thymus has been studied extensively in the mouse. This is due to the availability of antibodies to membrane macromolecules that serve as an index of the maturational stage of the cell. These surface antigens are polymorphic; they differ among the various strains of mice to the point where appropriate alloimmunization will give rise to specific antibodies (Chapter 6). These antigens include the H-2 antigens, the thymic-leukemia (TL) antigen, the GIX antigen, the θ (or Thy-1), and the Ly1, Ly2,3 antigens.

The H-2 antigens are found in thymocytes as well as in most other cells and will be described in Chapter 6. TL is not a single antigen but a complex of several. Some strains of mice lack identifiable TL; interestingly, if thymic leukemia develops in these strains, the leukemia cells will express TL on their membranes. Thus, the expression of TL antigens appears to be controlled by both structural and regulatory genes, the latter acting by repressing TL expression on thymocytes of some strains. The TL antigens have been identified as 40,000 to 50,000 molecular weight glycoproteins.

The GIX antigen is related to the 70,000 molecular weight class of glycoproteins that also form part of the envelope of certain murine leukemia viruses. The GIX molecule is thought to be coded by the viral genome integrated into the chromosome of the cell. Expression of GIX is inherited as a typical Mendelian trait. GIX antigens are found only in thymocytes and not in mature T cells.

The Thy-1 or θ is present on both mature thymocytes and mature T cells and also in brain cells, epithelial cells, and fibroblasts. The

Ly1,2,3 system includes three loci that control proteins found exclusively on lymphocytes of the T cell class. Ly2 and Ly3 are closely linked and are considered in our discussion as a single trait.

The process of thymocyte differentiation in the mouse can be followed by examining for the presence or absence of the alloantigens described above. The data so far supports the following sequence of maturation:

1. Stem Cell ---> Prothymocyte. Stem cell becomes committed to the T lineage and becomes a prothymocyte. Prothymocytes are found in bone marrow of adult mice, have H-2 antigens, but lack TL, GIX, and Thy-1.

2. Prothymocyte ---> Immature Thymocyte. This step takes place in the cortex of the thymus, to which the prothymocyte migrates. The immature thymocyte acquires the TL, GIX, Ly1,2,3, and Thy-1 alloantigens but is functionally immature and will not proliferate in response to the lectin PHA nor respond in a mixed leukocyte culture (MLC) (Chapter 6).

3. Immature Thymocytes ---> Mature T Cell. The cell acquires a higher content of H-2, loses TL and GIX, and reduces its content of Thy-1. At some step, T cells separate into subsets differing in the amounts of Ly1 or Ly2,3. The importance of these subsets is discussed later (Table 5.1 summarizes these points).

Table 5.1

Characteristics of the T Lineage

Cells	Alloantigens				Functional Assays		
	H-2	TL	θ	Tdt	Proliferation with PHA	MLC	Localization in Thymus
Prothymocyte	++	—	—	+	—	—	(Bone Marrow)
Immature Thymocyte	++	+	+++	+	—	—	Cortex
Mature T Cell	++++	—	+	—	+	+	Medulla

Another important marker of thymocyte differentiation is the enzyme terminal deoxynucleotidyl transferase (Tdt). Tdt is a unique enzyme capable of adding mononucleotides to a DNA segment in the absence of a template. Tdt is found in some bone marrow cells, in prothymocytes, and in immature thymocytes; it is absent in mature T cells. Tdt has also been found in cells of many of the acute lymphoblastic leukemias of children.

The control of differentiation within the thymus has been the subject of intense study. It is thought that this process may be regulated by "hormones" or factors synthesized by the epithelial cells. Various peptides have been isolated from the gland, some of which have been well characterized biochemically. Extracts of thymus glands or the purified peptides are capable of promoting part of the differentiation of thymocytes in vitro, for example, prothymocyte to thymocyte differentiation. Indeed, a proportion of the stem cells isolated from bone marrow when incubated with the thymic factors for just two hours will develop the Thy-1 surface alloantigen. The precise role and cellular source of the thymic factors still awaits more study.

Recent studies suggest that the stroma of the thymus may influence part of the differentiation of the thymocyte. The thymic stromal cells —epithelial and macrophages—are very rich in their membrane content of proteins coded in the I region of the Major Histocompatibility Gene Complex. These molecules termed Ia antigens are key molecules modulating all cellular interactions involving T cells (Chapters 6, 8, and 10). The interactions between thymocytes and Ia-bearing stromal cells may influence how the mature T cells interact with antigen.

<u>Secondary Lymphoid Organs: The Lymph Nodes.</u> The lymph nodes are small, round, or oval organs containing lymphocytes within a reticular stroma. The lymph nodes are usually found in groups in certain regions of the body, for example, along the large blood vessels in the abdomen, in the mesentery, axilla, or inguinal regions. The lymphatics are a network of channels paralleling the blood circulation. The lymphatics collect extravascular material, including fluids, extravasated from capillaries. Once inside the channels, the fluid is called lymph. The lymph nodes are positioned along the lymphatic channels. The lymph drains into the node via the afferent lymphatics and exits via efferent channels. The lymph eventually drains into the major lymphatic vessels such as the thoracic duct and the right lymphatic duct. These, in turn, empty into the blood circulation. Lymph and cells traveling in the lymphatics effectively become distributed throughout the body.

Lymph nodes contain lymphocytes distributed mainly into two areas: the <u>superficial cortex</u> and the <u>deep cortex</u>. In between the cells there is a system of lymphatic channels running from the cortex, where the <u>afferent lymphatics</u> empty into the subcapsular sinus, into the <u>medulla</u>, where they collect into the <u>efferent lymphatics</u>.

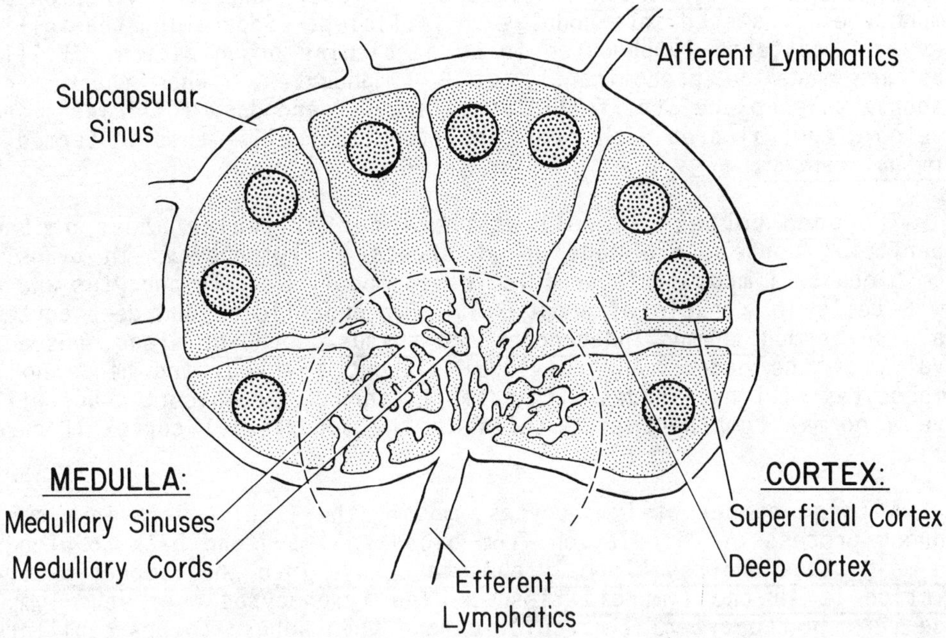

Figure 5.1. The description of the structure of the lymph node is given in the text.

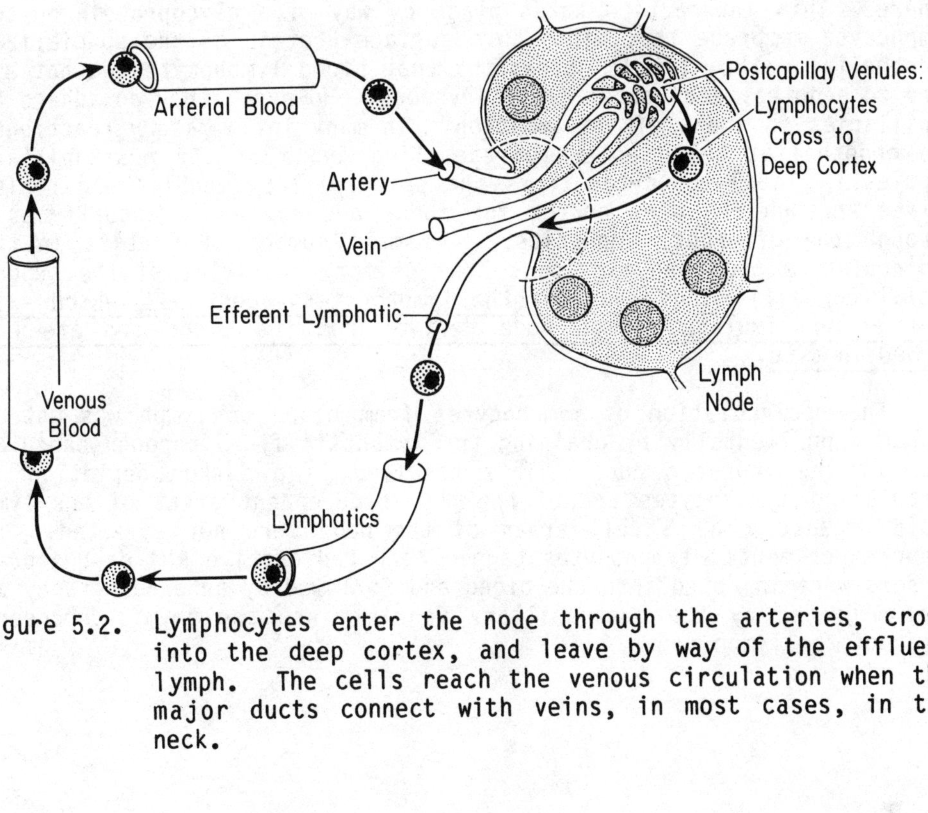

Figure 5.2. Lymphocytes enter the node through the arteries, cross into the deep cortex, and leave by way of the effluent lymph. The cells reach the venous circulation when the major ducts connect with veins, in most cases, in the neck.

The superficial cortex consists of a closely packed collection of lymphocytes clustered into nodules or follicles. Separating the follicles are scattered lymphocytes in no particular organization. Follicles are made up predominantly of B lymphocytes. When the immune response takes place, the follicles enlarge ("secondary follicles") and develop a central area with large proliferating cells—this is termed a germinal center.

The deep cortex, as well as the interfollicular areas of the superficial cortex, are made up of sheets of lymphocytes in transit from blood to lymph. This area is formed mostly by T lymphocytes and a few B cells in a ratio of about 3:1. The superficial and deep cortex are also termed thymus-independent and thymus-dependent areas, respectively, of the node. An individual without a thymus and hence no T lymphocytes will have nodes with a small, shrunken deep cortex but will have a normal component of B cells in the superficial cortex (Figure 5.1).

A large number of lymphocytes, mostly the T cells, are in a continuous process of circulation from blood to lymph and back to blood. The main place whereby blood lymphocytes cross into the lymphatic circulation is in the lymphoid tissue. The lymphocytes enter the lymph node through the arterial circulation and then adhere to postcapillary venules found abundantly in the cortex of the node, in the diffuse lymphoid tissue surrounding the follicles (Figure 5.2). The postcapillary venules have a tall, specialized endothelium to which the lymphocytes adhere. This interaction takes place by way of a glycoprotein on the lymphocyte membrane that binds to a surface protein of the specialized endothelial cell. (It is noteworthy that blood lymphocytes do not adhere to endothelia of other capillary beds. However, they do adhere to capillaries in areas of inflammation. In many inflammatory reactions, the endothelial cells enlarge, resembling those of the postcapillary venules.) The lymphocytes cross the postcapillary venules and recirculate through the deep cortex for about one day and eventually exit through the efferent lymphatics. (A small number of B cells in the recirculating pool can migrate to the primary follicles of the superficial cortex.) Thus, most of the lymphocytes--about 95%--which exit from an unstimulated lymph node derive from the blood and are not formed in situ.

The recirculation of lymphocytes from blood to lymph was established experimentally by draining the lymphatic fluid through cannulation of the thoracic duct. This resulted in a marked depletion of circulating lymphocytes and of the thymic-dependent areas of the lymphoid organs. The B cell areas of the node were not affected. In other experiments, lymphocytes tagged with radioactive RNA or DNA precursors were injected into the blood and followed by autoradiography as they migrated by the postcapillary venules into the thymic-dependent areas of the lymph nodes.

Trapping of Antigen. Antigens that enter a lymph node can be trapped in the two main areas of the node. The cells that trap the antigen are phagocytes (macrophages) or specialized kinds of reticular or dendritic cells. Antigen is readily trapped in the deep cortex, i.e., the thymic-dependent areas, and in the walls of the lymphatic sinuses, both of which contain phagocytes that avidly take up the antigen. The trapping of antigen in the deep cortex is thought to represent an early important step in immune induction. As soon as antigen is taken up by the phagocytes, inductive events are initiated whereby lymphocytes then recognize and interact with some of the antigen-trapped molecules. Trapping of antigen by the phagocytes is favored if the antigen is coated with antibody, but this is not a necessary prerequisite for all antigens. Most of the antigen taken up by the macrophages is readily digested by these cells; however, a few antigen molecules apparently escape total breakdown, and these are the ones involved in the interaction with the lymphocytes. The first evidence for antibody formation occurs outside the lymphoid follicles as a result of the meeting between B and T lymphocytes and phagocytes that have trapped the antigen.

A second area where antigen is trapped is the superficial cortex, in the lymphoid follicles. Antigen percolates through the follicle and is trapped there only in circumstances where an immune response has already been initiated and there is antibody to form antigen-antibody complexes. The antigen-antibody complexes—also containing complement proteins—become bound to the surface of specialized cells found inside the follicles called follicular dendritic cells. These cells have many thin cytoplasmic prolongations that extend among the lymphocytes of the nodule. The follicular dendritic cells contain very few lysosomes and pinocytic vesicles, and the antigen-antibody complexes are retained on their surfaces for long periods of time. Thus, the trapping of antigen in the superficial cortex results from an ongoing immune response since it will not take place in conditions where no antibody is made. The functional significance of antigen-antibody complexes' trapping in dendritic cells of the follicle is still unresolved since the localization appears not to be necessary for antibody production. Some think it may be related to the maintenance of immune memory.

The entrance of antigen leads to a marked series of changes in the structure and in the pattern of circulation of the lymph nodes:

1. First, as stated above, antigen enters the node by way of afferent lymph and is bound by macrophages. Shortly after the entrance of antigen (first twenty-four hours), there is a marked reduction in the number of lymphocytes leaving the node by efferent lymphatics, and a marked increase in the number of cells found in the deep cortex. Presumably, the lymphocytes keep on crossing from blood to the lymph node, but their exit is stopped by mechanisms not yet known, perhaps mediated by prostaglandins secreted by the macrophages. Neutrophils and eosinophils are also found in abundance at this time.

2. From two to five days later, there is an increase in lymphocytes leaving by way of the efferent lymphatics. At this time, more lymphocytes cross from blood into node, and the shut-off mechanism found in first twenty-four hours is no longer operative. The lymphocytes capable of reacting with the antigen in question (which is a small fraction of the total lymphocyte population) stay in the node during the period (presumably because they are interacting with the macrophage-bound antigen) and are not found in the efferent lymphatics. During this period of time, the cellularity of the node increases, and the distinction between deep and superficial cortex is obscured. Proliferation becomes abundant in the deep cortex. The first antibody-containing cells appear within the deep cortex and also in the superficial cortex.

3. After five days, the number of cells leaving the node by the efferent lymphatics is reduced, but not the lymphocytes that have reacted with the antigen (and thus are "primed" or activated); they now leave the node, disseminating the immune process throughout the tissues. At the end of the first week, the superficial cortex develops well, and germinal centers become evident. Plasma cells are abundant around germinal centers and in interfollicular areas. The medullary cords, which represent areas in between the sinuses of the medulla, contain many antibody-forming cells.

Secondary Lymphoid Organs: The Spleen: The spleen is an abdominal organ that functions both to clear particulate materials from blood and to concentrate blood-borne antigens. Indeed, the immune response to antigens in the blood takes place predominantly in the spleen. Histologically, the spleen is divided into the white pulp, comprising the lymphoid tissue, and the red pulp, an area rich in sinuses; so-called because of its abundant content of red blood cells. The lymphoid tissue of the white pulp is organized around small arteries and arterioles; it is also divided into a thymic-dependent and -independent area. The thymic-dependent area is the diffuse lymphoid tissue, rich in T cells, immediately surrounding the arteriole, so-called periarteriolar lymphoid sheath. The thymic-independent area comprises the follicular or nodular B cell areas which surround the T cell areas.

THE B LYMPHOCYTE

The B lymphocyte derives from a stem cell through a maturation process independent of antigen stimulation. Before birth, progenitors of B cells are found in the liver and in the spleen; after birth, the bone marrow becomes the major source. The B cell differentiates from a stem cell to an early immature cell that finally evolves to a late, mature B cell. The mature B cell is not an antibody-secreting cell but can readily differentiate upon antigen stimulation to an antibody-secreting cell. The end state of the antigen-driven differentiation process is a plasma cell. Plasma cells contain abundant cytoplasm rich in endoplasmic reticulum and do not divide, having a life of about two to three days. Between the end-stage plasma cell and the B cell, there are intermediate cells of large size, with abundant cytoplasm and active antibody secretion.

To summarize what will be described in Chapter 8, B cells respond to most antigens by proliferating as well as by differentiating to plasma cells. Such responses by B cells usually require cooperative interactions with T lymphocytes. In the absence of cooperative interactions, the result of the interaction of B cells with antigen depends on the class of antigens. Thymus-dependent antigens will not stimulate and may even tolerize, while the special class of thymic-independent antigens will stimulate a restricted response. The end result of B cell stimulation by antigen is the acquisition by the individual of circulating antibodies as well of the capacity to generate a secondary response (immunological memory).

Evidence that B Lymphocytes Initiate Immune Responses and Differentiate into Plasma Cells. Immune responses can be initiated by purified lymphocytes. This can be tested in experimental animals by transplanting purified lymphocytes, using genetically identical animals that do not reject transplanted cells or tissues, as follows:

a. Heavily irradiate a group of mice. The X-irradiation destroys the lymphocytes but not the macrophages. The X-irradiated mouse is immunoincompetent. If challenged with antigen, the mouse will not be able to mount an immune response.

b. Harvest lymphocytes from the spleen of a normal mouse. Perform cytochemical analysis and check for purity. The spleen of normal mice contains about equal number of T and B cells.

c. Transplant the lymphocytes from the normal to the immunoincompetent X-irradiated recipient.

d. Immunize the recipient with antigen.

The recipient will make an immune response identical in magnitude to that of a normal mouse. The injected antigen is trapped by the radioresistant macrophages of the recipient—the injected purified T and B cells interact with the antigen and proliferate and differentiate. Using appropriate alloantigens, the lymphocytes of normal mice can be "marked" and followed in their differentiation to plasma cells.

Surface Molecules of B Cells. Intense studies are now being carried out to characterize different surface macromolecules in B cells. The purpose of these studies is to try to identify surface molecules involved in key cellular interactions and/or as receptors for other mediators. The presence or absence of surface molecules may also serve to classify a subset of B cells. The following surface molecules have been identified in B cells:

1. Ig (described below)

2. Fc Receptor. Most B cells have Fc receptors which are surface structures that specifically bind to the Fc fragment of IgG. The Fc receptors are described in the next section dealing with mononuclear phagocytes. The Fc receptor of B cells is detected using an appropriately labeled antigen-antibody complex (usually, antibody-coated red cells, fluorescein-labeled polymerized IgG, or a soluble immune complex in which the antigen is a protein labeled with fluorescein). The detection of the Fc receptor in B cells requires a higher concentration of complexes as compared to macrophages, a reflection perhaps of a smaller number of surface sites. Monoclonal antibodies have now been produced against the Fc receptor. The function of the Fc receptor may be to aid the B cell in binding antigen bound to antibodies.

3. C3 Receptors. About one-half to three-fourths of B cells have a receptor for fragements of C3, enabling them to bind to antigen-antibody complexes containing bound complement. The C3 receptors are detected by using sheep erythrocytes coated with IgM anti-red cell antibody and C. (The Fc receptor of the B cell does not bind to mu chains.) The function of C3-positive or C3-negative B cells has been the subject of analysis in recent years. In the mouse, B cells from young mice (up to two to three weeks of age) lack C3 receptors. These young B cells are less responsive than their adult counterpart, but the relationship between this and the C3 receptor is not yet clear. Two distinct C3 receptors, CR1 and CR2, are found in B cells (described later with mononuclear phagocytes and in Chapter 12).

4. Histocompatibility Molecules. B cells express surface antigens coded in the major histocompatibility gene complex (MHC), including molecules coded in the I region. Most B cells have I-region-associated molecules (the Ia antigens or Class II glycoproteins), but there are a few which do not. The B cells that do not have Ia antigens, respond less well to thymic-dependent antigens, and show poor differentiation to IgG synthesis.

5. Lyb Antigens. In the mouse, a series of alloantigens have been identified in B cells using cross-immunization between appropriate inbred stains. Of particular importance are the Lyb3,5 and 7 system. A mutant strain of mice, the CBA/N, has been shown to have an X-linked recessive trait characterized by the absence of B cells lacking these three alloantigens.

Recognition of Antigen by B Cells. B lymphocytes interact with antigen via specific receptor molecules located on their plasma membrane. The receptor molecules for antigen are Ig molecules identical in specificity with those secreted when the B cells' progeny differentiates into plasma cells. Because T cells have no recognizable Ig molecules on their surface, the presence of Ig on the lymphocyte membrane can be used as a marker for B cells.

Identification of Surface Ig. The basic procedure that is used to identify and quantitate B cells consists of incubating freshly harvested lymphocytes at cold temperature with anti-Ig antibodies labeled with fluorescein isothiocyanate. The antibody will bind to the surface Ig of the B cell. After incubation, the cells are washed well in order to eliminate the antibody that is not bound and are then examined under the fluorescent microscope or by flow cytometry. The B cells are identified by the presence of small discrete dots of fluorescence over their surface. The number of B cells in peripheral blood of man ranges from five to twenty percent (Figure 5.3).

Surface Ig molecules can also be biochemically identified. The method that is most commonly employed consists of the isolation of proteins from the plasma membrane of B cells radiolabeled with I. Cells are first labeled with I, and the radiolabeled proteins are then extracted from the membrane using detergents. The extracted proteins are incubated with an anti-Ig antibody; the immune complex is separated from the rest of the labeled proteins; the labeled Ig is then dissociated from the antibodies and examined biochemically, usually by polyacrylamide gel electrophoresis using sodium dodecylsulphate (Figure 5.3).

Number and Class of Ig: B cells contain from 0.5 to 1.5 x 10^5 molecules of Ig per cell. The class of Ig displayed on the cell surface has been examined using class-specific antibodies. The majority of Ig-bearing lymphocytes shows both IgM and IgD on the cell surface. The IgM molecules found on the cell surface are monomers (and not pentameric molecules such as those found in secreted IgM). The presence of IgD serving as an antigen receptor was surprising, inasmuch as IgD is found only in trace amounts in serum (Chapter 3). Both the surface IgM and IgD are synthesized by the B cells. This can be tested by removing surface Ig from the membrane by proteolysis and showing that, upon culture, the lymphocytes can reexpress the Ig on their membrane. The number of B cells bearing surface IgG is very small.

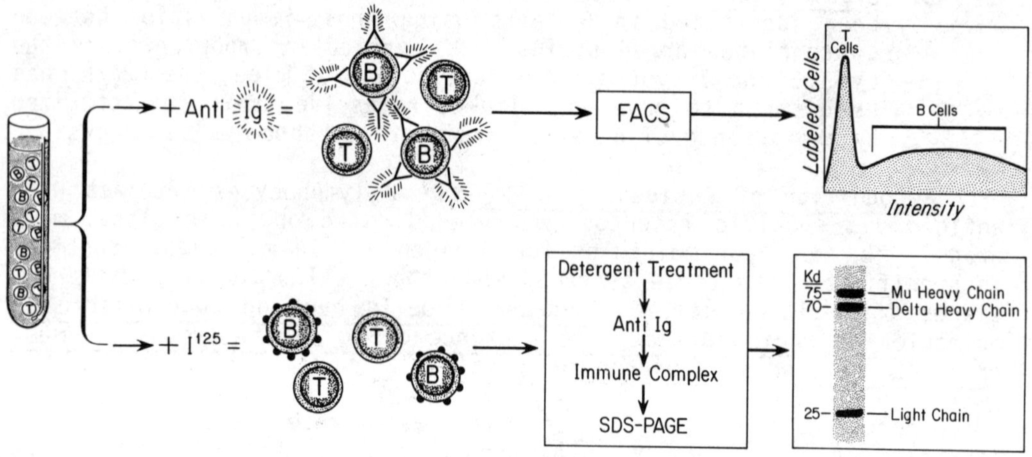

Figure 5.3. This figure depicts the techniques used to identify and to study B cells. In the upper section, the B cells are incubated with a fluorescein-tagged anti-Ig antibody. The B cells, now coated with anti-Ig, are examined in the fluorescence-activated cell sorter (FACS) (Chapter 4). The graph shown in the figure indicates that T cells have minimal fluorescence, while B cells comprise cells with different degrees of intensity. (Cells incubated with an unrelated antibody would have shown low fluorescent intensity and a single peak at the level of intensity found for T cells.) The FACS will give a precise estimate of the percentage of surface Ig-positive cells. In the lower section, all the membrane properties are labeled with I, including surface Ig (shown as dark circles). The cells are then treated as described, and the surface Ig identified by immunoprecipitation with anti-Ig and electrophoresis (using sodium dodecyl sulfate and polyacrylamide gels).

Ig molecules are unique in that they function both as soluble molecules, in serum and extracellular fluids, and as integral membrane proteins, serving in this instance as antigen receptors on B cells. Surface Ig is clearly an integral membrane protein: it cannot be solublized from the membrane by treatment with various salts; furthermore, when solubilized by non-ionic detergents, it becomes insoluble when attempts are made to remove the detergent. Surface Ig appears to be fixed to the membrane through its C terminal end that contains a small number of hydrophobic amino acids. Indeed, surface IgM is slightly bigger in size than the secreted counterpart.

As expected from the fluid mosaic model of membrane structure (Singer and Nicolson, Science, 175:720), surface Ig on the B cell is free to diffuse within the plane of the membrane. Interaction of antigens with the surface Ig produces a dramatic series of events both at the cell surface and in the cytoplasm (Figure 5.4). First, the antigen binds to surface Ig, forming complexes of various sizes. These complexes then move within the plasma membrane and rapidly coalesce to one pole or segment of the cell. The cell appears to have a "cap" of complexes. This process whereby surface complexes redistribute to one area of the cell surface has been termed capping. Ligand binding is accompanied by an association of surface Ig to cytoskeletal structures. Biochemically, surface Ig becomes insoluble in detergent, indicating a linkage to the detergent-insoluble cytoskeleton. The requirements for capping of surface Ig-ligand complexes are: 1) a multivalent ligand; 2) fluid membrane; 3) energy metabolism; and 4) the integrity of the cytoplasmic contractile elements.

Following capping, the B lymphocyte undergoes a brief episode of translatory motion. After this stage, the bulk of the surface complexes are eliminated from the cell by endocytosis and intracellular digestion. The cell is then bare of Ig receptors but expresses new receptors after a few hours. The outcome of this episode of antigen binding depends on various circumstances. Antigen binding in the absence of cooperative interactions with T cells will not stimulate differentiation to antibody formation except in the case of thymic-independent antigens. Figure 5.4 depicts the scheme of early events in B cells.

Antigen Binding to Surface Ig. The clonal selection theory was postulated by M. Burnet to explain, at the cellular level, the formation and specificity of antibodies (Chapter 1). It was postulated that lymphocytes would develop bearing unique antigen receptors. Antigen would bind to, and thus select, those cells having receptors for it. As the cell binding the antigen was stimulated, it would secrete an antibody molecule of the same specificity. The clonal selection theory has been substantiated. All the surface Ig molecules of an individual B cell have the same combining site, thus reacting with a unique antigen determinant. B cells binding antigen are found in an individual prior to exposure to antigen. After antigen stimulation, there is an increase in the number of B cells binding the antigen as well as a relative and absolute increase in the cells with receptors of high affinity for the antigen. Antigen binds preferentially to and, therefore, selects those B cells having receptors of high affinity. After binding antigen, the B cells, usually following cooperative interactions with T cells and macrophages, proliferate and differentiate into a plasma cell, which secretes an Ig molecule of the same specificity as the B cell.

The binding of antigen to B cells has been verified in experiments using radiolabeled antigen and the technique of autoradiography. The experiment consists of incubating lymphocytes with a highly radioactive

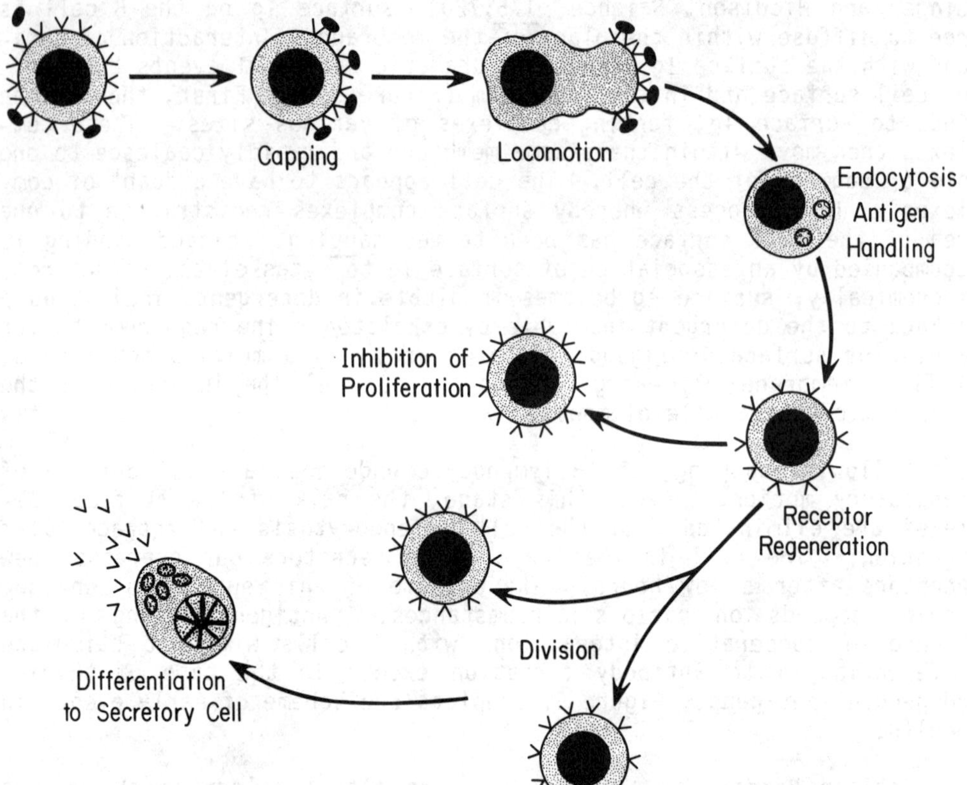

Figure 5.4. Interaction of B cells with antigen first results in capping, then stimulation of locomotion. Several cycles of capping and regeneration of receptors will induce proliferation. Very immature B cells, however, will not proliferate and may even be inhibited. The process of differentiation requires interaction with T cells, in the case of thymic-dependent antigens.

---

antigen. Only those lymphocytes having specific receptors will bind the radioactive antigen. The cells are then washed in order to eliminate non-bound antigen, smeared on a glass slide, and coated by a photographic emulsion. After a few days, the slides are processed and developed. Those cells binding radioactive antigen will show small grains of silver over the entire surface. Using this method, one finds very few lymphocytes binding a given molecule of antigen (one to ten per hundred-thousand) in accordance with clonal selection theories. If the B cells are treated with a proteolytic enzyme, the Ig receptors are stripped off, and the cell will no longer be able to bind the radioactive antigen.

The binding of antigen by B cells is essential for the development of an immune response. This point can be tested either by eliminating the specific antigen-binding cells ("negative selection") or by purifying them ("positive selection"). In a former case, the elimination of a clone of antigen-binding B cells results in no immune response to the antigen in question but a perfect response to unrelated antigens. In the latter, "positive selection", the immune response is made only to the antigen used in the selection.

Example of a Negative Selection Experiment. The clones of antigen-binding cells can be eliminated in the following experiment:

1. Harvest lymphocytes from the spleen of a mouse.
2. Prepare two columns of dextran beads, one having covalently bound the protein antigen BSA (bovine serum albumin); the other with bound BGG (bovine gamma globulin).
3. Pass lymphocytes through each column.
4. Test the lymphocytes that pass through the column for their capacity to make a response to both antigens (this can be done by injecting with cells into X-irradiated mice, challenging the mice with the antigens, and then testing for production of antibody).
5. Results:

Lymphocytes Passed Through	Antibody Response to: BSA	BGG
BSA column	—	+
BGG column	+	—

6. Interpretation: The B lymphocytes with Ig receptors for BSA attach to the BSA beads and are retained in the column. Those lymphocytes having receptors for BGG are not retained in the BSA-bead column, pass through, and are capable of mounting an antibody response to it. The same holds true for the BGG column, which retains the BGG-cloned cells and not the BSA-binding lymphocytes.

Example of a Positive Selection Experiment. These experiments are more difficult to perform because of the difficulties in purifying cells binding a given antigen. Progress has been made in recent years using a number of technical approaches. One such approach is now described:

1. Conjugate gelatin to the hapten, DNP. The DNP-gelatin complex is layered on culture dishes. The gelatin solidifies at cold temperature.

2. Layer on top of the DNP-gelatin plates a suspension of lymphocytes (in the cold). Wash the plates very well after one hour of incubation.

3. Remove the cells bound to the gelatin (this is done by warming the dishes to 37°C, melting the gelatin, and then digesting it with collagenase).

4. Test the response of the lymphocytes.

5. The results show that only DNP-specific cells are bound to the gelatin and that only anti-DNP antibodies are produced by these cells.

Restrictions in the Expression of Surface Ig. The expression of Ig is restricted in the B cell. Of the extensive library of variable genes, the cell selects only one set of H chain and L chain V genes. Thus, one B cell will bind only one kind of antigen and no other. There is, likewise, restriction in the expression of constant H chain genes, The majority of B cells have surface IgM and IgD but no other Ig classes. Few B cells bear IgG. During antigen stimulation, the B cell switches the constant H chain class synthesized without a change in variable portion (see below). Finally, the cell demonstrates allelic exclusion; that is, it reads the genetic information for Ig genes of only the maternal or paternal chromosome (Chapter 10).

Changes in Ig During Ontogeny. The development of mature B cells bearing IgM and IgD is preceded by an early immature stage where the cells have predominantly IgM. The best evidence for this sequence comes from studies of B cell development during ontogeny in the mouse. During fetal life and approximately during the first week of neonatal life, the B cells have IgM, lack the C3 receptor, and are highly sensitive to tolerance induction. Tolerance induction is simply tested *in vitro* by incubating the B cells with a protein antigen for a brief period of time. Several days later, the number of antibody-forming cells is tested in a plaque assay. Under these conditions, neonatal B cells are found not to respond, apparently as a negative result of exposure to the antigen during the brief period of incubation.

By the second to fourth week of life, murine B cells bearing both isotypes appear, together with the presence of some cells bearing C3 receptors. Functionally, these mature B cells are now resistant to tolerance. It should be noted that the immature type of B cell is also found in the *adult* mouse, in the bone marrow. During adulthood, the bone marrow becomes the source of B cells that develop first through an immature stage similar to that found in neonates. Later, the B cells home to lymphoid organs and acquire the mature characteristics.

The generation of the repertory of recognition by B cells during fetal and neonatal life has been examined in the mouse. The mouse is born with few B cells and consequently has a limited number of different clones. We emphasize again that each clone exhibits sepcificity for only one antigenic determinant. During the first ten days of neonatal life, there is a marked proliferation of lymphoid cells in general and particularly of B cells, as each cell divides every twenty-four hours. Consequently, with time, not only new clones of B cells appear, but the number of cells forming each clone enlarges. The interesting point is that the emergence of various different clones, with time, is not random, but rather follows an apparent program. For example, at birth, many B cells are found reactive to the haptens DNP or TNP (trinitrophenyl) but few to the hapten fluorescein. The fluorescein-reactive cells do not appear until a week later. This pattern of development is consistent and unrelated to antigenic stimulation.

The Question of B Cell Subsets. The issue has been raised on whether the B cell lineage is made up of distinct and stable subsets or by cells in different stages of maturation and activation. The most provocative studies suggesting the presence of distinct sublines involves the mouse strain CBA/N. This strain of mice has an immunological defect linked to the X chromosome consisting of an impaired response to some selected polysaccharides. The B cells of the defective mice lack three surface markers, the b3, b5, and b7 antigens. The CBA/N mouse may lack a stable subset of B cells (those that are Lyb5+) or may have a problem in B cell maturation (implying that Lyb5- develop into Lyb5+).

Changes in B Cells During Antigen Stimulation. In the small resting B lymphocyte, most of the synthesized Ig is transported to and inserted in the plasma membrane to serve as a receptor protein. About ninety percent of the synthesized Ig remains surface bound after a four-hour period of labeling with radioactive leucine: the half-life of the cell-associated surface Ig has been estimated to be about twenty to thirty hours. The B cell also sheds small amounts of IgM into the medium, but this secreted material has a size of 7S to 8S instead of the 19S size of serum IgM. The shed IgM is presumably derived from membrane IgM. Indeed, cells that have their surface proteins radiolabeled with I release radioactive monomeric IgM into the medium. The mechanisms involved in the spontaneous release, or shedding, of IgM must lead to a change whereby Ig, as an integral membrane protein insoluble in aqueous milieu, now becomes soluble in serum. This may be due to limited proteolysis at the cell surface.

Stimulation by antigen, together with some signal from T cells, results in a dramatic alteration of B cell physiology, inducing cell division and differentiation. Differentiation entails:

1. the development of endoplasmic reticulum;

2. increased biosynthesis of Ig;

3. secretion of Ig at a high rate;

4. a change in the Ig class secreted by the cell; and

5. a high turnover of surface Ig.

These changes are found not only in the plasma cells but also in large lymphocytes that develop from the small B cells. The turnover of surface Ig markedly changes to a half-life of two to four hours, about one-tenth of that found in the resting cell. The Ig that is secreted by the stimulated B cell or its derivatives is now 19S IgM or the other Ig classes. This IgM secreted by the cell cannot be radioiodinated at the cell membrane, clearly indicating that the pathway of secretion is independent from that of transport of Ig to the membrane.

As noted earlier, the bulk of surface Ig receptors belongs to the IgM or IgD class. Yet, when differentiation takes place, there is secretion of IgG or other classes, indicating that differentiation entails preservation of the recognition site to which the cell is precommitted, together with profound structural changes as the secreted Ig evolves into different structures and classes. Thus, the cell, with a 7S monomeric IgM on its surface, begins to secrete a 19S soluble IgM, an IgG, IgA, or IgE. The change in expression of H chain implies a switch in the genes coding for the different H chains while maintaining its previous reading of H genes coding for the variable portion of the same polypeptide chain (Chapter 10).

Evidence in favor of a genetic switch comes from a number of observations. For example, the immune response *in vitro* of murine spleen cells to foreign red cells was studied in the presence of an excess amount of various anti-Ig antibodies. The antibodies, by reacting with the B cells and covering and/or clearing surface Ig, would stop the cell from interacting with antigen. Exposure to anti-IgM antibodies stopped cells from making not only antibodies of the IgM class but also antibodies of the IgG or IgA class. Thus, the indications were that the precursor cells of plasma cells secreting gamma or alpha chain Ig must have been derived from the IgM-bearing cells. In other experiments, it was found that in *immune* animals (i.e., in spleen cells of animals previously immunized) IgM was not as effective in stopping IgG production, suggesting that some of the precursor B cells—which had immunological "memory"—must have had IgG-bearing receptors. This observation was confirmed in another system in which murine spleen B cells incubated with lipopolysaccharide were stimulated to differentiate by secreting IgM or IgG antibodies. Exposure of these B cells to anti-Ig could shut off this differentiation process by ways not yet clear—anti-mu chain antibodies stopped the differentiation to <u>both</u> IgM and IgG secretion.

A second line of evidence in favor of class switch comes from cytological studies in which plasma cells have been found to contain IgG in their cytoplasm while exhibiting IgM on their membranes.

The precise function of surface Ig when interacting with antigen and each of the two main surface isotypes has been the subject of intense study. One school of thought is that membrane Ig may have only a passive role, which is to focus antigen. Others, however, argue that Ig plays a more important function of signalling metabolic changes that, together with the cooperative influences from T cells, result in proliferation and differentiation. In favor of this interpretation are the results showing that antigens or antibodies to surface Ig—alone, without any other cells—can induce profound changes in B cells such as efflux of intracellular Ca, stimulation of motility, and regulation of DNA synthesis (Figure 5.4).

<u>Plasma Cells.</u> Plasma cells derive from B cells. They do not divide but actively secrete Ig molecules synthesized in their endoplasmic reticulum. Plasma cells, in contrast to B lymphocytes, have very few Ig molecules on their membrane (remember that with B cells 90% of Ig goes to the membrane to serve as an antigen receptor; in plasma cells, more than 90% of the Ig molecules are secreted). Plasma cells secrete antibody molecules of identical chemical structure having the same antigen specificity and, as a rule, the same Fc portion. Plasma cells are markedly increased in lymphoid tissues during the secondary immune response but are not normally found in blood. Some patients with Ig deficiencies lack plasma cells (Chapter 15). In Chapter 3, we discussed that multiple myeloma is a neoplastic condition of plasma cells that can be diagnosed by an examination of the serum Ig. Normal serum Ig is heterogeneous in an electrophoretic field and can be identified as a broad band of protein. In multiple myeloma, all plasma cells derive from a single malignant cell producing a homogeneous antibody that can be identified as a sharp peak in an electrophoretic field.

T LYMPHOCYTES

T lymphocytes, the other major lymphocyte class, are cells essential for the full expression of immunity and, as such, are involved in many functions:

1. T cells function as regulatory cells modulating the activities of B cells (or other T cells). The regulatory function of T cells can be positive or negative. Helper T cells are those that cooperate with B cells—or other T cells—to bring about an effective response. Suppressor T cells, as their name indicates, are capable of suppressing a given immune function (Chapters 8 and 9).

2. T cells are involved in cellular immunity reactions, which include reactions of delayed sensitivity, contact sensitivity, and resistance to infection with certain bacteria, such as the facultative intracellular bacteria, and viruses. T cells carry part of these functions by elaborating a number of molecules that can affect the inflammatory response or behavior of other inflammatory cells, principally, macrophages. Such molecules are termed lymphocyte mediators or lymphokines (Chapter 7).

3. T cells are the major cells involved in transplantation immunity and, as such, are involved in allograft rejection and graft-versus-host reactions which consist of the reaction of a set of immunocompetent T cells against cells or tissues bearing different histocompatibility antigens (Chapter 6).

4. T cells can act as cytotoxic T cells; that is to say, they have the capacity to kill other cells. This phenomenon is best seen as part of the immune response against viruses or tumors. The name, cytotoxic T cells, is synonymous with cytolytic or killer T cells (Chapters 7 and 11).

A question of major importance is whether these various functions of T cells are carried out by a single T cell with various functional capabilities or, on the contrary, by defined subsets. It is now accepted that there are three major stable sets of T lymphocytes:

T helper cells (also called inducers by some; these are the cells involved in regulating B cells and in cellular immunity reactions).

Cytolytic T cells: involved in killing.

Suppressor T cells: involved in inhibition of the response.

By the use of different alloantigens, again in the mouse, it was possible to identify discrete T cell subsets having different functions. The most significant information has come from studies of the Ly antigens, a system found in the mouse on T lymphocytes and referred to before. To recapitulate, the Ly system comprises three loci: Ly1,Ly2, and Ly3. Ly2 and Ly3 are very closely linked. Each Ly locus has two allelic forms. By using appropriate stains of mice and antibodies to Ly1, or Ly2, 3 and complement, one can kill the T cells bearing one or another specificity. Three sets of T cells are found, those having Ly1, Ly2,3 (called Ly1+, Ly2+); those having Ly1, but no Ly2,3 (Ly1+, Ly2-); and those having Ly2,3 and small amounts of Ly1. Because these latter cells have such a limiting amount of Ly1, they are not killed by anti-Ly1 (and complement) (we will name them Ly1-, Ly2+).

The immature thymocytes in the thymus cortex (those bearing TL) bear both the Ly1 and the Ly2,3 antigens. This is not the case with mature T cells in the lymphoid tissue or in the recirculating pool where the distribution is as follows:

Ly1+, Ly2,3+ = 50%

Ly1+, Ly2,3- = 33%

Ly1-, Ly2,3+ = 17%

The Ly1+, Ly2,3- or the Ly1- Ly2,3+ phenotypes of the mature T cells are stable; that is to say, each cell will not give rise to the other. This would indicate that each cell belongs to a particular line of differentiation and is not a sequential stage of a single differentiation line.

The model of differentiation currently proposed envisions the following:

Thymocyte		Mature T Cell
Ly1+, Ly2,3+	--->	Ly1+, Ly2,3+
		Ly1+, Ly2,3-
		Ly1-, Ly2,3+

By killing T cells of one subset with the appropriate anti-Ly antisera, one can explore whether a given T cell function is carried out by a given subset of T cells. Indeed, it has been found that certain T cell functions are associated with cells bearing a particular Ly phenotype, as shown in Table 5.2.

Table 5.2

Markers of Mature T Cells

	Mouse		Human	
	Ly1	Ly2	T4	T8
Helper T cells	+	--	+	--
Suppressor T cells	--	+	--	+
Cytolytic T cells	--	+	--	+

Subsets of T cells analogous to those described in the mouse have now been identified in humans using monoclonal antibodies raised in mice against human T cells. These monoclonal antibodies identify two major sets of mature T cells in blood and secondary lymphoid organs. The T4 subset includes the helper T cell, while the T8 subset includes the suppressor and cytolytic T cell subsets. The ratio of T4/T8 in circulating blood is about 2. The T4 and T8 subsets are stable lineages that do not interconvert (Table 5.2).

Receptor for Antigen in T Lymphocytes. The study of the T cell receptor has been the subject of many studies, many of which have led to diverse and controversial findings. At the present time, the consensus is that the receptor is not conventional surface Ig as found in B cells. Surface immunoglobulin is not detected on T lymphocytes by conventional procedures which readily detect it on B cells. Thus, the presence or absence of surface Ig can serve in the identification of cells as B or T.

Recent studies have apparently identified structures on T cells associated with a receptor function. Monoclonal antibodies (Chapter 4) have now been raised against a structure on antigen-reactive helper or cytolytic T cells which inhibits their specific interaction with antigen presented on antigen-presenting cells (Chapter 8). These monoclonal antibodies are believed to react with the T cell receptor for antigen because they affect the response only to the specific antigen. For example, antibodies raised to T cells that are reactive with ovalbumin only block the response to ovalbumin but not to various unrelated antigens. (The antibodies are raised by immunizing mice with purified T cells reactive to antigen. These T cells are pure clones of antigen-reactive cells produced by the method elaborated in Chapter 8.) The surface protein reactive with the antibodies is dilsulphide-linked protein made up of two different chains of about 45,000 and 42,000 daltons. The thinking at present is that the dimer is part of the T cell receptor, although it has not been ruled out whether other proteins may form part of the receptor.

There are also some indications that the T cell receptor may contain an antigen-combining site having an idiotypic determinant related to, or shared with, the Variable Heavy chain of Ig. To recapitulate, idiotype refers to an antigenic determinant on Ig molecules localized to the antibody-combining site (Chapter 3). Limited experiments have found that both T and B cells reactive against some antigens share similar idiotypes. This finding was thought at first to indicate coding of the T cell receptor by immunoglobulin V genes. However, the recently verified absence of rearranged V genes in antigen-specific T cell cloned lines is not compatible with this conclusion. In B cells, the variable portion of Ig is encoded in different gene segments that are rearranged during B cell maturation (Chapter 10). Another mechanism must, therefore, account for the sharing of some idiotypic specificities by B cells and T cells.

One very important characteristic of the T cell receptor for antigen is that it must interact not only with antigen but also with an MHC-encoded glycoprotein. Both the antigen and the MHC molecules are presented to the T cell on the surface of an antigen-presenting cell (Chapters 6, 7, and 8). Thus, the helper T cells recognize antigen in the context of Class II molecules (or Ia antigens), while most of the cytolytic T cells recognize antigen in the context of different MHC molecules, the Class I glycoproteins. Some T suppressors can interact with antigen directly.

A second set of observations related to the T cell receptor are the findings of soluble molecules derived from T cells capable of binding antigens. These antigen-specific factors of about 40,000 to 50,000 daltons have been obtained from T lymphocytes and have three properties:

a. They bind antigen specifically, i.e., T cells from mice immunized with a given antigen release a product that interacts specifically with the antigen. The degree of antigen specificity has not been extensively analyzed. Very recent studies suggest that these molecules may have the same idiotype as an antibody reacting with the same antigen.

b. They contain determinants coded by genes in the major histocompatibility complex. This is to say, antibodies to the gene products of the I region of the MHC bind to the factor, indicating a shared antigen between factors and MHC I region gene products of the histocompatibility gene complex (Chapter 6).

c. <u>They mediate regulatory functions</u>; some factors added to lymphoid cell suspensions can increase helper function of T cells, while others mediate suppressor function. Suppressor and helper factors can be differentiated on the basis of the antigen coded by the MHC contained in the factor. Helper factors react with anti-I-A antisera, while suppressor factors react with anti-I-J antisera (Chapter 7). These are antigens encoded in the major histocompatibility gene complex of the mouse.

The <u>antigen-specific factors</u> have been interpreted by some to represent the T cell antigen receptor. Their biochemical structure is not yet resolved. Their precise biological role <u>in vivo</u> has not been determined, although their powerful effect <u>in vitro</u> suggests that they may be involved in physiological processes. The suppressor factors, which are the best studied so far, contain two disulphide-linked peptides. One chain is about 40,000 daltons and appears to react with the antigen. the second chain, about 20,000 daltons, contains the I-J-reactive determinant.

<u>Markers of T Lymphocytes: Human</u>. The monoclonal antibodies to T4 and T8 identify T cell subsets. The helper T cells are T4 positive. The cytolytic and suppressor T cells are T8 positive. The radio of T4 to T8 in blood of normal individuals is about 2. Different monoclonal antibodies identifies antigen found in all circulating T cells (T3 and T12). The T lymphocytes of man can also be identified by the <u>E rosette test</u> (E = sheep red cells). This is because T cells bind in a non-immunological way to <u>sheep</u> red cells (and not to other red cells). The percentage of T cells binding E is usually about sixty to seventy percent of peripheral blood lymphocytes.

<u>Mouse</u>. Mouse T cells can be identified by various alloantigens. The Thy-1 or Θ antigen is one of the most commonly tested in experimental work. The treatment of murine T cells with an appropriate anti-Θ antibody in the presence of complement results in death of most T cells with abrogation of their function. This approach has been used extensively in order to determine which immunological function is dependent on the integrity of T cells.

The antigen-driven activation of T lymphocytes is explained in Chapters 6, 7, and 8.

RESPONSE OF T AND B CELLS TO MITOGENS

A number of molecules—plant proteins or bacterial products—have the capacity to interact with, and stimulate, the cells of the immune system. These mitogens, which have been very useful for studying the biochemistry of cell stimulation, have the following general characteristics:

1. They usually bind to many classes of lymphoid cells, although only some classes will respond, while others do not.

2. They are polyclonal; that is to say, they stimulate a substantial number, if not most, of a given class of cells.

The most widely used mitogens include the plant lectins, a series of proteins extracted from various seeds, which have specificity for carbohydrates. The plant lectins most commonly used include phytohemagglutinin (PHA) and Concanavalin A (Con A). PHA and Con A in short-term cultures (i.e., three to four days) stimulate mostly the T cells to proliferate. Some B cells proliferate, at least in humans, in long-term cultures (of more than five days, for example). In the mouse, PHA and Con A are selective T cell mitogens (Chapter 4 analyzed the technique for assaying lymphocyte transformation).

Bacterial products such as the lipopolysaccharides (LPS) from gram-negative organisms stimulate only B cells to proliferate and differentiate to plasma cells (Table 5.3).

ARE THERE MORE THAN TWO MAJOR CLASSES OF LYMPHOCYTES?

The bulk of lymphocytes have surface markers for T or B cells; however, a small number have been found to lack them. The lymphocytes lacking T or B cell markers have received various names; some have used the term "null". Null lymphocytes probably encompass a number of different cell lines, perhaps in some stages of differentiation. Among the null lymphocytes are included K or NK cells (K = killer; NK = natural killer); for brevity, we will call them NK. These are cells of size slightly larger than a lymphocyte with one or two prominent cytoplasmic granules and a kidney-shaped nucleus. The NK cells have a strong Fc receptor for IgG and will bind to indicator particles or cells coated with antibody. The NK cell can kill antibody-coated nucleated cells, most likely by a process involving the release of oxygen-derived compounds. (This is the phenomenon called "antibody-dependent cellular cytotoxicity".) NK cells can also bind—and kill—some tumor cells or virally infected cells <u>in the absence of antibody</u>. The molecular basis of the binding and recognition by NK cells of diverse cellular targets is not clear. Because NK cells have a strong Fc receptor, they can bind circulating IgG and can be confused with B cells. In contrast to true B cells, NK cells do not synthesize IgM and IgD and lose, with time in culture, the IgG bound by way of their Fc receptors.

Table 5.3

DNA Synthesis of Murine B and T Cells Stimulated by Con A and LPS

Cells	Mitogen Added	Tritiated Thymidine Incorporation (Counts per Minute)
Spleen	None	1,200
Spleen	Con A	120,500
Spleen	LPS	35,000
Isolated T cells	Con A	115,000
Isolated T cells	LPS	1,700
Isolated B cells	Con A	2,300
Isolated B cells	LPS	43,000

Table 5.3 Cells are cultured with mitogens for three days, during the last twelve hours in the presence of 1 uc of tritium-labeled thymidine. After three days, the amount of thymidine incorporation in the cells' DNA is determined. Con A stimulated only the T cells, while LPS affected the B cells.

The exact lineage of NK cells is far from established. Some human and mouse NK cells appear to have low levels of some T cell markers as well as to share some surface antigens with macrophages. Yet true differentiation to classical T cells or to macrophages has not been found. NK cells are found in athymic mice. They increase in number by the action of interferon and can be inhibited by E class prostaglandins.

Table 5.4

	B Cells	NK Cells	T Cells
Amount in blood	5 - 10%	5 - 10%	80-90%
IgM and IgD on their Membranes	+	—	—
IgG on their membranes	(very few)	+	—
E rosette	—	—	+
T4/T8 ratio	—	—	2
Binding of monomer IgG	—	+	—
Binding of polymer Ig	+	+++	±
Stability of surface Ig	Stable	Labile	—
Reexpression of surface Ig	Reexpresses IgM and IgD	Will not reexpress IgG	—

Table 5.4 is a summary of the three major lymphocyte classes found in blood of humans.

THE MONONUCLEAR PHAGOCYTE SYSTEM

Mononuclear phagocytes are widely distributed throughout the body in blood, bone marrow, liver, lymphoid tissue, connective tissue, nervous tissue, and serous cavities. They form an important part of the defense mechanism by removing microorganisms from blood and tissue. Phagocytes are highly avid in phagocytosis and pinocytosis. They engulf many different kinds of antigen and thus participate in early immune inductive events. Mononuclear phagocytes also respond to external stimuli coming from activated lymphocytes and/or microorganisms and participate in cell-mediated types of immune reactions. Elie Metchnikoff in 1892 named them "macrophages" because they were capable of ingesting large particles. In 1924, Aschoff introduced the name "reticuloendothelial system", a term which is still widely used to group various kinds of cell capable of taking up vital dyes. The phagocytes have been identified as a cell line originating from a dividing precursor which, after a time, matures, spending a brief time in

Table 5.5

Classification of the Mononuclear Phagocyte System

Cells	Localization
Stem cells (committed)	Bone marrow
Monoblasts	Bone marrow
Promonocytes	Bone marrow
Monocytes	Bone marrow Peripheral blood
Macrophages	Tissue Connective tissues (histiocytes) Liver (Kupffer cells) Lung (alveolar macrophages) Lymph nodes (free and fixed macrophages) Bone marrow (macrophages) Serous cavities (pleural and peritoneal macrophages) Bone tissue (osteoclasts?) Nervous system (microglial cells)

the circulation, then settles in the different tissues. The phagocytes have received different names, depending on their tissue localization and/or state of maturation.

Origin and Maturation. The earliest recognizable precursor is the promonocyte found in the largest number in the bone marrow. Promonocytes are rapidly dividing cells and, as such, are radiation sensitive. Promonocytes enter the blood, becoming monocytes, which circulate for twenty-four or forty-eight hours after which they migrate randomly to different tissues, and there mature to macrophages. Macrophages are highly phagocytic cells and contain numerous lysosomes and endocytic vesicles. Monocytes and macrophages divide infrequently and are radioresistant. The factors that regulate the entrance and exit of macrophages from tissues are not well known.

The mature macrophage is distinct morphologically from the lymphocyte. The macrophages are larger cells (about 15 to 20 u in diameter) with abundant cytoplasm and a relatively small indented nucleus. The cytoplasm contains pinocytic vesicles and lysosomes. The lysosomes contain a variety of digestive enzymes.

Interaction with Antigens. Mononuclear phagocytes have the capacity to bind to and engulf numerous particulate materials (phagocytosis). Also, a number of soluble molecules can be taken up to variable degrees (pinocytosis). Usually, the extent of polymerization or aggregation of the soluble molecules favors their uptake. For example, macrophages will bind very weakly monomer albumin molecules, whether autologous or foreign, but will bind strongly to the same molecules if polymerized. The biochemical basis of the interaction with particulate of soluble molecules is partially known. Phagocytes can bind to carbohydrate residues in glycoproteins such as mannose, n-acetylglucosamine, and fucose. The binding of mannose takes place by a specific receptor protein. Regardless to the extent to which a particulate or soluble material binds by itself to the macrophage, the binding increases by many fold if the material in question is coated with antibody and complement. This is because the phagocytes have at least two distinct sets of surface receptors, the Fc receptors and the C3 receptors.

The Fc receptors bind specifically to the heavy chain of IgG and not to other Ig classes. Among the human IgG subclasses, macrophages bind to IgG1 and IgG3, very weakly to IgG2, and not at all to IgG4. The physical state of Ig is important for forming a stable complex with the Fc receptor. In its normal monomeric form, the serum Ig will bind to it but readily dissociates. However, in the situation where the antibody is complexed to an antigen in an immune complex, the binding of the antibody to the macrophage Fc receptor is more stable because of cooperativity among the invididual binding sites. Recent studies have established the presence in most species of two distinct Fc receptors coexpressed on the macrophages. These two receptors differ in their binding specificity, in their sensitivity to trypsin, and in their reactivity to monoclonal antibodies (directed to the receptor). In the mouse, where most of the studies have been done, one Fc receptor (termed FcR I) binds to IgG2a and is trypsin resistant; the other (termed FcR II) binds to IgG1 and IgG2b, is trypsin sensitive, and reacts with a monoclonal antibody (2.4.G2). Initial structural studies indicate that both receptors are integral membrane proteins with molecular weights of 67,000 for FcR I and 50,000 to 60,000 for FcR II.

The C3 receptor recognizes C3 after cleavage by the C3 convertase, i.e., the C3b protein (Chapter 12). There are three distinct C3 receptors now recognized, the CR1, CR2, and CR3 receptors. CR1 is a 205,000-dalton membrane protein that binds to C3b preferentially. It is found on monocytes, macrophages, B cells, neutrophils, and glomerular epithelial cells. CR2 is a protein of 148,000 daltons that strongly interacts with C3d. It is found in B cells. Finally, CR3 is a dimer composed of chains of 175,000 and 95,000 daltons that binds preferentially iC3b. CR3 is found on monocytes, macrophages, and neutrophils.

Table 5.6

Binding of Red cells to Macrophage Monolayers at Room Temperature

Treatment of Red Cells	Content of Culture Media	Binding
1. No treatment	Regular medium	(±)
2. IgG antibodies	Regular medium	++
3. IgG antibodies	Excess aggregated HSA	++
4. IgG antibodies	Excess aggregated IgG	±
5. IgM antibodies	Regular medium	±
6. IgM antibodies and complement	Regular medium	++++
7. IgM antibodies and complement	Fresh serum	+++
8. IgM antibodies and complement	Excess C3b	±

Both Fc and C3 receptors are tested by adding an indicator particle, red cells or bacteria, coated with antibody and complement to a monolayer of macrophages and observing the binding by microscopy. Table 5.6 shows a number of experimental manipulations that indicate the specificity of binding sites for IgG or complement. In Group 2, red cells opsonized with IgG antibodies (of all subclasses) bind to the macrophage. This binding is not inhibited by adding an excess of polymerized albumin to the medium (Group 3). On the other hand, aggregated IgG will inhibit, indicating the specificity of interaction between the Fc receptor and IgG (Group 4). Red cells opsonized with IgM antibodies bind poorly (Group 5). However, the addition of small amounts of fresh serum brings in C3 to the red cells and, with it, the binding to macrophages (Group 6). The binding cannot be competed by native C3 but only by C3b (Groups 7 and 8).

Endocytosis: After the antigens bind to the membrane, the macrophage interiorizes them in vesicles in an energy-requiring process (the term endocytosis is used to include both phagocytosis and pinocytosis). The endocytic vesicles are invaginations of the membrane which seal off and then flow into the cytoplasm. There is evidence that the process of endocytosis is dependent on the integrity of cytoplasmic microfilaments. Microtubules are also involved perhaps by directing the flow of endocytic vesicles into the perinuclear area where the lysosomes are found in abundance. The endocytic vesicles eventually fuse with the primary lysosomes to form the phagolysosomes. As the two vesicles fuse, the contents of the lysosomes spill into the endocytic vesicle to start the process of intracellular digestion.

The lysosomes of the macrophage contain a number of enzymes with specificity for proteins, polysaccharides, lipids, and nucleic acids: acid phosphatase, beta glucuronidase, glucosaminidase, beta galactosides, acid ribonuclease, acid deoxyribonuclease, cholesterol esterase, etc. This large variety of enzymes make the process of intracellular digestion extremely efficient. For example, a radioactive protein taken up by macrophages is rapidly degraded at an exponential rate so that, after a few hours, most of the protein has been catabolized to the level of amino acids. Residual undigestible material may remain in phagolysosomes for long periods of time.

The mechanisms of the microbicidal action of macrophages is not completely elucidated. Many bacteria are rapidly killed following ingestion, but others remain and multiply in the phagocytic vacuoles. These are the intracellular pathogens (Chapter 6). <u>The intracellular pathogens are killed or inhibited in their growth when the macrophage becomes activated by cellular immune reactions.</u> The killing of bacteria appears to be unrelated to the effects of lysosomes. Lysosomal enzymes serve primarily for the degradation of dead organisms.

At present, there is great interest in the microbicidal effects of products of oxidative metabolism. In the neutrophil, it is known that hydrogen peroxide is generated as a result of a respiratory burst following phagocytosis and that, in the presence of myeloperoxidase and halide, it will halogenate bacteria. The incorporation of iodine or chlorine into the cell wall disrupts its integrity by mechanisms not well known. With respect to macrophages, phagocytosis produces an increase in oxygen consumption and in glucose oxidation by way of the hexose monophosphate shunt (in the shunt, glucose is oxidized to carbon dioxide and a 5 carbon sugar). All these effects are markedly increased in the activated macrophages. Macrophages lack myeloperoxidase—monocytes do have it—but contain catalase which may well substitute for myeloperoxidase. Crucial in the generation of hydrogen peroxide, and in itself a highly reactive free radical with potential microbicidal effects, is the superoxide anion. The superoxide anion is generated by an enzyme that catalyzes the one-electron reduction of molecular oxygen using a pyridine nucleotide as the electron donor (some claim it to be NADPH, others to be NADH). The reactions are:

1. $O_2 + O_2 + NADPH \dashrightarrow 2O_2^- + NADP^+ + H^+$
2. $O_2^- + O_2^- + 2H^+ \dashrightarrow O_2 + H_2O_2$

The enzyme that catalyzes reaction No. 2 is superoxide dimutase which may be responsible for protecting the cell from its own superoxide anion. Macrophages, after phagocytosis and especially if activated, have an increased production of superoxide anion. Whether superoxide anion, hydrogen peroxide, or other free radicals account for all microbicidal effects of macrophages is not known.

Secretory Function of Phagocytes. Besides the functions of pinocytosis, phagocytosis, and intracellular digestion, the phagocytes are actively secretory cells that synthesize and secrete a large number of materials. The materials secreted by the phagocytes can be grouped into three categories:

A. Enzymes capable of affecting extracellular proteins. Included are:

1. Plasminogen activators: species of 28,000 and 48,000 daltons have been identified; the plasminogen activators are serine proteases capable of converting plasminogen into plasmin. Plasmin is involved in the lysis of fibrin. Thus, the secreted plasminogen activators, together with plasminogen from blood, result in a fibrinolytic system.

2. Collagenase and elastase: These two enzymes are capable of attacking collagen and elastic tissue, respectively.

3. Lysosomal proteases: a number of hydrolases such as acid phosphatases, beta glucuronidase can also be secreted into the extracellular environment.

B. Products involved in defense processes, which include:

1. Lysozyme: a protein of 14,000 daltons active against the peptidoglycan of bacterial cell walls (hydrolyzing specifically the 1-4 glycosidic linkages between n-acetylmuramic acid and n-acetyl-glucosamine).

2. Complement proteins: C2, C3, C4, C5, and Factor B are made and secreted by phagocytes.

3. Interferon: Interferons are a family of anti-viral proteins (Chapter 7). The interferon released by macrophages has a molecular weight of about 45,000 daltons.

C. Factors capable of modulating function of surrounding cells; most of these factors have not been characterized biochemically. Included are:

1. Interleukin-1 (IL-1): IL-1, also known as lymphocyte-activating factor, is a protein of about 15,000 daltons secreted by the macrophages, particularly after interaction with immune complexes, bacterial products, or T cells. IL-1 has an important number of biological effects: it can stimulate thymocytes to proliferate and mature T cells to release their own

growth-promoting molecules and also has a direct potentiating effect on B cells (Chapter 8). IL-1 can stimulate liver cells to secrete a number of proteins following infections—these proteins, called acute phase reactants, include haptoglobin, C-reactive protein, and C3. Finally, IL-1 induces fever. It is the main molecule responsible for the fever response following infection and immunological reactions. Curiously, T cells proliferate and secrete proteins more strongly at 39 degrees C or 40 degrees C than at 37 degrees C. Fever could be considered an acute response to antigen that results in a higher T cell activity.

2. Other growth and differentiating factors: Macrophage culture fluids contain a protein needed for the in vitro differentiation of bone marrow stem cells to granulocytes (colony-stimulating factor). A second factor is capable of differentiating immature thymocytes. The relationship between these two factors is not known. Macrophages also secrete growth factors for fibroblasts, endothelial, and smooth muscle cells.

3. Cytotoxins: Some investigators claims that macrophages, under special circumstances, secrete materials that can kill some tumor cell lines. These materials have been poorly characterized.

4. Low molecular weight products: A large number of small metabolites can be released by macrophages. These include cyclic AMP, prostaglandins, and purine and pyrimidine nucleosides. Phagocytes are major secretors of arachidonic acid metabolites, which include various prostaglandins as well as the leukotrienes.

Conditions for Increased Secretion. The majority of the materials listed above are destined for secretion, being released by the cell shortly after being synthesized. These include the plasminogen activators, collagenase, elastase, and lysozyme. The lysosomal proteases, in contast, are destined for intracellular digestion, although part of them are released during phagocytosis (i.e., about 10 to 30%). (The release of lysosomal enzymes takes place at the time that a particle is being phagocytosed. The primary lysosomes can fuse with endocytic vesicles that are not completely closed but are still open to the outside.)

The conditions for secretion vary depending upon the physiological state of the phagocytes:

1. Some materials are released continuously regardless of the functional state of the cell. Example: lysozyme.

2. Others are released only subsequent to phagocytosis. The act of phagocytosis serves as a stimulus for the cell to make and

release the products. Example: plasminogen activators, collagenase, elastase.

3. Others depend on the state of activation of the phagocyte. Macrophages can become highly active as occurs during various types of infections. These activated macrophages can be triggered very rapidly to secrete large amounts of some of the materials.

Functional Significance of the Secretory Function: The secretory function of macrophages gives the phagocytes the potential to exert a regulatory influence on its surrounding environment, in inflammation and tissue repair, in infection, perhaps in the control of hematopoiesis, and in critical steps in immunity. The release of enzymes, some of which have powerful effects on connective tissue proteins, could play a critical role in inflammation, in particular, as it pertains to the clearing of inflammatory sites. One can envision that, at the same time that the phagocyte is participating as a scavenger, it helps in the elimination of unwanted proteins by secretion of the various proteolytic enzymes. Along these lines, it is interesting to note that the phagocytes are prominent cells in various processes of collagen resorption. Abundant numbers of phagocytes are found in the postpartum uterus at the time of intense collagen resorption and in granulomas. In many of these examples, there is some evidence of phagocytosis of collagen fibers.

The range of secretory products of phagocytes attests to their obvious importance in the defense mechanisms. Phagocytes appear in evolution before lymphocytes. Thus, their non-specific contribution to defense against exogenous invasion—the release of enzymes, interferon, complement protein, lytic and growth factors—is protean. As lymphocytes emerged in evolution as cells capable of directing specific immune responses, the multifaceted properties of the phagocyte were adapted to the more complex requirements of specific immunity. Phagocytes indeed contribute to lymphocyte activation by intracellular processing as well as by releasing lymphostimulatory molecules.

Function of Phagocytes in Immunity. There are two stages in the immune response where phagocytes play an important role:

1. In immune induction: Phagocytes concentrate and trap the antigen molecules. Most of the antigen molecules taken up are degraded, except a few that are presented to the lymphocytes. Phagocytes, therefore, serve as an antigen-processing cell for B-T interaction (Chapter 8).

2. In cell-mediated immunity: Phagocytes respond to lymphocyte products and accumulate at sites of ongoing reactions. They form the main component of the inflammatory response of cellular immunity reactions. (Phagocytes are also an important

component of chronic inflammatory reactions not involving immunological mechanisms.) (Chapter 6).

Inductive Events Involving Antigen and Macrophages. The cellular interactions involving macrophages, B cells, and T cells are detailed in Chapter 8. Some of the phenomena involving macrophages are introduced now. Immune responses develop best if antigens are concentrated in lymphoid organs by phagocytes. It is well known that antigen molecules that are poorly taken up by phagocytes, i.e., not concentrated because of their physicochemical properties, induce poor immune responses. This is one example of the cell cooperation so common in immunity. B and T lymphocytes respond only if they recognize antigen in close proximity to each other and to the phagocytes that trap the antigen. The best way to illustrate this phenomenon is to study the immune response to different physical forms of a protein antigen. Some protein antigens can be tested in an aggregated or polymerized form, or in a non-aggregated or monomeric form. The polymers circulate poorly and are avidly taken up by macrophages. The monomers remain in the circulation and bind weakly to the phagocytes.

Experimental Protocol No. 1. Immunize a rabbit intravenously with bovine serum albumin (BSA). BSA preparations are made up of unaggregated, monomeric albumin, and a variable amount of polymerized albumin of different sizes. Polymers and monomers can be separated from each other, isolated, and tested for their immunogenicity.

	Concentrated by Phagocytes of Lymphoid Organ	Time in Blood	Immunogenicity
Polymer BSA	++++	Short	High
Monomer BSA	±	Long	Poor

This experiment shows that the polymerized BSA is highly immunogenic in contrast to monomer BSA. If a mixture of polymer or monomer BSA are injected, one finds the monomers circulating in the blood with a half-life of about four days and the polymers taken up by the macrophages. The rabbits respond with anti-BSA antibodies by seven to ten days. If the rabbit is bled a day or two after injection of BSA (and before antibodies appear in blood), the circulating monomer BSA molecules can be purified and used to immunize a second unrelated rabbit. This second rabbit will not mount an anti-BSA response. In contrast, if the macrophages that ingested the polymer BSA are isolated and transplanted with their content to a normal animal, a strong immune response develops to the macrophage-associated BSA. (This part of the experiment, transferring macrophages, has not been done in the rabbit but instead with genetically inbred strains of mice where cells can be transplanted without being rejected.) The overall conclusion is that the pathway of antigen, first taken by macrophages and from the macrophage "presented" to lymphocyte, is the most effective way to stimulate a response.

Experimental Protocol No. 2. This same kind of experiment can be done completely in vitro by mixing macrophages containing the antigen with T and B lymphocytes and culturing the mixture for four to five days, at which time the culture is titrated for number of antibody-forming cells. Example:

	Culture	Antibody-Forming Cells at Day 5
No. 1	10^7 lymphocytes, no antigen	40
No. 2	10^7 lymphocytes, 0.1 ug of soluble antigen	260
No. 3	10^7 lymphocytes, 0.01 ug of soluble antigen	75
No. 4	10^7 lymphocytes, 0.1 ug of antigen bound to 10^5 macrophages	3,950
No. 5	10^7 lymphocytes, 0.01 ug of antigen bound to 10^4 macrophages	1,875
No. 6	0.1 ug of antigen bound to 10^5 macrophages	0

The culture containing the lymphocytes has a small number of antibody-forming cells (background of 40). The lymphocytes respond to soluble antigen but do much better to macrophage-bound antigen.

In summary, one of the very earliest inductive events consists of the uptake of antigen by macrophages of lymphoid tissues. The macrophages take up a number of antigens mainly if these are large polymers or if the antigens are coated with antibody and complement. The macrophages serve an important role not only by destroying the bulk of the antigen molecules but, at the same time, by presenting a few antigen molecule to the lymphocytes, particularly to the T lymphocyte. The antigen presented to the T lymphocytes is represented by a very small number of molecules that have not suffered extensive catabolism. The antigen is always presented together with Ia antigens on the macrophage membrane. The T lymphocytes react only to the antigen associated with the macrophages (Chapter 8). In the presence of an excess of soluble antigen, the lymphocyte response to antigen is not strong (Experimental Protocol 1). Besides the presentation of antigen, the macrophages secrete products that stimulate the lymphocyte for a better response. Thus, macrophage function may result from a combination of three properties:

1) Removal of excess antigen; 2) antigen presentation; and 3) secretion of stimulatory molecules.

OTHER ACCESSORY CELLS

So far we have mentioned two cells in lymphoid organs involved in antigen-handling events: the mononuclear phagocytes and the follicular dendritic cells. A third family of cells recently recognized also appears to participate in some immune inductive events. These cells are the Langerhans-dendritic cells found in abundance in the epidermal layers of the skin and also in the deep cortex of lymph nodes. Langerhans cells derive from stem cells found in bone marrow and migrate to the epidermis where they are found squeezed between the keratinocytes. The cells show a low level of Fc and C3 receptors, can bind to antigen, and exhibit Ia antigens on their membranes. Langerhans cells can bind to antigens deposited in the skin and then move from there by way of the efferent lymphatics to the deep cortex of the lymph nodes. In spleen and lymph nodes, a dendritic cell akin to the Langerhans cell can be isolated and studied for its immunological reactivity. Langerhans cells isolated from the skin and dendritic cells isolated from spleens are active in presenting some antigen to T cells and are very effective stimulators of the "mixed lymphocyte reaction" (Chapter 6).

EFFECTOR CELLS

A number of leukocytes and connective tissue cells participate as effector cells in immunological reactions. These include the granulocytes and the mast cells. Each of the three kinds of granulocytes participate: neutrophils in reactions mediated by antigen-antibody-complement complexes, eosinophils, and basophils in reactions involving IgE antibodies. An essential connective tissue cell in reactions mediated by IgE antibodies is the mast cell. Complete description of these various cells will not be given here. Students are encouraged to review standard textbooks on histology for detailed information. However, a few comments on these various cells are necessary in the context of their role in immunity.

Neutrophils are the most abundant leukocyte in blood of humans, representing about 50 to 60% of the total white cells. They are an important cellular component in acute non-infectious inflammation, in inflammation mediated by pyogenic bacteria, and in reactions involving antigen-antibody complexes. Neutrophils in blood are capable of marginating to the wells of endothelial cells, adhering to these, and crossing into the sites of the lesion. The neutrophils are attracted to the sites of inflammation by chemotactic factors. These factors direct the cell to move directionally to an area where the factors are concentrated. Somehow the neutrophil can recognize concentration gradients of the chemoattractant and reorient its directionality in accordance with the gradients. This process has been studied extensively *in vitro* by using two-compartment chambers separated by a filter. The cells are placed on the top and the chemoattractant on the bottom. The neutrophils respond by penetrating into the filter. The known chemoattractant substances for neutrophils include host factors and bacterial products. The most active host factors are the *chemotactic peptides* derived from cleavage of C3 and C5. Proteolytic cleavage of these two proteins not only results from activation of the complement sequence but also from the action of tissue proteases and proteases derived from the clotting system (thrombin). Neutrophils themselves release a factor chemotactic for other neutrophils. Another potent chemotactic factor is *leukotriene* B_4 (Chapter 14). The *bacterial chemotactic factors* have been obtained from a number of organisms. Their biochemistry is now being investigated. The evidence so far available is that the bacterial factors have a "site" of action on the cells distinct from the complement peptides. A common structure in all bacterial chemotactic factors is a sequence of amino acids made up of formyl-methionine-leucine-phenylalanine. The neutrophils have surface receptors for this sequence and, in fact, can respond chemotactically to synthetic polypeptides made of F-Met-Leu-Phe.

The interaction of neutrophils with microorganisms is similar in some regards to what was described for the macrophage. The neutrophil contains receptors for Fc fragments of IgG and for C3b, which enables them to engulf opsonized organisms. The process of ingestion is similar to that of macrophages. Neutrophils kill bacteria probably by oxidative mechanisms, also mentioned in the context of the macrophages. The neutrophils contain primary, azurophilic granules rich in myeloperoxidase. This enzyme, together with hydrogen peroxide generated during the respiratory burst that takes place after phagocytosis, and halides from the halogenating system. Other molecules have been identified in bacterial killing, such as cationic proteins and lactoferrin. Neutrophils also participate in tissue pathology involving antigen-antibody complement. Chapter 14 deals with this point.

The eosinophil is found in blood in small numbers, 1 to 5%. It is a frequent cellular component in allergic reactions (Chapter 14), perhaps attracted by a tetrapeptide chemotactic factor released from mast cells during anaphylactic reactions. The eosinophils are abundant also during parasitic diseases, where it is thought that they may play an important role. Chemotactic factors derived from immunological reactions may be instrumental in their accumulation at sites of parasitic infestation. Eosinophils can bind to the surface of some parasites and kill them. This has now been well studied with the larva (Schistosumala) of *Schistosoma mansoni*. Schistosomiasis is characterized by the presence of worms attached to the portal and mesenteric veins. The worms release eggs which become trapped in tissues, like the liver, resulting in severe inflammation and fibrosis. Eosinophils can bind to the larva in the presence of antibodies and degranulate, releasing some very basic proteins that are lethal for the parasite.

Finally, basophils and mast cells are essential components for the function of IgE antibodies since they are the cells that contain granules with the vasoactive amines (Chapter 14 considers the biology of these cells). From the point of view of their origin and morphology, both cells are distinct. Basophils are circulating blood cells, polymorphonuclear granulocytes formed in bone marrow, and capable of emigrating to sites of inflammation. Mast cells are mononucleated connective tissue cells not found in blood.

REFERENCES

Inglis, J. R. (ed). B Lymphocytes Today. Elsevier Biomedical Press, Amseterdam, 1982.

Katz, D. H. Lymphocyte Differentiation, Recognition, and Regulation. Academic Press, Inc., New York, 1977.

Moller, G. (ed.) Functional T Cell Subsets Defined by Monoclonal Antibodies. Immunol. Rev., 74, 1983 (contains seven articles reviewing T cell subsets in humans and experimental animals).

Nabholz, M., and MacDonald, H. R. Cytolytic T lymphocytes. Ann. Rev. Immunol., 1:273, 1983.

Rosenthal, A. S., Lipsky, P. E., and Shevach, E. M. Macrophage-lymphocyte interactions and antigen recognition. Fed. Proc., 34:1743, 1975.

Schreiner, G. F., and Unanue, E. R. Membrane and cytoplasmic changes in B lymphocytes induced by ligands—surface Ig interactions. Adv. Immunol., 24:38, 1976.

Unanue, E. R. Secretory function of mononuclear phagocytes. Am. J. Immunol., 83:396, 1976.

CHAPTER 6

Histocompatibility

All species contain a gene segment termed the Major Histocompatibility Gene Complex (or MHC) coding for cell surface glycoproteins that regulate the recognition of antigen by T lymphocytes. The molecules coded for in the MHC are termed histocompatibility molecules. The MHC includes several genetic loci that code for two distinct kinds of cell surface histocompatibility molecules—the Class I and the Class II molecules. Class I and Class II molecules are different from each other, structurally, antigenically, as well as from a functional point of view. Most subsets of T lymphocytes do not recognize antigen molecules directly; they do so only when the antigen is presented on the surface of an appropriate cell—the antigen-presenting cell. The antigen-presenting cell must "present" to the T cell at least two molecules—the antigen (or a fragment thereof) and one of the histocompatibility molecules. To a great extent, the class of histocompatibility molecule dictates the kind of T cell involved in the interaction. Thus, Class I molecules regulate the interaction between cytolytic T lymphocytes and target cells bearing usually a virus or a tumor antigen; Class II molecules, on the other hand, regulate the interactions between the helper T cells and the antigen-presenting cell containing the foreign protein. Because the generation of T helper cell is a crucial event in the initiation and development of an immune process, it follows that Class II molecules are essential elements for the responses to all polypeptide antigens.

In each species, the MHC comprises several loci that code for distinct Class I or Class II molecules. A most important characteristic of these MHC molecules is their extraordinary degree of polymorphism. Indeed, each locus has several allelic variants (usually twenty to forty forms). The distinguishing feature in the physiological interactions between the T lymphocyte and the histocompatibility molecules is the necessity for the T cell to interact with identical Class I or II molecules as expressed on its own cells. Thus, T cells will not recognize foreign antigens on the surface of antigen-presenting cells from other members of the species expressing a different histocompatibility allele. This results in the phenomenon termed MHC restriction; that is to say, the histocompatibility glycoproteins impose restrictions on the recognition of foreign antigens by T cells. Simply stated, in order for the T lymphocyte to recognize foreign antigens, they must, at the same time, recognize their own Class I or II molecules as self. The experimental evidence for these MHC restrictions are described in Chapters 7 and 8. As an introduction, we can now state that the MHC restriction is best shown using combinations of T cells with antigen-presenting cells derived from inbred strains of mice that differ only at the MHC. Thus, for example, a T helper cell from a given inbred line will recognize the protein diphtheria toxin as a foreign antigen when presented by macrophages of the same strain but not by macrophages of a different inbred line. T cells do not respond to the toxin unless it is in the context of its own Class II molecules.

The functions of the MHC gene products are described in four separate chapters. The present chapter deals with the genetics and chemistry of the MHC molecules and their function in transplantation immunity. Indeed, the histocompatibility molecules were discovered by immunologists studying transplantation of allogeneic tissues and cells. The only apparent exception to the rule that T cells recognize foreign antigens, only in the context of syngeneic histocompatibility molecules concerns their interactions with foreign histocompatibility molecules. Indeed, T cells can react directly with cells carrying allogeneic Class I or II molecules. (Concerning nomenclature, the Class I antigens are termed the classical transplantation antigens, while the Class II are termed the Ia antigens; the letter "I" stands for Immune response region. "Ia" equals I region-associated antigens. The Ia antigens are also synonymous with I-region gene products.) Chapters 7 and 8 describe the physiological interactions between T cells, Class I or II molecules, and antigen. Lastly, Chapter 10 examines further the function of Class II molecules as the products of Immune response genes, in their control of the responses to different protein antigens. The physiological role of the Class I and II molecules in immune responses to protein antigens were, in fact, discovered in early studies on the genetic control of responses of inbred animals to various protein antigens. We shall now give a brief historical review of the major findings that led to the seminal discoveries in histocompatibility.

HISTORY

The discovery of histocompatibility molecules and their physiological function came from two different fields—transplantation and immunogenetics. The first transplantation phenomena that were seriously examined used tumor cells, in mice, in an attempt to study cancer biology. It was perceived that a tumor arising spontaneously in a mouse could not be transplanted into a different mouse from an outbred colony. In contrast, tumor cells could "grow" if transplanted within colonies of mice. The pioneering work of Peter Gorer in England using inbred strains of mice established the immunological basis of transplantation reactions and called attention to cell surface proteins as the antigens responsible for such reactions. (Inbred strains of mice are developed by repeated matings of brother and sister; after twenty generations of such inbreeding, more than 98% of the genetic material is completely identical in all offsprings.) Gorer identified antigens in red cells from different mouse strains using serological methods and rabbit antibodies. He observed that the transplantation of tumor cells derived from an inbred mouse strain (the A strain) into mice of a different inbred line (the C57BL/6) resulted in rejection of the tumor and the production of antibodies. These antibodies (BL/6 against A tumor cells) were not specific for the tumor but reacted with all the tissues of the mouse strain from which the tumor derived (A), including the antigen (termed antigen II), identified previously on red cells. Gorer went on to establish that the F1 offspring (first filial generation) between the two inbred strains (A x BL/6) did not reject the A tumor—the F_1 cells, moreover, contained antigen II. Thus, the basic laws of transplantation immunity were established. The tumor cells were behaving as a graft, and this graft, containing histocompatibility antigens, would be recognized as foreign (an allograft) and rejected by inbred strains that lacked the antigen. In contrast, an inbred line having the same antigen recognized the tumor cells as self and would not reject them. (Tumor cells can have tumor-associated antigens to which an individual can respond under appropriate conditions described in Chapter 11.)

Subsequently, Peter Medawar and his associates, also in England, extended these observations to skin grafts, and showed that skin allograft, although inducing antibodies, were rejected as a result of cellular immunity. Further progress in the field came from studies in inbred mouse strains and by the development, by G. Snell and associates, at The Jackson Laboratory (Bar Harbor, Maine) of congenic strains. The congenic strains of mice are identical to an inbred partner strain except for a segment of chromosome which has been "inserted" using appropriate breeding programs. Snell and associates produced strains that differ only at the MHC and were thus able to obtain invaluable information on the role of this defined gene segment in transplantation immunity. For example, the B10 and the A are two inbred strains of mice, each with its own MHC allelic form. The B10.A strain was developed by a special breeding program. It contains the MHC of the A inbred strain, while the rest of its genome is identical with that of the B10 mouse. A B10.A accepts skin from an A mouse and rejects that of the B10 mouse; while a B10 rejects skin from the A mouse.

Using inbred and congenic strains, Snell identified a major gene locus responsible for strong graft rejection (termed H-2, for the antigen II described earlier) and minor loci of weaker antigenicity. The analysis of inbred strains also disclosed a very puzzling feature of the MHC which was its extraordinary polymorphism. This caused considerable confusion for many years, particularly as concerns the serological reactions using antibodies to the MHC-encoded antigens. Subsequently, the perceptive studies of D. Shreffler and J. Klein simplified the H-2 system and identified that more than one locus was responsible for the various reactions. It is now established that, in the mouse, the K and D loci and, in man, the A, B, and C loci code for distinct Class I molecules (Figures 6.1 and 6.2).

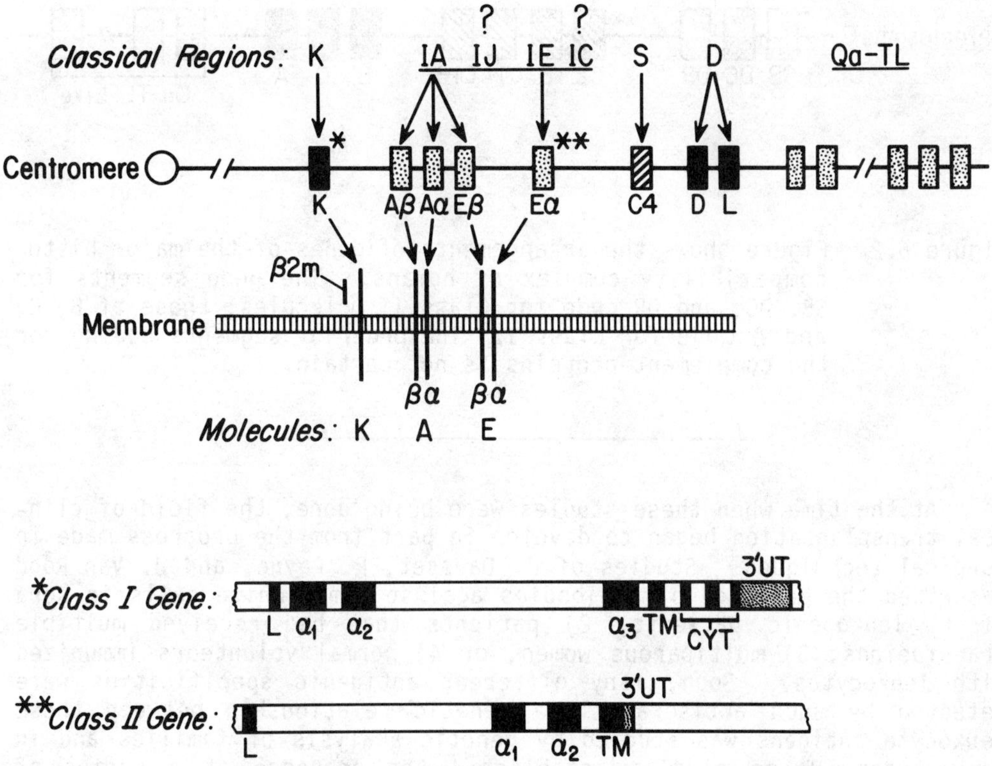

Figure 6.1. The figure depicts the Major Histocompatibility gene loci of the mouse and its gene products. The classical regions of the murine MHC are K, I, S, and D; K and D code for Class I molecules; I encompasses several subregions, two of which code for Class II molecules; the S region codes for C4 (see text). Represented in the figure are the arrangements of the various gene segments shown as boxes. A representation of a gene segment into exons (dark) and introns (clear) for a Class I or II gene is shown in the lower part. L refers to the exon encoding the leader sequence; alpha-1, alpha-2, and alpha-3 refer to the exons coding for the external domains; TM refers to the trans-membrane exons, CYT to the exons that code for the cyto-plasmic domain, and 3'UT refers to the 3' untranslated regions. This graph is modified from diagrams published by L. Hood, et al., in Ann. Rev. Immunol., 1:529, 1983.

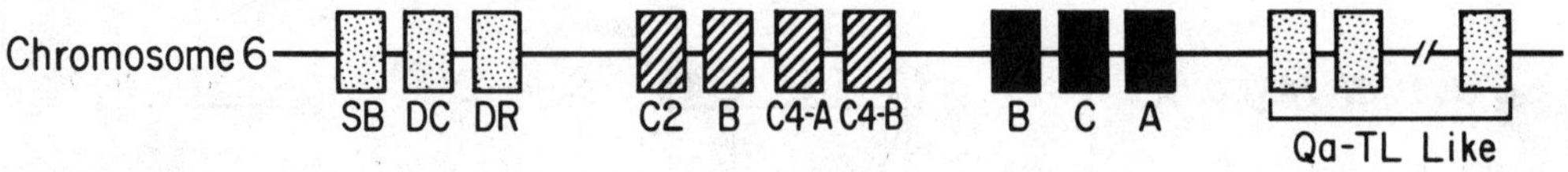

Figure 6.2. Figure shows the arrangements of genes of the major histocompatibility complex of humans. The gene segments for SB, DC, and DR code for Class II molecules; those of B, C, and A code for Class I. The order of segments coding for the complement proteins is not certain.

At the time when these studies were being done, the field of clinical transplantation began to develop in part from the progress made in surgical techniques. Studies of J. Dausset, R. Payne, and J. Van Rood described the presence of antibodies against human white cells in sera of 1) leukopenic patients, 2) patients that had received multiple transfusions, 3) multiparous women, or 4) normal volunteers immunized with leukocytes. Soon, many different antigenic specificities were detected by such antisera. The genetic relationship between these leukocyte antigens was studied by genetic analysis of families and in populations. These studies established the presence of a series of closely linked genetic loci in man. Furthermore, as in the mouse, the genetic studies demonstrated a relationship between the tissue alloantigens defined by serological methods and those detected by tissue transplantation. This resulted in the indentification of the major histocompatibility complex of man termed the <u>HLA complex</u> (human leukocyte antigens) (Figure 6.2).

For many years, the physiological significance of the MHC went unnoticed until, by the middle of the 1960's, when several observations started to indicate its possible regulatory effect in physiological interactions. F. Lilly reported that the development of resistance to leukemia virus depended on the H-2 of the mouse strain. Subsequent studies in the human discovered a curious relationship between the presence of a given HLA antigen and susceptibility to some diseases. Several quite disparate diseases showed this association. A most striking example was <u>ankylosing spondylitis</u>, a chronic inflammatory disease of the spine, in which about 90% of white patients have the HLA-B27 antigen. At the same time, B. Benacerraf and H. McDevitt discovered the role of the MHC in the responses of inbred animals to protein antigens (Chapter 10). Benacerraf and associates identified two inbred guinea pig strains, only one of which responded by making antibodies or delayed sensitivity to DNP-poly-l-lysine (PLL). They went on to show that the recognition of the PLL by the T cell was the crucial event regulated by the MHC. McDevitt made studies of the response of inbred mouse strains to (T-G)A-L (Chapter 2). Some strains made a strong response, and others were low responders. The responder status was linked to the H-2 gene segment. Furthermore, he identified, in strains of mice having recombination at the H-2, a new gene locus controlling the response. This genetic region was termed the I region. Following the Benacerraf-McDevitt studies, the fields of immunogenetics and cellular immunology exploded with new observations that led to a clear understanding of the role of histocompatibility molecules in the cell interactions that regulate immune responses. Chapters 7 and 8 detail these experiments. Advances in cell culture and in cell isolation techniques, the availability of cells from the inbred strains, and the use of antibodies to the Class I or Class II antigens were essential to progress in understanding the role of the MHC in cell interactions regulating immunity. As expected, the histocompatibility molecules did not evolve for the purpose of rejecting grafts but for physiological reasons, i.e., to exercise a fine regulation in the discrimination of foreigness by the individual. Thus, the seminal finding that resulted in the discovery and elucidation of the MHC gene products came from investigators in widely disparate fields: mouse geneticists, serologists, transplantation and cancer biologists, and cellular immunologists.

BIOCHEMISTRY

Class I polypeptides are integral membrane glycoproteins consisting of two chains linked by non-covalent interactions. The heavy chain contains about 345 amino acids and one to two carbohydrate side chains for a molecular weight of about 45,000 daltons. It contains three functional portions: an extracellular, a hydrophobic or transmembrane, and a cytoplasmic segment. The extracellular segment consists of three domains, of about ninety amino acids each, two of which —second and third—contain a disulphide-linked bridge. (The first domain, or alpha-1, is at the N terminus of the molecule.) The disulphides in the second and third domain (alpha-2, and alpha-3) are located at about their ends, resulting in a folding of the molecule with a loop of about sixty amino acids. One to two carbohydrate chains of about three thousand molecular weight are attached by N-linked glycosyl units to the first and second domain. The transmembrane segment, which is about forty amino acids long, crosses the membrane and is rich in non-polar amino acids. The cytoplasmic portion of the molecule contains about thirty amino acids. The second chain is the beta-2 microglobulin, of about 12,000 daltons. It is not directly attached to the membrane but associates with the third domain of the heavy chain. There is a precise relationship between the domain structure and the gene segments coding for them with exons coding for each of the three external domains, one for the intramembranous one and three small ones codings for the cytoplasmic portion. The Class I polypeptide can be envisioned folded into the membrane as in Figure 6.3.

The heavy chain of the molecule is solely responsible for the genetic polymorphism, while the beta-2 microglobulin is highly conserved. The heavy chain does not contain areas of variability restricted to one segment as, for example, with the constant and variable regions of the immunoglobulin molecule. Rather the amino acid changes within the various allelic forms are spread within the three extracellular domains, although predominating in certain stretches of the molecules (for example, for mouse Class I polypeptides, position 61 through 83 of the first domain, and 95 through 99 exhibit a strong degree of variability, while the third domain is more conserved). Overall, there is a great degree of homology (about 80%) within the different Class I loci

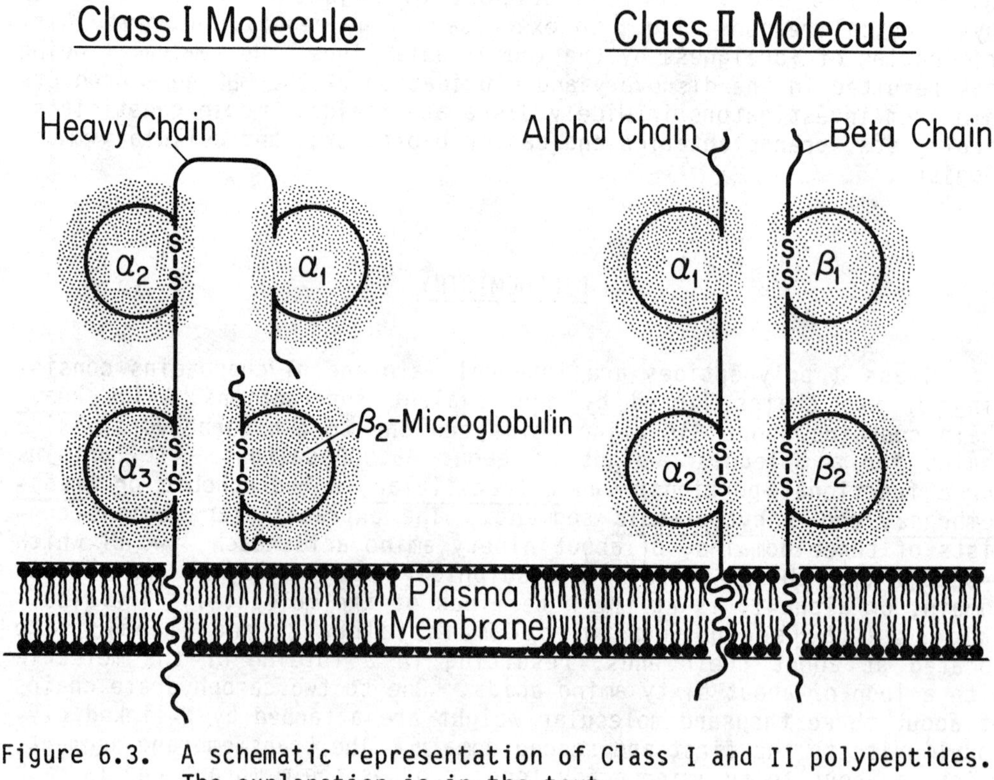

Figure 6.3. A schematic representation of Class I and II polypeptides. The explanation is in the text.

(A and B in the human or K and D in the mouse) and between different alleles of a given locus. The fact that Class I polypeptides encoded in different loci are so similar supports the hypothesis that they have arisen by duplication of a common ancestral gene.

The structure of Class II polypeptides is quite different from Class I. Class II molecules consist of two chains with approximately equal number of amino acids, non-covalently linked, and each attached to the membrane by a transmembrane segment. The alpha chain has about 230 amino acids, 30,000 to 33,000 daltons; the beta chain is smaller, about 220 amino acids, 27,000 to 29,000 daltons. Each chain comprises an external portion, each with two domains of about ninety amino acids, a hydrophobic segment (thirty amino acids), and a short cytoplasmic portion (of about ten to fifteen amino acids). The second domain of the alpha chain and both domains of the beta chain contain disulphide bonds. Short polysaccharide chains of about 3,000 daltons are attached to each chain—two with the alpha and one with the beta chain (Figure 6.3).

The extent of amino acid variability in the alpha and beta chain among the different alleles is now being studied. The alpha chain has limited variability, while, in contrast, the beta chain shows significant number of different amino acid changes among the different alleles. The relationship between the protein structure and the gene segments encoding them are shown in Figure 6.1.

Sequence analysis of MHC molecules has revealed that the domain structures of Class I and II molecules have a great degree of homology. Moreover, the molecules display significant structural homology with the immunoglobulin's basic domain, suggesting that all these immunologically important molecules may be derived from a common gene by duplication and diversification.

GENETICS

The first MHC to be studied and the best known is that of the mouse. In the mouse, the H-2 gene complex is located on chromosome 17, in between the centromere and the telomere. The beta-2 microglobulin chain is encoded in chromosome 2. The H-2 gene complex is classically divided into four major regions, the K, I, S, and D, spanning the length of about 0.3 centimorgans: the K and D regions, located at both ends, contain loci that code for Class I polypeptides, the I region has loci coding for Class II molecules, while the S region codes for the C4 component of complement. The significance of genes coding for complement components within the MHC is not known. The K region contains a locus that codes for the H-2K Class I polypeptides, while the D region contains two closely linked loci coding for D and L Class I molecules.

The three Class I polypeptides are co-expressed on the membranes of all cells.

The I region in the mouse was discovered as a genetic region governing the immune response to synthetic polypeptides (Chapter 10). It has been historically divided into five subregions: I-A, I-B, I-J, I-E, and I-C. Only in I-A and I-E have the gene products been identified. These are the A and E Class II molecules. The existence of I-B and I-C as distinct regions coding for well-defined protein is in doubt at present. (I-B was defined using two recombinant inbred strains as a region controlling immune responses to a few selected antigens. I-C has been defined as controlling the generation of T suppressor cells.) Also controversial is the mapping of the I-J region which was identified by the use of antibodies made between two recombinant inbred strains. These antibodies react with T suppressor cells and their factors. The mapping of the I-J subregion within the MHC has been seriously questioned based on gene analysis of the corresponding MHC gene segment. No membrane molecule coded in the I-J has yet been identified. Despite the present uncertainties about the mapping of the I-J region, nevertheless the anti-I-J antibodies have been extremely useful reagents for identifying T suppressor cells and their polymorphic products.

The I-A subregion contains three loci coding for the A-alpha (the alpha chain of A), A-beta, and E-beta chains, while the I-E subregion contains the locus coding for the E-alpha chain. (A complete A or E Class II molecule is formed by its respective alpha and beta chains, A-alpha and A-beta form the A molecules, and E-alpha and E-beta form the E molecules.) A cell from an inbred strain potentially co-expresses two different Class II polypeptides, one A-alpha-A-beta, a second E-alpha-E-beta. In an F1 hybrid from two inbred lines, each allelic form of the alpha and beta chain of the A molecules, can intermix to form functional molecules. The same applies to the E polypeptides. A few strains of mice lack representation of the E Class II polypeptides. At this point, we should introduce the term haplotype, meaning the entire combination of alleles of the various MHC loci in a given individual or strain of mice. The A and E Class II molecules are expressed on B cells, macrophages, and other antigen-presenting cells as well as activated T cells.

Distal to the K region there are a number of loci coding for other Class I-type polypeptides (the Qa and TLa loci). These Class I polypeptides are structurally similar to the K and D encoded molecules in the sense of having a heavy chain linked to a beta-2 microglobulin chain. The TLa locus codes for the TLa antigens (antigens expressed exclusively on the surface of thymocytes, not in mature T cells, and in some leukemias; hence, Thymus Leukemia antigen). The five Qa loci (Qa1 to Qa5) are expressed in low amounts on the surface of lymphocytes. Their degree of polymorphism is limited, and their function is not known. Some cytolytic T cells have been found to be directed to allogeneic Qa antigens. Only two loci, Qa1 and Qa2, have been characterized as separate loci encoding for a distinct polypeptide. By methods of molecular genetics, thirty-one different genes have now been mapped to the Qa-TL region, a surprising finding since their function is mostly unknown. Whether all these genes are expressed on the cell is not known; the impression at present is that many are not functional.

The HLA gene complex is found on Chromosome 6. The gene for beta-2 microglobulin is on chromosome 15. The four major regions in man, in order, from the centromere, are D-B-C-A. The A, B, and C contain loci that code for distinct Class I polypeptides. The D region codes for Class II molecules. (This pattern of gene distribution seems to be the rule in most species and is found also in monkeys and rats. The mouse may be the exception where the loci for Class II are inserted in between those for Class I.) Three loci have been identified in the D region coding for Class II polypeptides, the SB, DC, and DR. The SB and DC loci have been identified by serological means and have recently been studied by techniques of gene cloning. The initial studies indicate that each locus codes for distinct alpha and beta chains. In fact, the first gene analysis discloses three distinct beta genes in D and two in DC. The Class II molecules encoded in DC appear to be the equivalent of the A molecules in the mouse, while those encoded in DR show sequence homology to the E polypeptides of the mouse. As in the mouse, genes coding for complement are found within the human MHC, although their exact position has not yet been established. The genes for C2, C4, and factor B may be located somewhere in between the D and B loci (Figure 6.2).

The various genes in the MHC are inherited as Mendelian codominant traits. One major characteristic is their great polymorphism. In the mouse, in which most studies have been directed to inbred lines, each locus contains twenty to forty allelic forms. Studies of wild mice show that the alleles recognized in inbred mice represent a fraction of the total. In human studies, the degree of polymorphism is also extensive with eight to forty alleles per each of the loci. Population studies in man have shown variation in the prevalence and frequency of HLA antigens from one population to another. Furthermore, the frequency of certain haplotypes is in excess of what would be predicted by random association. This indicates <u>linkage disequilibrium</u> for the inheritance of some haplotypes. This linkage disequilibrium implies that there is a selective advantage to inhibit recombination at this gene segment and for the genes to remain <u>en bloc</u>. Close to the H-2 gene complex in the mouse (about 5 cm) is located the T/t complex, a series of loci that are involved in embryonic differentiation. Evidence indicates that the t complex may contain a suppressor of crossing-over and that this may include the H-2 complex (i.e., some H-2 haplotypes occur repeatedly with certain combinations of t genes).

There is much discussion concerning the origins of the polymorphism in MHC. There is no evidence to indicate that the polymorphism has arisen from diversification or increased rate of mutation in a given locus. Rather, the polymorphism may have appeared very early in the speciation and was then maintained through evolution. The genetic mechanisms generating polymorphism are not known. Studies of mice with mutations at H-2 show many amino acid substitutions, a pattern which is not consistent with point mutations. Mutations in Class I loci have been explained by gene conversion in which there is exchange of genetic material between one gene and another related gene in a different portion of the chromosome. Regardless of the mechanism, the polymorphism may be construed as functioning to allow the species to have immunological reactivity to a very wide range of antigenic molecules.

CELLULAR REPRESENTATION

Class I polypeptides are expressed on the surface of all cells although they are most heavily represented in lymphoid cells. Red blood cells have a very low content and, in some species, lack Class I molecules. The expression of Class II molecules, on the other hand, is restricted, particularly to lymphoid cells. In humans, early undifferentiated hematopoietic cells express Class II molecules. Monocytes and macrophages express Class II to a variable degree; Langerhans cells have a high content, while most B cells have low to moderate amounts. Activated T cells can also express them. Lymphokines can promote the expression of Class II molecules on monocytes and macrophages, increasing their capacity for antigen presentation. Interestingly, cells known not to have Class II molecules can synthesize them after interaction with T cells or with their secreted lymphokines; these include some endothelial cells, keratinocytes, and fibroblasts. These recent findings suggest that the potential to express Class II molecules is present in many cells, but its expression is under fine regulation.

FUNCTION OF HISTOCOMPATIBILITY MOLECULES: TRANSPLANTATION

The physiological role of the Class I and II polypeptides is discussed in Chapters 7, 8, and 10.

Transplantation. Transplantation involves the transfer of live cells or tissues from one individual to another (Figure 6.4). The term graft is used to denote transplanted cells, tissues, or organs, which can be:

An autograft, from one site to another of the same individual.

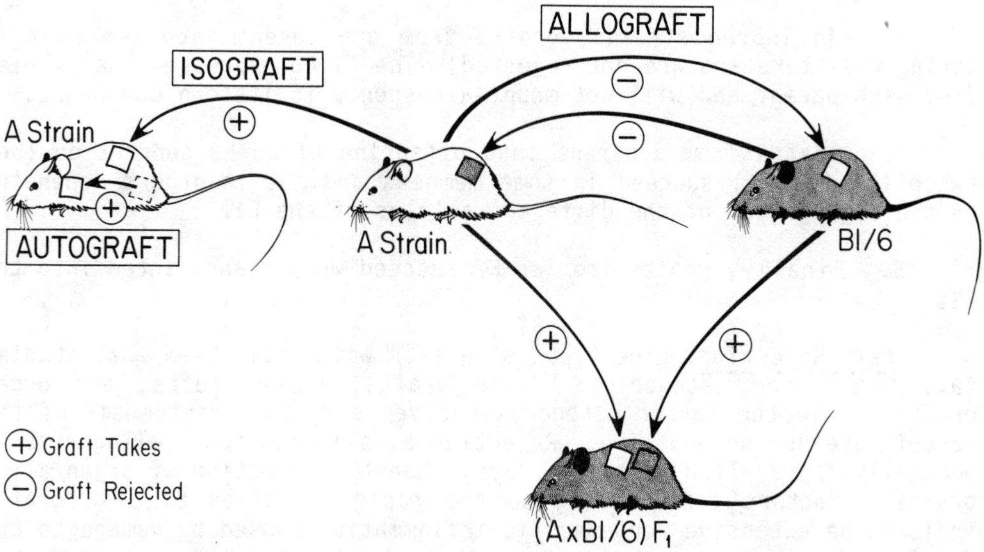

Figure 6.4. The graph illustrates some of the basic laws of transplantation.

An isograft or syngeneic graft, from one member to another of an inbred strain.

An allograft, among individuals of the same species that are genetically disparate, or,

A xenograft, from one species to another.

Some of the classical laws of transplantation that apply among inbred strains were discussed in the Historical section. These laws show the inheritance of the histocompatibility antigens as Mendelian codominant traits. They also demonstrate the fact that individuals are unresponsive to transplantation antigens expressed on their cells or tissues (Chapter 9). These laws are:

1. Isografts are not rejected and will take without problems.

2. Allografts are rejected; the rapidity by which they are rejected depends on the differences in histocompatibility antigens. Differences at the MHC induce strong graft rejection in comparison to differences at the minor histocompatibility loci. (The minor histocompatibility loci code for polymorphic cell surface molecules that play

some role in transplantation rejections. These molecules are weak antigens and require strong immunization measures to be detected.)

3. In inbred strains, grafts from one parent into the F1 offspring will take and are not rejected. The F1 co-expresses the alleles from each parent and will not mount a response to its own component.

4. Grafts from a parent into offspring of an F2 generation (between the two F1) succeed in some members and not in others depending on the segregation of the different alleles of the F1.

5. Finally, grafts from an F2 succeed when transplanted into the F1.

Graft Rejection. The types of grafts which have been most studied fall into three categories: skin grafts, tumor grafts, and organ grafts. Only the latter category involves surgical anastomosis of the vasculature during grafting. Rejection of skin and tumor allografts is generally faster (ten to twelve days) than the rejection of organ allografts. Factors contributing to the rapid rejection of skin grafts include the extensive non-specific inflammation caused by damage to the dermis and the greater degree of ischemic necrosis which occurs during the hours post-grafting. Lymphatic drainage is apparently necessary to initiate rejection of skin, but not to initiate rejection of organs. The large vascular area of organs may be the reason why lymphatic drainage appears unnecessary to initiate organ rejection.

Most types of solid tissue allogeneic grafts, including skin and kidney grafts, show similar histological changes. During the first few days, the graft heals in and vascularization begins. A small number of hematogenous leukocytes may be seen infiltrating the perivenous tissue in the first few days, especially in grafts with surgically connected vasculature (kidney, lung, liver). A massive cellular infiltration of the graft tissue usually begins between the fifth and seventh days. The majority of the infiltrating cells are mononuclear cells (lymphocytes and mononuclear phagocytes), and a minority are polymorphonuclear granulocytes. Increasing amounts of tissue damage and necrosis are seen during the next few days until the rejection process is completed.

After an individual has rejected an allogeneic graft, a second graft of the same genotype will be rejected with a similar sequence of events but with an accelerated tempo, rejection usually being complete a few days earlier than a primary graft. This "second set" rejection rate can be used to detect specific transplantation immunity.

Individuals who have had repeated or prolonged exposure to allogeneic antigens may develop a state of hyperimmunity characterized by large amounts of circulating antibody. When such individuals receive allografts, an accelerated rejection occurs. Under these conditions, in the case of skin grafts, vascularization never takes place, since healing is interfered by immune complex formation and inflammation. After two to three days, the skin appears white instead of the usual pink color seen during vascularization of primary grafts; hence, the term white graft. If a kidney is transplanted into a recipient who has preexisting immunity to the HLA antigens on the graft, the transplanted kidney may suffer immediate vascular damage and become ischemic. Therefore, to avoid such hyperacute reactions, serum from the recipient patient is always tested for cytotoxic antibodies to donor cells prior to grafting.

Transplantation immunity can be transferred to a non-immune recipient by intravenous injection of living lymphoid cells from an immune donor. During active immmunization by grafting, the cells that transfer immunity are found first in the lymph nodes draining the graft area and later in the thoracic duct, peripheral blood, spleen, and peritoneal exudate. When immune lymphocytes tagged with tritiated thymidine are used to transfer transplantation immunity, very few labeled cells are found among the many mononuclear cells infiltrating the rejected graft. Lymphocytes from a sensitized population accumulate in somewhat higher numbers in rejecting grafts than in grafts to which no immunity has been transferred, but this may be largely a non-specific response to inflammation. Thus, a very small number of specific lymphocytes can initiate the rejection process.

T lymphocytes are responsible for allograft immunity. These lymphocytes are specific for the allogeneic MHC gene products found in the transplanted cells. At least two functionally different subclasses of effector T lymphocytes are have been identified playing important roles in the destruction of grafted tissue: the cytolytic T lymphocytes and the helper T lymphocytes capable of releasing lymphokines (Chapter 7). Monocytes attracted and activated by the lymphokine may well collaborate with cytolytic T cells.

In graft rejection, the T lymphocytes of the cytolytic class are directly mainly to the Class I alloantigens which serve as the main stimulus for their generation. In contrast, the helper T cells are reacting mostly with the Class II alloantigens found in cells of the graft. Following an allograft, both cytolytic and helper T cells can be found in the draining lymph nodes with reactivity to Class I or II alloantigens, respectively, of the grafted cells. There is synergy between each set of lymphocytes both in the inductive phase of immunity, i.e., during the generation of the response, as well as in the effector state. During the inductive phase, the helper T cells activated by their interaction with Class II alloantigens collaborate via their secretion of lymphokines with the cytolytic T cells interacting with Class I molecules (Chapter 7). This results in an optimal generation of T cytolytic cells, while, at the same time, the T helper clones are expanding in number and secreting lymphokines that then recruit and activate macrophages. Graft rejection and generation of cytolytic T cells, however, can take place using inbred strains that differ only at the K or D locus, indicating that these alloantigens are sufficient to activate cytolytic T cells.

Graft-Versus-Host Reactions. Grafts which contain significant numbers of immunocompetent lymphoid cells can mount destructive reaction against the host, i.e., graft versus host (GvH) reactions. Apart from noting the possible dangers associated with the use of grafts of lymphohematopoietic tissue for therapeutic purposes, GvH reactions have provided simple assays for demonstrating the presence of immunocompetent cells in normal components of blood, peritoneal exudates, and thoracic duct lymph. GvH reactions take place when the recipient is unable to reject the transplanted lymphocytes, as in immunologically crippled patients, X-irradiated animals, and in F1 recipients of immunocompetent parental cells. These reactions are extremely important, since they may take place when bone marrow is transplanted in immunologically deficient children. (Note in Chapter 15 the case of the patient with severe combined immunodeficiency.)

The GvH disease results from the presence of T lymphocytes in the grafted cells that react primarily with Class II alloantigens of the host. The T helper cells interact with the Class II alloantigens, multiply, and secrete the various lymphokines that result in severe inflammation. A prominent feature of GvH disease is an enlarged spleen (splenomegaly). This enlargement is caused primarily by proliferation of host cells, probably mononuclear phagocytes. Moreover, most of the damage in GvH disease is mediated by those host inflammatory cells activated by the reaction of transferred immunocompetent cells with histocompatibility antigens. Other symptoms of GvH are enlarged liver and lymph nodes, hemolytic anemia, reduced immunoglobulin and complement levels, reduced immunocompetence, skin rash, inflammation of the intestinal mucosa, and weight loss. Death can ensue in severe GvH cases. Chronic GvH is associated with activation of C type viruses and increased incidence of malignancy.

The mixed leukocyte reaction (MLR). The mixed leukocyte (or lymphocyte) reaction is produced by culturing the lymphocytes from two genetically disparate individuals. The lymphocytes from one individual (responder) will recognize primarily the Class II alloantigens on the cells from the second individual (the stimulator cells) and will proliferate. The stimulator cells are represented by cells having Class II antigens on the membrane such as monocytes and Langerhans-dendritic cells. A few days later, the degree of proliferation is measured usually by the incorporation of radioactive thymidine into the DNA of the responder cells. Two-way MLR occurs when the lymphocytes in each individual respond against the stimulator cells of each other. In the one-way reaction, one set of cells is treated in such a way as to inhibit their division (by giving drugs or X-irradiation); these treated cells will not respond yet will contain the stimulator cells (i.e., the cells bearing Class II molecules). In this way, the MLR is limited only to the lymphocytes of the untreated set reacting with the treated stimulator cells. As mentioned, the Class II molecules are by far the strongest stimulator of the MLR. The MLR can be used as a clinical transplantation test to examine for alloantigeneic differences unrelated to the classical transplantation antigens that are detected by typing with alloantibodies. During the MLR, the cytolytic T cells are generated against Class I alloantigens of the stimulator cells.

Comments on Human Transplantation. Today organ transplantation represents an important alternative for the treatment of several diseases, especially for disorders involving an irreversible loss of organ function. Kidney transplantation constitutes the most common form of organ transplantation. Transplantaton of bone marrow, cornea, heart, liver, and pancreatic islets are also performed in a more limited number of patients, in selected institutions. Prognostic factors that have important roles in organ transplantation are HLA matching, HLA and non-HLA (ABO) antibodies, and pretransplant blood transfusion.

Evidence that HLA antigens are important in allotransplantation is derived from tissue matching and subsequent graft survival rates. In the absence of preimmunization, allografts are rejected more slowly in HLA-matched pairs of donors and recipients. Within a family, skin grafts among siblings who share both HLA haplotypes survive considerably longer than grafts between individuals who differ at one haplotype. They, in turn, do better than grafts exchanged between related individuals with two haplotype differences. The evaluation of preimmunization in the recipient as determined by the crossmatch procedure is critical, since allografts are rejected in an accelerated manner or do not become vascularized when performed in recipients with alloantibodies against donor antigens.

HLA matching consists of identifying alleles of the HLA loci (A, B, C, and D) by serotyping HLA antigens in unrelated individuals (phenotypes). Family studies characterize the inheritance of these antigens in such a way that the genotypes can be identified. A transplant between parent and offspring or between siblings that share one HLA haplotype is said to be HLA haploidentical. A transplant between sibling HLA genotypically identical or different at both haplotypes are said to be either HLA identical or HLA different. In unrelated individuals, the degree of matching is assigned by the number of HLA antigen matches and mismatches. HLA matching influences the outcome of an unrelated kidney allograft.

The actual matching of donor and recipients in renal transplantation is commonly expressed by the degree of identity according to HLA phenotypes or genotypes. Although the role of HLA matching in renal transplantation between related individuals is undisputed, the effect of matching for HLA phenotypes on the survival of cadaver transplantation is not clear. The cadaver-matching correlations reported in recent surveys range from good in France and England, to moderate in Scandinavia, to fair in the United States. The data presented in Figure 6.5 illustrate the long-term survival rates for cadaver, parent-to-child (one-haplotype identical), and two-haplotype-identical sibling kidney transplants. Part of the reason for these discrepancies is due to an incomplete definition of the HLA region and the possible role of additional unknown histocompatibility loci.

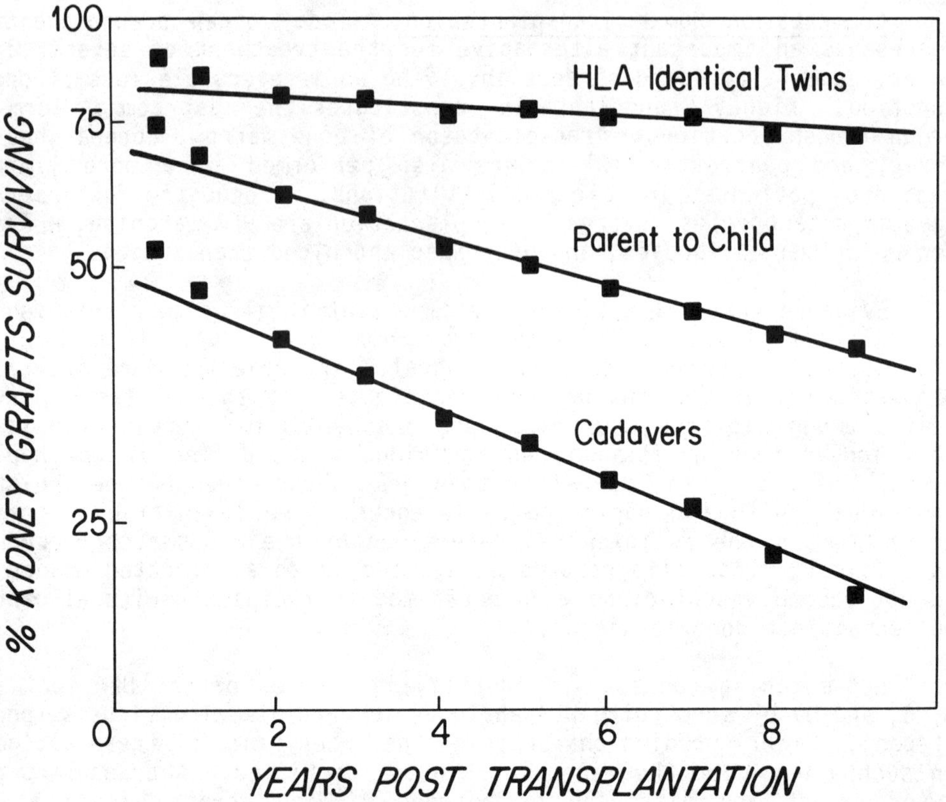

Figure 6.5. The role of HLA in renal allograft survival. Comparisons of graft survival times in two haplotype-identical siblings, one haplotype-identical parent-child combination, and cadaver transplants without any haplotype identity.

Problems of bone marrow transplantation include: 1) the control of host immunologic reactions directed against the alloantigens of the bone marrow cells, and 2) the reactivity of the donor's immunocompetent cells in the bone marrow graft directed against the recipient. The resulting GvH reaction, plus the likelihood of infections make bone marrow transplant difficult. In bone marrow transplantation, the donor, in most cases, is a sibling with two HLA-identical haplotypes. Rarely is an HLA-identical, mixed lymphocyte reaction-negative, unrelated donor used. It appears that HLA-D identity is most important in prevention of GvH reaction, but there are many other non-HLA factors that are also important.

The usual indications for marrow grafting are immune deficiency diseases, aplastic anemias (anemias where there is a central failure of bone marrow to produce red cells) and some leukemias. Among the immunodeficiencies, the most commonly treated by bone marrow transplantation is the severe combined immunodeficiency states (Chapter 15). In severe combined immunodeficiency disease, there is a high rate of bone marrow engraftment (takes of 88%).

There has been recent progress in bone marrow transplantation. Early studies in the mouse had indicated that the GvH disease was caused by the very few mature T cells in the marrow inoculum. Their elimination using specific antibodies (with complement) resulted in the elimination of GvH: the stem cells homed to the thymus of the irradiated recipient and matured, becoming tolerant to the host histocompatibility antigens. Recent extension of this protocol to humans has met with remarkable success: bone marrow cells were treated with a very efficient monoclonal antibody (anti-T12) that killed the mature T cells and then were transplanted into the mismatched irradiated recipient. There was complete reconstitution of hematopoiesis and lymphocyte function without GvH disease.

Although tissue matching improves the outcome of allotransplants, the success of clinical transplantation is directly related, in part, to the development of good methods of immunosuppression. In general, it is known that HLA-identical and haploidentical transplants require less immunosuppression than the unrelated grafts given to patients. Most protocols consist of a combination of corticosteroids, azothioprine, and cyclosporin A. Cyclosporin A is a fungal product that appears to inhibit the function of helper T cells. Recent trials are evaluating the use of monoclonal antibodies directed to T cell subsets.

REFERENCES

Bodmer, W. F. HLA: A super supergene. Harvey Lect., 72:91, 1978.

Dausset, J, and Svejgaard, A. HLA and Disease, Munksgaard, Copenhagen; Williams and Wilkins Company, Baltimore, 1977.

Hood, L., Steinmetz, M., and Malissen, B. Genes of the major histocompatibility complex of the mouse. Ann. Rev. Immunol., 1:529, 1983.

Klein, J. Biology of the Mouse Histocompatibility-2 Complex. Springer-Verlag, New York, 1977.

Klein, J., et al. The traditional and the new version of the mouse H-2 complex. Nature, 291:455, 1981.

Nathenson, S. G., et al. Primary structural analysis of the transplantation antigens of the mouse H-2 histocompatibility complex. Ann. Rev. Biochem., 50:1025, 1981.

CHAPTER 7

Cellular Immunity and Delayed Hypersensitivity

In this chapter, we shall consider some of the functions of the helper T cells and the cytolytic lymphocytes in the context of cellular immunity to infectious agents. The next chapter discusses the role of helper and suppressor T cells in the regulation of cellular interactions. Cell-mediated immunity, or cellular immunity, are processes specifically initiated by T lymphocytes and characterized by an inflammatory reaction rich in highly activated macrophages. Cellular immune reactions occur: 1) during infection by microorganisms; 2) in the course of immunity to soluble protein antigens; 3) as a component of immune reactions against tumors and transplanted tissues; 4) in contact sensitivity; and 5) as components of some autoimmune diseases.

This chapter reviews cellular immunity to microorganisms and delayed hypersensitivity reactions to soluble antigens. Both of these processes are characterized by an inflammatory response involving the mononuclear phagocytes.

CELLULAR IMMUNITY IN INFECTIOUS DISEASES

The respective roles of antibody and leukocytes in combating bacterial infections generated intense controversy at the turn of the century. Elie Metchnikoff was the first to propose that phagocytes were capable of ingesting and killing viable organisms. However, concomitant studies of P. Ehrlich, R. Bordet, R. Pfeiffer and others also indicated an important fole for "humoral immunity" mediated by antibody and complement. It soon became evident that both interpretations were correct: leukocytes—neutrophils, in particular—were required to kill some types of bacteria, but antibody and complement were required for their ingestion by the leukocytes. It later became apparent that resistance to infection was highly complex and, in many cases, required another element besides antibody for "opsonization", and leukocytes to ingest and kill the organisms. This conclusion was reached in chronic infections like tuberculosis. The tubercle bacilli were ingested by phagocytes but were not killed, and infection persisted for long periods of time. The tubercle bacilli have the potential to grow inside macrophages—and are considered facultative intracellular microbes. Resistance to infection with the tubercle bacillus depends on the acquisition by the phagocytes of microbicidal properties as a result of T cell stimulation. However, the intricate and complex relationship between T cell immunity and macrophage activation for resistance to infection by intracellular pathogens took many years to unravel; in fact, it is only very recently that all the interactions were understood.

In general terms, resistance to microorganisms may be mediated by antibody—humoral immunity—or by T cells through cellular immune reactions:

1. <u>Antibody-mediated immunity</u>: The formation of antibodies that bind to the antigen results in the fixation of complement. The antigen-antibody complex is then phagocytized by neutrophils. Humoral immunity plays a major role against infection with most gram-positive organisms, and some gram-negative organisms, all of which are rapidly killed once taken up by the leukocytes. In these instances, the critical step in stopping microbial growth is the rapid ingestion of the organisms, which depends on their opsonization by antibody and complement. However, leukocytes phagocytize poorly many bacteria that have a thick capsule of carbohydrate. The pneumococcus is a classical example. The rate of phagocytosis of pneumococci by neutrophils is increased one-thousand- to ten-thousandfold in the presence of antibody and complement. In this infection, once antibody is made by the host, the bacteria are rapidly eliminated. Furthermore, protection can be transferred by injection of serum containing specific antibodies.

Humoral immunity is also effective against bacteria that release highly powerful <u>toxins</u>, such as diphtheria and tetanus. The antibodies bind to the toxins and block their interaction with the target organs. Antibodies also play a role in neutralizing some viruses—such as the polio viruses—during the early period of infection, when viremia is present. Chapter 15 gives examples of infectious diseases in children with genetic defects of B cells or of complement proteins.

2. <u>Cellular immune reactions</u>: Cell-mediated immunity plays a major role in the resistance to many bacteria, viruses, fungi, and protozoa, all of which have the capacity to live and multiply in the cells of the host, mainly in mononuclear phagocytes. The growth of these microorganisms is not stopped by their phagocytosis, and further steps are required to inhibit their multiplication and spread. These steps involve the accumulation, and activation, of phagocytes in foci of infection. The phagocytes, once activated, stop the growth of the pathogen. In these infections, the helper T lymphocytes play the central role in the activation of the phagocyte system that results in the destruction of the pathogen. In viral infections, the cytolytic class of T cells with specificity for viral antigens stops the virus from

propagating by killing the infected host cells as well as by secreting gamma-interferon. Below are listed some intracellular pathogens, the immunity to which is thought to depend on cellular mechanisms:

Intracellular Pathogens of Man

Bacteria:	Mycobacterium tuberculosis Salmonella typhosa Brucella abortus Listeria monocytogenes
Fungi:	Candida albicans Cryptococcus neoformans Histoplasma capsulatum
Viruses:	All
Protozoa:	Toxoplasma gondii Malarial plasmodia Leishmania donovani Trypanosoma cruzi

Let us consider some typical examples of humoral and of cellular immunity to infectious agents. Staphylococcal infection can trigger antibody formation as well as a variable degree of cellular immunity. However, all that is required for the control of the infection is for the bacteria to be opsonized (i.e., bound to antibody and complement) in order that the neutrophils can engulf them. Once phagocytized, these organisms are highly sensitive to the bactericidal effect of the neutrophils, and are killed. In contrast, bacteria of the type listed above (i.e., the tubercle bacilli, for example) are not killed after phagocytosis, even if bound to antibody and complement. This is a case that requires T cell-macrophage interactions for their elimination.

CELLULAR IMMUNITY REACTIONS MEDIATED PRIMARILY BY HELPER T CELLS

The cellular landmark in immune reactions involving cellular immunity is the presence of activated phagocytes, in large numbers in the infective foci, sometimes forming granulomas. A granuloma is a collection of phagocytes, many of which have phagocytized the infectious agents. The macrophages forming the granuloma adhere closely to each other, adopting epithelial-like characteristics; these altered macrophages are termed epithelial cells. Some of the macrophages fuse with each other, forming multinucleated giant cells.

The role of cellular immunity in infection is apparent in the description of experimental tuberculous infection in the guinea pig by Robert Koch in 1891. Inoculation of virulent tubercle bacilli in the skin of unimmunized guinea pigs led to severe infections that rapidly disseminated, extending to draining nodes and beyond, to other organs. Such severe systemic infections frequently produced death. However, infection of a previously inoculated, immune guinea pig resulted in absence of dissemination of the bacteria and in the formation of a large localized, indurated nodule in the skin at the site of the inoculation. This nodule could progress to necrosis and ulceration. The immune guinea pig was then able to curb the dissemination of the virulent bacteria. The tuberculous nodule was composed of large, activated phagocytes. The phagocytes contained tubercle bacilli, many of which were dead or inhibited in their multiplication.

Insights into what occurred in the tuberculous granuloma came from studies of M. Lurie in the rabbit. In 1942, Lurie cultured tubercle bacilli with phagocytes in the anterior chamber of the rabbit's eye. He found that the bacilli grew in the phagocytes from normal, uninfected, rabbits but did not grow in phagocytes from infected, immune rabbits. Furthermore, serum from the infected rabbits did not stop the multiplicaton of bacteria in normal phagocytes; the tubercle bacilli was ingested readily by the phagocytes in the absence of serum and even better in its presence, but subsequent growth was not inhibited. The concept began to emerge that, for microbicidal action, a particular state of macrophage activation was required. This interpretation gained strenth following the studies of G. MacKaness and associates who outlined the role of lymphocytes in immune recognition and in activating macrophages for bacterial action. Also crucial in the understanding of the macrophage-T cell effects were the studies of delayed hypersensitivity which highlighted the role of lymphocytes (see below).

Cellular immune reactions are not only found against the microbes listed above but are also generated against microbial products or to soluble proteins. Take the example of the tubercle bacilli. Infection with the tubercle bacilli produces a state of cellular immunity. A challenge of the infected individual with the bacilli results in the activation of the cellular immune process described above. The immune individual, however, can also respond to bacterial products. The intradermal injection of the immune host with soluble products of the tubercle bacilli results in the formation of an indurated type of lesion characterized by the presence of lymphocytes and macrophages in the dermis. This is the delayed hypersensitivity lesion that is equivalent to the reaction previously described against the live organisms. The production of the delayed sensitivity lesion denotes a state of cellular immunity to the tubercle bacilli. In practical terms, the production of a delayed sensitivity reaction is of great importance inasmuch as it permits a physician to determine if a patient has an active state of immunity to the microorganisms in question. For example, a diagnosis of tuberculosis may be made if a suspected patient develops a strong delayed sensitivity reaction to an intradermal injection of tuberculin or purified protein derivative (PPD). Tuberculin is a crude heat-concentrated filtrate of a liquid culture of the tubercle bacillus. PPD is a preparation containing mostly proteins from the culture fluid. Skin tests of these types are also employed for the diagnosis of other bacterial, viral, and fungal infections.

Delayed sensitivity reactions, therefore, are inflammatory reactions characterized by infiltration predominantly with phagocytes, resulting from a specific state of T cell immunity. As mentioned earlier, the state of cellular immunity (or T cell immunity) that allows the individual to manifest a delayed reaction can also be produced by immunization with soluble protein antigens. In experimental work, in order to produce strong cellular immune reactions, the proteins are injected mixed with a water-in-oil emulsion (Freund's adjuvant). The water-in-oil emulsion may contain dead tubercle bacilli (complete adjuvant equals water-in-oil emulsion that contains the antigen plus dead tubercle bacilli; incomplete Freund's adjuvant equals water-in-oil emulsion with the antigen but no tubercle bacilli). The Freund's adjuvant produces a very strong inflammatory reaction that is conducive to the generation of a strong T cell immunity. Delayed sensitivity reactions to soluble proteins administered without adjuvants contain a conspicuous infiltration by basophils, together with the usual macrophages. These reactions develop very early after immunization and also depend on specific immune T lymphocytes.

Why is the term "delayed" used for characterizing these cellular reactions? Delayed sensitivity reaction elicited in the skin of immune individuals start developing after six to eight hours, increasing in size and intensity for twenty-four to forty-eight hours. The histological picture is a diffuse infiltration of the deep and superficial areas of the dermis by mononuclear cells. The mononuclear infiltrate consists mostly of macrophages with some lymphocytes. The infiltrate is more conspicuous around small vessels and varies in severity depending on the state of immunization. Severe reactions may be accompanied by damage to the blood vessels with thrombosis and necrosis of the tissue. In delayed reactions, there is also an increase in vascular permeability.

What is the difference between the granuloma produced in the skin by infection with live tubercle and the diffuse delayed sensitivity lesion produced in the same individual by injection with tuberculin? Both reactions result from the same pathogenetic mechanism. The main difference is the amount and form of presentation of the antigen. In the granuloma, the cellular reactions center around the foci of infectious organisms that are in the process of multiplying. Hence, there is a high concentration of antigen in discrete spots, and the inflammation reaction surrounds them. In the reaction to the soluble tuberculin, the antigen is spread through the dermis; and the inflammation, therefore, is diffuse. If, for example, instead of injecting soluble tuberculin, one injects the same amount but conjugated to small, insoluble polyacrylamide beads, then the tuberculin elicits a granulomatous reaction centered around the bead.

What happens when antigen is injected into the skin of an immune individual with circulating antibodies? If the immune individual has a high titer of IgG antibodies, then an Arthus reaction develops prior to the delayed sensitivity reaction. Arthus reactions result from the deposition of antigen-antibody-complement complexes along vessel walls and are characterized by: 1) their early development (approximately two to four hours); 2) the presence of hemorrhage because of severe damage to vascular basement membranes; and 3) infiltration by neutrophils (see Chapter 13). The development of the Arthus reaction requires the injection of a relatively large amount of antigen into the skin. By injecting very small amounts of antigen, the degree of "Arthus reactivity" can be minimized, yet the delayed hypersensitivity component may still be apparent. Arthus reactions denote the presence of circulating antibodies in contrast to delayed reactions which indicate cellular T cell immunity.

Another important component in the inflammatory reponse elicited by antigen is the increase in vascular permeability elicited by antibodies of the IgE class (Chapter 14). These antibodies bind to tissue mast cells and, upon interaction with antigen, induce the release of vasoactive amines. IgE-mediated increase in vascular permeability can be elicited with very small amounts of antigen and take only a few minutes to develop. Table 7.1 compares these three types of immunological inflammatory reactions.

Table 7.1

Immunological Reactions Induced in the Skin

Reaction	Time	Histology	Pathogenesis
Arthus	2 to 4 hours	Infiltration by neutrophils	Antigen-antibody complexes ⟶ PMN
Delayed sensitivity	24 to 48 hours	Infiltration by macrophages and some lymphocytes	T cell ⟶ lymphokines ⟶ macrophages
Anaphylactic	First few minutes	Edema, few cells	IgE ⟶ mast cells

What happens when antigen is injected intravenously into an immune animal displaying strong delayed sensitivity to the antigen? A systemic delayed sensitivity reaction will be produced. This reaction is characterized by fever, a drop in circulating monocytes, and by a skin rash. The fever is caused by the production of an endogenous pyrogenic substance by the macrophages (interleukin-1) (see Chapter 5). The monocytopenia is transitory and is caused by a loss of monocytes to the extravascular tissue. The skin rash is produced by multiple reactions involving antigen and the lymphoid cells.

MECHANISMS

Let us analyze both the cellular immune reactions in bacterial infections and in delayed hypersensitivity skin reactions. Cellular immune reactions involve two components: 1) a specific component, represented by the T lymphocytes that specifically recognize the antigen; the antigen is presented to the T lymphocyte by a macrophage having Class II molecules on its membrane; and 2) a non-specific component, represented by the macrophages which, as a result of T cell stimulation, are recruited into immune sites and become activated. Therefore, T lymphocyte-macrophage interactions take place at two distinct stages of immunity: first, in the immune induction or recognition state in which the T cell becomes stimulated by antigen bound to local macrophages in association with an MHC gene product; second, during the effector phase of cellular immunity in which the antigen-activated T lymphocyte then recruits and activates new macrophages for cytocidal activity.

The specific component of cellular immune reactions. The classical experiments of K. Landsteiner and M. Chase established the existence of specific cellular immunity and demonstrated that delayed hypersensitivity is mediated by specifically immune lymphocytes and not by serum antibody. These experiments were carried out prior to the time when immune T cells were known to be the specific mediators of the reactions. These investigators transferred tuberculin-delayed sensitivity adoptively in guinea pigs from an actively immune animal to a normal recipient, by peritoneal exudate cells, but not by antisera. Such transfers were carried out successfully between random-bred histoincompatible animals because: 1) large numbers of cells from several donors were transferred, and 2) the recipient animals were tested within twenty-four hours of the cell transfer previous to the immune rejection of the transferred cells. Subsequent studies not only confirmed the findings of Landsteiner and Chase in both delayed sensitivity and in resistance to intracellular pathogens, but established that T cells were responsible.

More recent studies carried out with inbred mice indicated that effective transfer of delayed sensitivity or of antibacterial immunity requires identity at the major histocompatibility gene complex (MHC) between donor cells and recipient for optimal transfer. As was mentioned briefly in Chapter 6, this restriction is due to the fact that genes in the MHC control the critical presentation of antigen to T cells by macrophages required for the induction of cellular immunity reactions. Indeed, activation of T lymphocytes for the initiation of cellular immune reactions requires the interaction with local macrophages that take up the antigen. Moreover, the macrophages interacting with the lymphocytes must express on their surface the Class II molecules encoded in the I region of the MHC (Chapter 6). In Chapter 5 we analyzed several examples indicating that immune induction was particularly effective if antigen was presented to lymphocytes in association with macrophages bearing Ia antigens. This phenomenon of lymphocyte-macrophage interation becomes particularly important in the generation of helper T lymphocytes that are responsible for cellular immunity. In Chapter 8 the details of macrophage-helper T cell interaction involving MHC molecules will be given.

Once the local macrophages and T cells have interacted, the T cells elaborate a variety of proteins (lymphocyte mediators or lymphokines) that recruit and activate new phagocytes derived from bone marrow stem cells.

What is the form or state of the antigen recognized by T cells in cellular immune reactions? We described in Chapter 2 that the antigen "recognized" by T cells may be partially denatured or altered by the host. This conclusion was based on studies of the specificity of delayed sensitivity to globular and denatured proteins. Immunization with a native protein in Freund's adjuvant results in delayed sensitivity; intradermal injection of the native antigen will elicit a delayed reaction. However, intradermal injection of the denatured antigen results in the same delayed reaction as the injection of the native antigen. This experiment implies that the antigen underwent some metabolic changes prior to recognition by T cells.

The following experiments illustrate the role of specific lymphocytes in cellular immunity to facultative intracellular bacteria.

Experiment 1: Immunity to facultative intracellular bacteria involves a specific component (= T lymphocytes) and a non-specific component (= phagocytes). Immunologic memory is a property of the T lymphocytes. In the following experiment by George Mackaness and associates at the Trudeau Institute, it was shown that lymphocytes are involved in specific protection against *Listeria monocytogenes* infection in mice:

1. Infect inbred mice with a small dose of virulent Listeria organisms.

2. Several days later sacrifice the mice and obtain serum and spleen lymphocytes. At this time, the mouse is immune and contains active lymphocytes capable of resisting infection.

3. Inject normal mice with spleen cells or serum from the immune or normal mice and then challenge with a lethal dose of virulent Listeria or virulent tubercle bacillus or both.

Results:

Transfer	Bacterial Challenge: Listeria	Mycobacteria	Listeria and Mycobacteria
Normal spleen cells	No resistance	No resistance	No resistance
Normal serum	No resistance	No resistance	No resistance
Listeria-immune spleen cells	Resistance	No resistance	Resistance to both
Immune serum	No resistance	No resistance	No resistance

Serum from immune mice does not confer protection—i.e., this infectious process does not involve an antibody-dependent mechanism. However, immune spleen cells contain lymphocytes with increased anti-Listeria immunity. These are triggered only by the specific agent (Listeria) but not by an unrelated bacteria (mycobacteria). However, if the immune events are triggered by the specific bacteria, then a concomitant infection by an unrelated organism is also curbed. This is because the specific anti-Listeria lymphocytes triggered activation of phagocytes, which then can kill unrelated organisms.

Experiment 2: Demonstration of immunity in culture:

1. Harvest macrophages from a normal guinea pig and place them in culture.

2. Add lymphocytes from animals immune to DNP-BGG (dinitrophenylated bovine gamma globulin) or BSA (bovine serum albumin) with or without the specific antigen. Infect cultures with Listeria organisms and measure growth of the Listeria in the macrophages.

Results:

Lymphocytes From	Challenge with DNP-BGG	Challenge with BSA
DNP-BGG immune	Growth is reduced	Normal growth rate
BSA immune	Normal growth rate	Growth is reduced
Non-immune	Normal growth rate	Normal growth rate

Interpretation: The immune lymphocytes were triggered by the specific antigen to activate the phagocytes. Once activated, the phagocytes stopped the growth of *Listeria*. Further developments of this culture system have shown that lymphocytes first interact with Ia-bearing macrophages containing the antigen after which the T cell releases protein mediators that then activate the macrophages for enhanced microbicidal activity.

Finally, the class of lymphocyte involved in cellular immunity is the T lymphocyte. Resistance is transferred only by the thymic-derived cell as shown in Figure 7.1. Animals thymectomized at birth offer little resistance to these infections.

The same kind of experiment can be done with regard to delayed hypersensitivity skin reactions. Purified T lymphocytes from an experimental animal immunized with a protein antigen and displaying a positive delayed skin reaction upon inoculation to a normal animal will transfer the delayed sensitivity state. It has been established that the helper T cell is responsible for cellular immunity to infection and for delayed sensitivity.

The inflammatory reaction. The histological hallmark of these reactions is the infiltration by macrophages that are highly activated and display increased microbicidal properties. Early investigators of cellular immune reactions questioned whether the infiltrating cells were lymphocytes or macrophages. The concensus at present, based on morphological and kinetic data, is that the bulk of infiltrating cells are bone marrow-derived macrophages together with a few T lymphocytes. One experiment that was instrumental in clarifying this issue is the following, based on protocols originally devised by R. T. McCluskey and B. Benacerraf. Guinea pigs were immunized with an antigen in Freund's adjuvant, resulting in the development of a strong state of cellular immunity. Two manipulations were carried out:

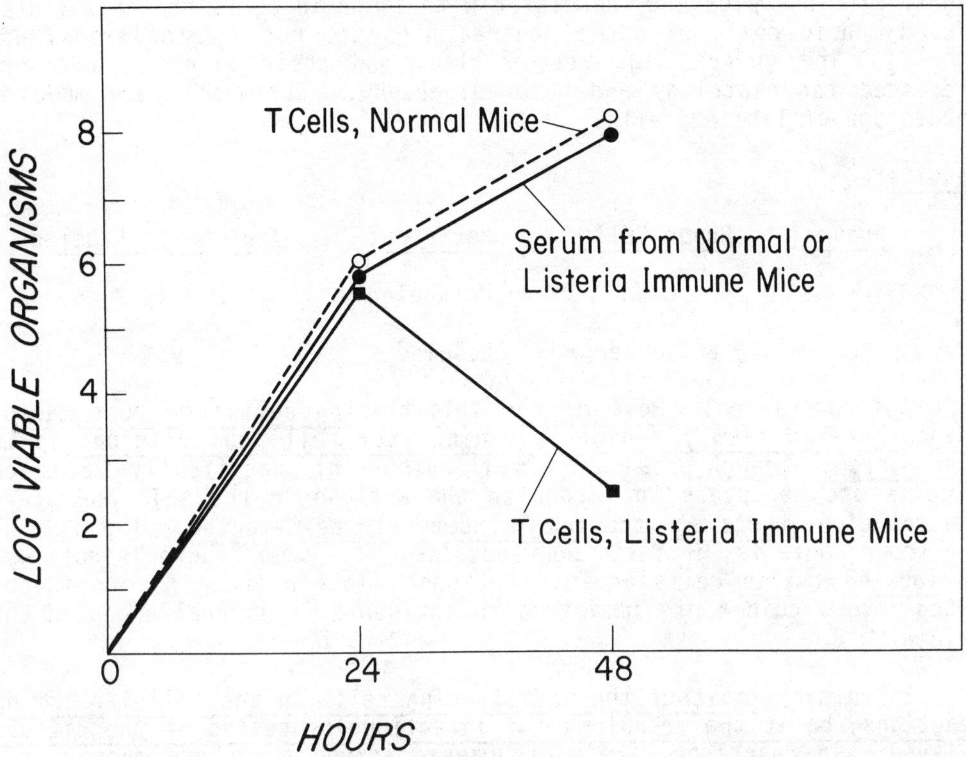

Figure 7.1. The curves show the growth of Listeria organisms in spleen of normal mice. Mice received serum of normal or Listeria-immune mice, or immune T cells. Only immune T cells stopped the multiplication of bacteria in the spleen.

A. Twelve days after immunization, one group of immune guinea pigs received tritiated thymidine, which was incorporated into lymphoid cells undergoing DNA synthesis, including the specifically immunized T lymphocytes. The lymphoid cells were harvested and injected into normal guinea pigs, which were then challenged in the skin with the antigen.

B. A group of normal guinea pigs received tritiated thymidine for three days, and then were injected with lymphoid cells from the immune group. These immune cells, in contrast to those of Group A, were not labeled with tritiated thymidine.

Both groups of guinea pigs were challenged by injecting antigen into the skin, and both developed positive delayed sensitivity reactions. (Guinea pigs not inoculated with lymphoid cells or transplanted with lymphoid cells of normal guinea pigs did not develop skin reactions.) The guinea pigs were killed, and their skin lesions were processed for histology and autoradiography. Estimates were made of percentage of labeled cells.

Results:

Group	Donor Cells	Recipient	% of Cells Labeled
A	Labeled	Unlabeled	4%
B	Unlabeled	Labeled	85%

Interpretation: Most of the infiltrating cells are host macrophages derived from a rapidly dividing stem cell pool originating in bone marrow. Though presumably small numbers of specifically immunized T cells are necessary to recognize the antigen in the skin and start the reaction, these are too few in number to be detected. The 4% figure shown above is, in fact, non-specific. The same figure is obtained if labeled immune cells against antigen 1 (as in Group A) are inoculated into a guinea pig immunized to antigen 2, then challenged in the skin with 2.

In summary, most of the infiltrating cells in the cellular immune reactions, be it the granulomas of infectious processes or the diffuse delayed skin reactions, are macrophages derived from bone marrow precursors.

Activated macrophages are phagocytes of very large size containing a large number of lysosomes and having increased phagocytic capacity. The activated macrophages rapidly spread in culture and adhere tenaciously to the culture dish. Table 7.2 compares the properties of macrophages residing in tissues to those activated by cellular immunity reactions. The most important feature of the activated macrophages is their enhanced microbicidal activity. During infection with a facultative intracellular bacteria, these activated macrophages are capable of either inhibiting the growth of, or killing the microorganism, in contrast to the macrophages from non-immunized individuals which do not. The microbicidal activity of activated macrophages has been attributed to the release of oxygen intermediates such as hydrogen peroxide, the hydroxyl radical, and/or superoxide anion. The oxygen-derived products at high local concentration have deleterious effects on various cells or microbes. In some instances, proteases released from the activated macrophages could be playing a cytocidal role. The process of activation requires an interaction of the macrophage with at least two sequential stimuli—first with the T cell lymphokines (see below) followed closely in time by one of a number of "triggering" stimuli such as bacterial products. The requirements for two sequential stimuli may

Table 7.2: Comparison of Resident and Activated Macrophages

	Resident Macrophages	Activated Macrophages
Attachment to surfaces	++	++++
Rate of pinocytosis	++	++++
Number of lysosomes	++	+++
Release of oxygen-derived products	±	+++
Release of neutral proteases	+	+++
Surface Fc receptors	++	+++
Surface Ia antigens	±	++++
Surface 5' nucleotidase	++++	+
Microbicidal and tumoricidal activity	±	++++

Table 7.2. Resident macrophages refers to macrophages that are normally found in tissues. Activated macrophages are macrophages activated by lymphokines secreted by T cells.

be one way to control that the activated macrophages do not cause inflammation except at the site of bacterial infection.

The action of the activated macrophage is non-specific; that is to say, the macrophages will inactivate bacteria or virus regardless of the organism that induced the infection. For example, infection with tubercle bacilli will produce activated macrophages which, when harvested, will have effect on the growth of tubercle bacilli as well as many other bacteria. See the example in Experiment 1, previous section.

Mechanisms of Macrophage Activation. The recruitment and activation of macrophages in cellular immunity reactions appears to take place via soluble mediators produced by the T lymphocytes. Culture fluids of T lymphocytes with antigen contain a number of active molecules termed lymphocyte mediators or lymphokines, that can reproduce aspects of the reaction. Some of these molecules have been partially characterized.

The following are the most important T cell mediators so far identified:

1. MIF: One of the first lymphocyte mediators to be studied is the macrophage inhibitory factor (or MIF) described originally by J. David and B. Bloom. MIF is assayed as follows: a capillary tube containing a suspension of macrophages is placed on a culture dish containing a suitable culture medium. With time, the macrophages come out of the capillary tube and migrate out into the dish. An area of migration of several mm can then be identified. If the medium contains MIF, the macrophages are inhibited in their migration. The extent of inhibition depends on the amounts of MIF. MIF is a molecule that increases the level of intracellular cyclic AMP, resulting in increased polymerization of microtubules and in a cell that migrates poorly. Perhaps the function of MIF is to stop the phagocytes from leaving the sites of cellular immune reactions.

The phenomenon of macrophage inhibition was first studied by taking peritoneal exudate cells from an immune guinea pig (containing T cells and macrophages) and placing them in capillary tubes containing media with the antigens. MIF was elaborated by the T cells and stopped the macrophages from migrating. For example, in the experiment of Figure 7.2, the peritoneal cells from a guinea pig immune to DNP-GPA (dinitrophenylated guinea pig albumin) or DNP-BGG (bovine Ig) were mixed with DNP-GPA, DNP-BGG, or DNP-albumin (DNP-BSA). Note the specificity of the reaction.

MIF has been studied in cultures of mouse, human, and guinea pig T lymphocytes and partially purified. It is a glycoprotein of about 20,000 to 40,000 molecular weight.

MIF can be generated *in vitro* by at least two manipulations: 1) interacting immune T cells with antigen; and 2) interacting T cells with lectins; for example, T cells incubated with PHA or Con A produce the factor. MIF can also be produced by B cells and some tissue culture lines of non-lymphoid cells. Although the B cells produce MIF *in vitro*, *in vivo* the T cells are the main component of the cellular immune reactions. This can be explained by the observation that T cells readily recognize macrophage-associated antigens and are the major component of the recirculating lymphocyte pool.

2. A Macrophage-Activating Molecule: This important molecule has properties very similar to MIF and appears to be identical with it. Macrophages cultured with this mediator become activated and develop microbicidal and tumoricidal properties.

3. A Chemotactic Factor: A chemotactic factor for macrophages different from MIF has also been identified. Perhaps this is the molecule responsible for recruiting phagocytes to sites of cellular immunity.

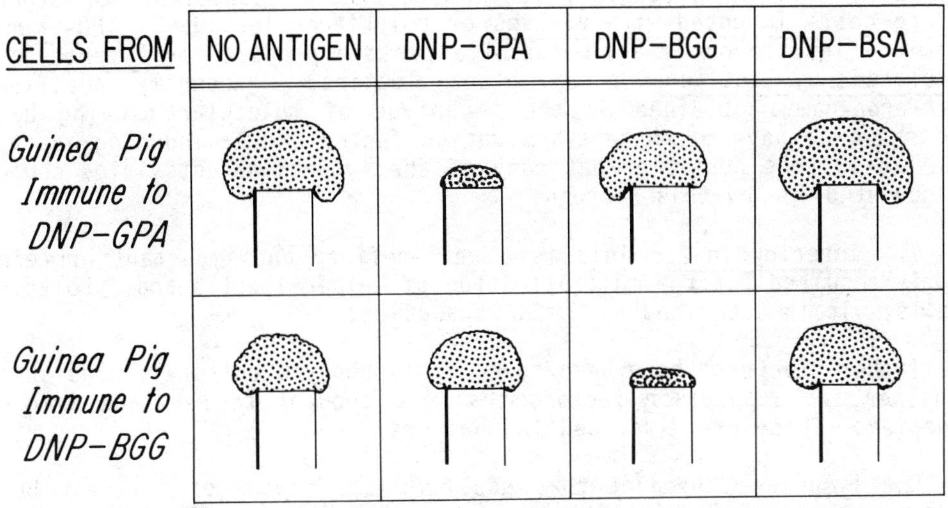

Figure 7.2. Guinea pigs were immunized with DNP-GPA or DNP-BGG. Two weeks later their peritoneal cells were collected. These cells contained about 10% T cells and 90% macrophages. The cells were placed in capillary tubes and placed into culture together with antigen. The immune T that made MIF inhibited the macrophages from "fanning" out into the dish.

---

4. Lymphotoxin: This is a protein that can kill very selected tumor cells in vitro. It is distinct from MIF. Its role in vivo remains unexplained.

5. Ia-Inducing Factor: These are 50,000-dalton proteins that both in vivo and in vitro induce macrophages to express I-region-associated (Ia) antigens (Chapters 5 and 7).

6. Interferon: Interferons are anti-viral proteins originally discovered by Isaacs and Lindemann in 1957. Interferon induces in infected cells the synthesis of an anti-viral protein that interferes with the assembly and multiplication of the virus. Interferons may also activate macrophages in tissue culture for increased cytocidal activity and enhance both in vivo and in vitro the function of natural killer cells (Chapter 11). Thus, interferons not only have an anti-viral effect but may have anti-tumor activity as well. Three classes of interferon have now been identified. IFN-alpha or leukocyte interferon is a protein stable at pH 2 produced by macrophages during their

interaction with particles or lymphocytes. IFN-beta or fibroblast interferon is a pH 2 stable protein produced by fibroblasts or other culture cells infected with viruses or polyribonucleotides. IFN-gamma or immune interferon is a pH 2 labile protein produced by lymphocytes stimulated by antigen or by plant lectins. Recently purified interferon-gamma obtained by the technique of molecular cloning has been shown to have macrophage-activating factor and Ia-inducing activity. It is thus possible that many of the lymphokine activities could be accounted for by this protein.

7. Interleukin-2: This is a well-defined and important protein that is required for the multiplication of helper T cells and cytolytic T cells. It is described in the next section.

(Other "factors" have been found in lymphocyte culture fluids such as helper and suppressor factors that are thought to regulate immune induction. These are discussed in Chapters 5 and 8.)

One lymphocyte product that has been the center of interest but which is still clouded in mystery is transfer factor. Transfer factor was originally described by S. Lawrence and has been studied mainly in humans. It is found in extracts of peripheral blood leukocytes of individuals exhibiting delayed sensitivity to tuberculin. The extract is dialyzed against water; and the active moiety, of small size, is recovered from the dialysate. Inoculation of tuberculin-negative individuals with the active moiety results in the acquisition of tuberculin sensitivity. Transfer factors for other bacterial and fungal products have been described. Transfer factor has not been characterized biochemically, and its mode of action remains unknown. Recent studies indicate that several molecules are found in the preparations of transfer factor, some of which have non-specific enhancing effects. It is possible that a small fragment of antigen may be responsible for some of the results.

Finally, are lymphocyte mediators the molecules responsible for the cellular immune reactions in vivo? The evidence so far obtained strongly suggests that this may be the case. Injection of crude preparations into the skin produces an inflammatory reaction with all the characteristics of a delayed hypersensitivity reaction. Further evidence in favor of a role of the lymphocyte mediators in vivo comes from analysis of serum, lymph, or tissue secretions of animals undergoing immunization. In limited experiments, MIF activity has been found in serum of mice infected with tubercle bacilli or in the efferent lymph from lymph nodes following antigen injection. These latter experiments were carried out in sheep where the lymphatics are large enough to cannulate. Extracts of skin of guinea pigs with a delayed reaction contain macrophages chemotactic factor.

PATHOLOGY OF CELLULAR IMMUNITY REACTIONS: CONTACT SENSITIVITY

Cellular immune reactions are essential for immunity against certain microorganisms. It is also thought that resistance to some tumors may involve a similar mechanism (Chapter 11). There are several instances in which cellular immunity may cause injury to the individual. For example, in rare autoimmune reactions, T lymphocytes react to self components and produce an inflammatory reaction identical to the delayed reaction (Chapter 13).

The most frequent examples of delayed reactions involving a host component are those of "contact sensitivity". Various chemicals have the property of binding to host proteins and forming antigenic compounds that are particularly effective in stimulating T lymphocytes. Many cases of eczema and dermatitis in man are delayed sensitivity reactions to chemicals that interact with skin proteins. Many of the "sensitizers" are represented by simple chemicals, metal ions, or lipid compounds to which the individual is exposed by skin contact. One example is contact with the poison ivy plant. This plant contains a catechol that binds to the skin proteins, forming a neoantigen which can induce a strong delayed sensitivity reaction. Many other examples of skin sensitizers have been reported: chrome, nickel, and beryllium ions form insoluble complexes with skin proteins and can immunize, a problem that is frequently observed in industrial workers handling these compounds. Also included as sensitizers are some hair dyes. A common characteristic of skin sensitizers is their small size, which allows them to diffuse into the epidermis, and their capacity to bind to proteins.

The specificity of contact sensitivity can be studied in experimental animals. The best studied model is the guinea pig immunized by skin painting with picryl chloride. Picryl chloride is trinitrochlorobenzene, which conjugates covalently to a number of skin proteins, forming trinitrophenylated-autologous protein conjugates. A guinea pig is exposed to this compound by "painting" the skin, becomes "sensitized", and is subsequently tested by intradermal injections with various foreign proteins conjugated to TNP. The immune, sensitized, guinea pig will react weakly or not at all to injection with TNP bound to conventional proteins but strongly if rechallenged with picryl chloride painted on the skin. Hence, in this situation, the T cell is mainly recognizing the complex of TNP with the autologous proteins rather than the chemical (i.e., the TNP) by itself. As expected, contact specificity can be transferred from an immune to a normal individual by T cells. Interestingly, the first transfer of a cellular immunity reaction by lymphoid cells was that of contact sensitivity to chemicals, a classical experiment done by K. Landsteiner and M. Chase using the guinea pig.

Contact sensitivity is best produced by the introduction of the chemical by way of the skin. There the chemical is eventually taken up by the Langerhans cells of the epidermis (Chapter 5). These cells then migrate into the dermis, enter the lymphatics, and end up in the deep cortex of the lymph nodes where they then present the antigen to the T lymphocyte. Introducing the chemical in areas of skin devoid of Langerhans cells does not result in sensitization and, moreover, can produce specific immunological tolerance. (This can be done in the mouse either by applying the chemical to the skin of the tail, which is naturally poor in Langerhans cells, or by deleting Langerhans cells by local ultraviolet irradiation.) To note is that one of the earliest examples of tolerance was the introduction of picryl chloride into the animal orally or intravenously (Sulzberger-Chase phenomenon). Guinea pigs fed or injected with picryl chloride were no longer able to develop contact sensitivity upon exposure to the chemical applied to the skin. Presumably, the exposure to the antigen in the absence of a presenting accessory cell produced a specific state of unresponsiveness due to suppressor T cells (Chapter 9).

CELLULAR IMMUNITY TO VIRUSES: THE CYTOLYTIC T LYMPHOCYTE (CTL)

Viral infections activate both B and T lymphocytes, resulting in the production of anti-viral antibodies and reactions of cellular immunity. As expected, no single cell type is responsible for the elimination of the virus—B cells are involved by producing antibodies, macrophages by presenting viral antigen and also by becoming activated, T helper cells by secreting lymphokines that regulate CTL and macrophages, and CTL by killing virally infected host cells. The relative importance of antibodies or T cells depends, in part, upon the biology of the particular virus and the stage of the infection. At an early stage, the antibodies are able to neutralize viruses in the blood and in extracellular fluids. The actual elimination of the infection from the host's cells depends mainly on the CTL. The CTL are generated within four to nine days after viral infection, decreasing in activity by fourteen days. They then maintain a state of immunological memory and readily become re-activated upon a new infection. The CTL act in two possible ways, first by binding to virally infected host cells and killing them, therefore, stopping the production and spread of new viral particles; second, by secreting lymphokines and, in particular, gamma-interferon following their interaction with the virally infected cell. The lymphokines stimulate the production of activated macrophages, while the gamma-interferon induces a state of anti-viral activity in the cells of the host. Recent studies using completely purified clones of CTL to influenza virus have shown their capacity to limit this infection *in vivo* in the mouse.

Let us consider the major characteristics of the CTL: their assay, the mechanism of killing, their generation, and their interactions with antigens and the Class I polypeptides of the MHC. CTL are generated in vivo, particularly in viral infections, during tumor growth, and during allograft rejection. CTL can also be generated against small reactive chemicals that bind to surface proteins of antigen-presenting cells.

The CTL Assay. CTL activity is measured in culture by exposing a target cell suspension, labeled with chromium-51, to the immune lymphocyte population at an appropriate ratio; this ratio varies from one to one-hundred lymphocytes per target cell, depending upon the activity of the immune cells. The cell mixture is gently centrifuged and the cells allowed to interact in the bottom of a test tube in culture medium for a period of four to twenty-four hours. When the assay is terminated, the cells are centrifuged, and the radioactive chromium released in the supernatant is measured and compared with the radioactive chromium released in the absence of immune lymphocytes (spontaneous release). A typical CTL assay is shown in Figure 7.3.

Mechanism of CTL-Mediated Lysis: The first stage in the interaction is the contact between the CTL and the target cells, the recognition by the CTL receptor of the antigen, and the establishment of a strong adhesion between the two cells. Adhesion formation takes place within a few minutes, at 37 degrees C, in the presence of Mg ions. It is blocked by most drugs which inhibit cytolysis, including cytochalasin B, inhibitors of ATP production, and local anesthetics. Research in progress has identified three surface structures of the CTL involved in the first state of adhesion. This has been examined by the finding that some selected monoclonal antibodies can inhibit the binding of CTL to target cells. One major key protein is the receptor for antigen itself to which antibodies have now been produced (Chapter 5). The other two surface structures represent molecules that are, either close to the receptor, or, most likely, involved in promoting the adhesion to the target and thus a stable cell interaction. One of them is the murine Ly2 antigen (Chapter 5), a protein made of subunits of 30,000 and 35,000 daltons. (Although the Ly2 polypeptide may contribute to the adhesion, it is not a necessary molecule: a limited number of CTL have the Ly1+Ly2$^-$ phenotype.) The second polypeptide, termed Lymphocyte Functional Antigen-1, is made up of two chains, 95,000 and 180,000 daltons. This protein is found on the membranes of most lymphocytes.

The second step following adhesion formation has been termed the "lethal hit". During this stage, the CTL imparts an irreversible lesion to the target cell. The lethal hit requires about ten minutes, is the most temperature-sensitive stage (being inhibited tenfold at room temperature, relative to 37 degrees C), and requires calcium ions (unlike adhesion), but not protein synthesis. No drugs have been shown to inhibit the lethal hit directly. This lethal hit state is detected by detaching the CTL from the target. This detachment does not prevent

T LYMPHOCYTE-MEDIATED LYSIS

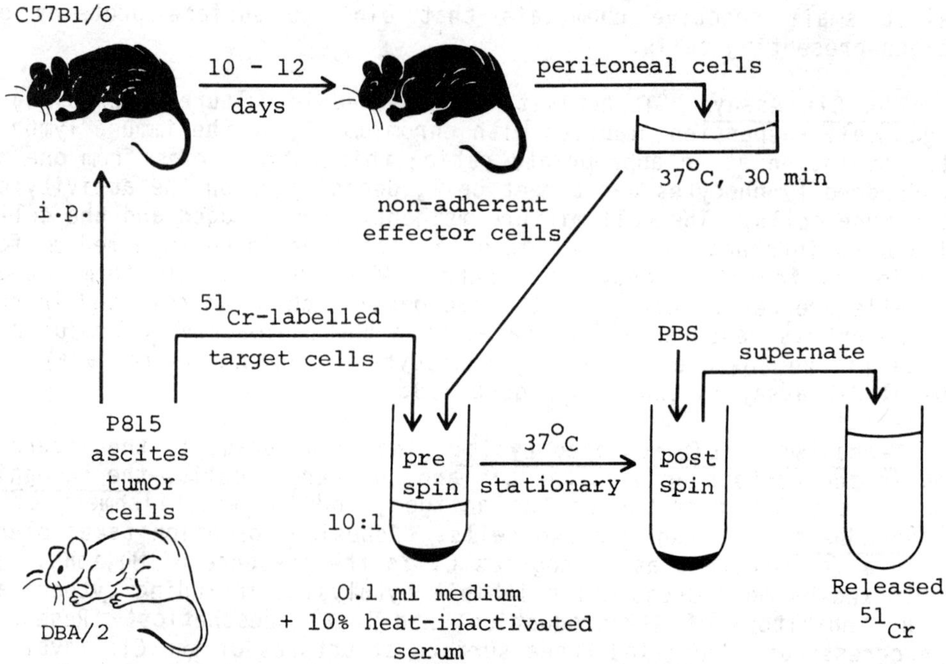

Figure 7.3. The graph shows the method for assaying CTL against an allogeneic tumor. An allogeneic cell is injected into mice, and the peritoneal cells are collected ten to twelve days later. The cytolytic T cells are found among the cells that do not adhere to the dishes. These are mixed with the allogeneic tumor radiolabeled with chromium. The release of chromium is taken as an index of cell death.

---

the subsequent lysis of the target cell. CTL may be detached by the calcium ion chelator EDTA.

The third and last stage of CTL-mediated lysis is "killer cell-independent lysis". This usually requires an hour or more, is weakly temperature dependent (inhibited tenfold at 0 degrees C relative to 37 degrees C), and is not inhibited by any drugs. Lysis is believed to be passive, possibly due to colloid osmotic swelling (water influx) resulting from membrane lesions produced by the lethal hit. Loss of electrolytes and some small metabolites occurs prior to loss of radiochromium, which is taken as the endpoint of lysis.

While the pharmacology of the CTL-mediated lysis suggests a secretory event, no direct support for this process has come forth. The selectivity of CTL-mediated killing speaks against a mechanism involving release of a non-specific toxin, nor have any toxins (specific or non-specific) been detected in supernatants or extracts from CTL. The primary site of attack is the target cell membrane. Evidence consistent with this mechanism is the finding that the electrolyte permeability of the target cell membrane increases during the lethal hit. The target cell probably plays a passive role, since glutaraldehyde-poisoned target cells can be lysed. However, the precise mechanism of the lethal hit remains obscure.

Generation of CTL. CTL are generated from precursor lymphocytes that are in an inactive state. Upon introduction of the virus, the first step in the process is the growth of the precursors and their differentiation into actively lytic cells. A number of cellular interactions are required for these events to take place. The two major interactions involve: 1) the helper T cells with Ia-bearing macrophages and 2) the CTL with the target cells bearing the viral antigen. The interaction between the helper T cells with the macrophage follows the same principles that we outlined for infections with intracellular pathogens, the details of which, with respect to MHC restrictions, are explained in Chapter 8. In brief, the helper T cells will recognize the antigen in the context of Class II polypeptides of the MHC. (Whether virally infected macrophages are as powerful as macrophages that have taken up proteins or bacteria is an issue that is not yet settled.) From this interaction, the helper T cells release a number of mediators, one of which is crucial for the CTL to proliferate. This lymphokine has been termed interleukin-2 (IL-2) or T cell growth factor.

IL-2 is a protein of 15,000 to 30,000 daltons, depending on the species. It will bind to specific receptors on the CTL (and also on helper T cells) and promote its growth. For the helper T cell to secrete IL-2, it needs the interaction with IL-1 secreted by macrophages. IL-2, once secreted, will not act on the CTL precursor because the precursor lacks a membrane receptor. These IL-2 receptors develop upon the interaction of the CTL precursor with the target cell. Once the CTL acquires the receptor and binds to IL-2, it changes from an inactive cell to a cell engaged in DNA synthesis. The final differentiation of the CTL to become a killer may involve a second lymphokine which has not yet been characterized. Figure 7.4 summarizes the interaction which necessitates two lymphocytes, each reacting with antigen in the context of Class I or Class II polypeptides of the MHC.

IL-2 has been used now to propagate CTL in culture. A single clone of CTL can be actually grown and maintained for long periods of time. The CTL clones are proving invaluable to study their biological role.

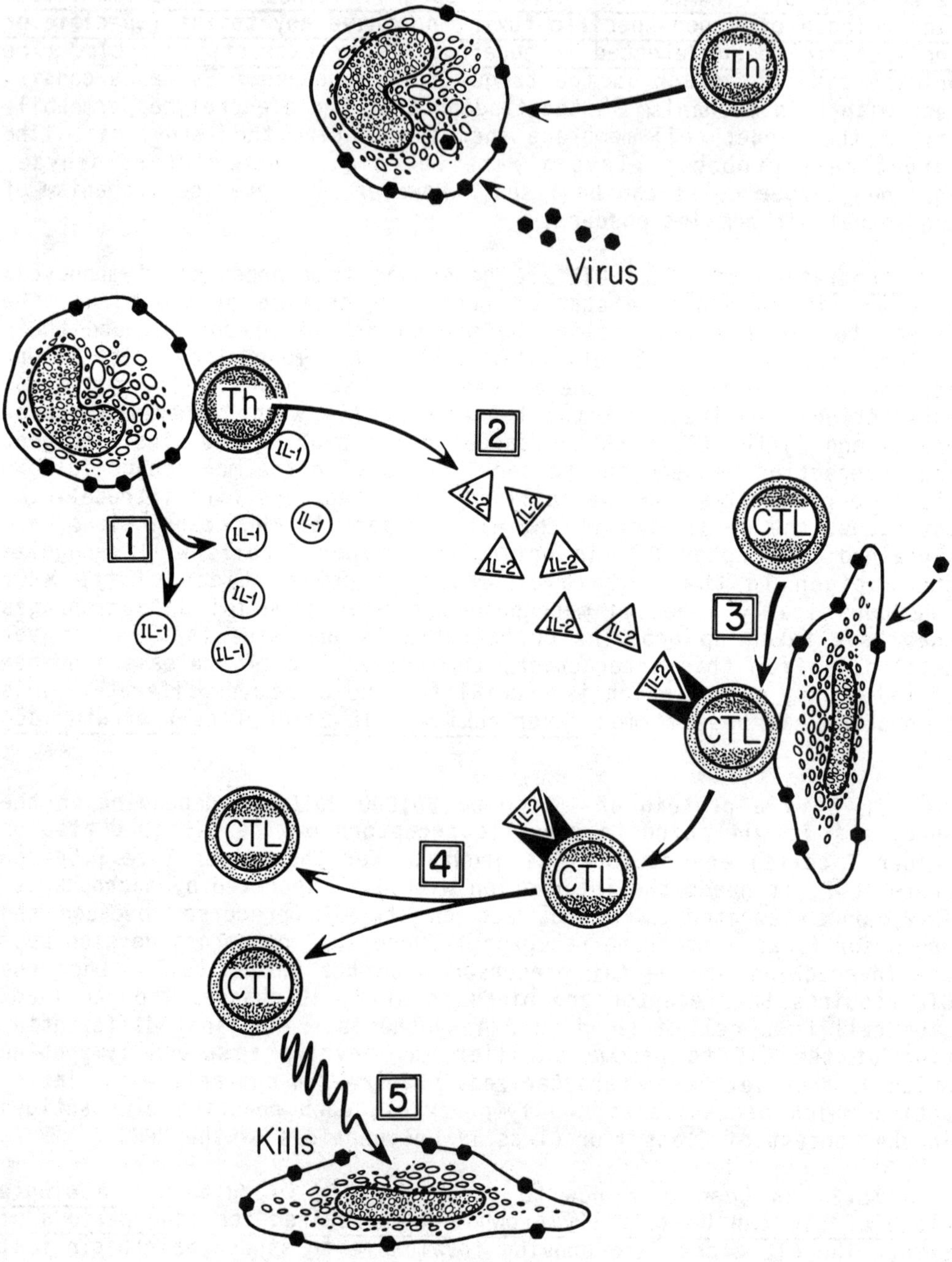

Figure 7.4. The explanation of this figure is on the following page.

Figure 7.4. The graph depicts some of the events leading to the generation and activation of cytolytic T cells (CTL). 1 = A T helper cell recognizes viral antigens in a macrophage; the macrophage releases IL-1. 2 = The activated T cell then releases IL-2. 3 = A CTL establishes contact with viral antigens displayed on a fibroblast and acquires receptors for IL-2. 4 = After binding to IL-2, the CTL proliferates. 5 = The expanded clone of CTL establishes contact with the virally infected fibroblast and kills them.

Recognition of Viral Antigen by CTL. CTL recognize foreign antigens (i.e., viral antigens) always on syngeneic target cells. The recognition is restricted by the Class I polypeptides of the MHC. The only apparent exception are the CTL directed to foreign alloantigens (Chapter 6) in which the CTL recognizes allogeneic Class I molecules directly. To show the MHC restriction, we will describe the specificities of CTL generated in the course of infection with a non-cytopathic RNA virus, the lymphocytic choriomeningitis virus (LCM), in the mouse. LCM produces a slow, persistent infection in mice.

Mice of different H-2 haplotypes are infected with the LCM virus. Several days later the mice are killed, and the lymphoid organs are harvested. The T cells of these LCM-immune mice in tissue culture will kill fibroblasts or macrophages freshly infected with LCM virus. Target cells not infected or infected with an unrelated virus will not be killed by the LCM-immune CTL. (The assay for estimating killing, as described before, uses radioactive Cr to label proteins in the "target" cell.) The striking observation is that T cells from a given strain will kill only LCM-infected target cells of the same strain and not of an allogeneic strain and vice versa (Table 7.3). Thus, CTL of the k haplotype will kill only fibroblasts of k infected with LCM and not fibroblasts from d.

Table 7.4 shows an analysis of this phenomenon generating CTL T cells in vitro. First, virally infected fibroblasts are incubated with T cells for a few days. This incubation generates CTL against LCM virus which are then assayed on fresh fibroblasts infected with LCM. The fibroblasts are of the same or from a different strain. The first four groups in Table 7.4 are self-explantory and show MHC restriction of cytolysis. Groups 6 and 8 show that the requirement is not for sharing the same MHC products of the CTL and the target cell. Rather, the requirement is that the target cell share MHC antigens with virus-bearing cells that originally stimulated the immune response which produced the CTL, i.e., Groups 5 and 7. Thus, while the killing is strictly dependent upon the virus antigenic specificities, these alone are not sufficient for CTL recognition. The virus specificities must reside on a cell membrane bearing the appropriate MHC specificities.

Table 7.3

Cytolytic T Cells		$H\text{-}2^k$ Targets		$H\text{-}2^d$ Targets	
H-2 Strain	LCM	LCM	No LCM	LCM	No LCM
k	-	0	0	0	0
k	+	30%	0	0	0
d	-	0	0	0	0
d	+	0	0	35%	0
k x d	-	0	0	0	0
k x d	+	25%	0	30%	0

Table 7.3. This table summarizes an experiment by R. Zinkernagel and P. Doherty (J. Exp. Med., 141:1427, 1975), who discovered the MHC restrictions in the CTL response. The "background" release of ^{51}Cr from targets, i.e., the release in the absence of CTL, has been subtracted from each point. The explanation of the experiment is in the text.

In the natural situation of an immune response to a virus infection or neoplasm, the target cell is a "self" cell bearing foreign antigens and, hence, is syngeneic to the CTL. Thus, the syngeneic MHC products serve as a component of the specificity recognized by the CTL. Unlike CTL, antibodies reacting with the foreign antigen recognize it as a separate entity independent from MHC products.

The CTL receptors for antigen appear to recognize a combined specificity of a foreign antigen (the virus in our examples) and the Class I polypeptides of the MHC. How both antigen and the Class I are associated is not clear at present. Regardless of this point, one issue that has become apparent is that MHC products serve as recognition structures for antigen in order for them to be identified as foreign by the T cells. Since all cells express Class I polypeptides, viral infections (or neoplasia) that occur in any tissue can be subjected to attack by the CTL.

Table 7.4

MHC Restriction of Virus-Specific Cytolysis

Group	Haplotype of CTL	Sensitizing Virus-Infected Cells	Virus-Infected Target Cells	Cytolysis
1	a	a	a	+
2	a	a	b	—
3	b	b	b	+
4	b	b	a	—
5	$(a \times b)F_1$	a	a	+
6	$(a \times b)F_1$	a	b	—
7	$(a \times b)F_1$	b	b	+
8	$(a \times b)F_1$	b	a	—

Table 7.4. The sensitizing virus-infected cells (Column 2) are used to elicit a primary CTL immune response. When sensitizing cells are not virus infected, no CTL are produced, since sensitizing cells are syngeneic to responder cells. The sensitized cells are then tested on target cells, also virally infected, of different haplotypes. When target cells are not virus infected, no cytolysis occurs.

Recent studies have indicated that the maturation of the early thymocyte may influence the pattern of MHC restriction. This has been done by producing "radiation chimeras": an inbred mouse with a given MHC haplotype is lethally irradiated and then transplanted with stem cells (from bone marrow). Some of the stem cells migrate to the thymus and there mature into T cells. Let A and B be two different MHC haplotypes. Stem cells of mice of haplotype (A x B), an F1 of two inbred strains A and B, are injected into an irradiated A. The CTL cells that eventually develop upon viral infection will be restricted primarily by A. In contrast, if stem cells from parent A are transplanted into the irradiated (A x B)F1, the CTL that develop are restricted by either the B or A haplotypes. Thus, during its development, the CTL precursors are generated that recognize as self those MHC antigens expressed on the cells of the host. Presumably, this learning experience is first obtained in contact with the stromal cells of the thymus.

REFERENCES

Bloom, B. R. In vitro approaches to the mechanism of cell-mediated immune reactions. Adv. Immunol., 13:205, 1971.

David, J. R., and David, R. R. Cellular hypersensitivity and immunity. Prog. Allergy, 16:300, 1972.

Gell, P. G. H., and Benacerraf, B. Delayed hypersensitivity to simple protein antigens. Adv. Immunol., 1:319, 1961.

MacKaness, G. B. The immunologic basis of acquired cellular resistance. J. Exp. Med., 120:105, 1964.

Moller, G. (ed.). MHC restriction of anti-viral immunity. Immunol. Rev., 58 (includes seven papers by the most active workers in the field), 1981.

Nabholz, M., and Macdonal, H. R. Cytolytic T lymphocytes. Ann. Rev. Immunol., 1:273, 1983.

Pick, E. (ed). Lymphokines, Volume 3 (an issue dedicated to an analysis of macrophage activation), Academic Press, New York, 1981.

Smith, K. A., and Ruscetti, F. W. T cell growth factor and the culture of cloned functional T cells. Adv. Immunol., 31:137, 1981.

CHAPTER 8

Regulation of Immune Responses by T Lymphocytes

Previous chapters considered the basic properties of lymphocytes and macrophages, the physiological changes taking place in lymphatic tissue after the entrance of antigen, the trapping of antigen by macrophages, and some of the cellular interactions taking place during the immune response. We have discussed that B cells include a wide diversity of antigen-specific clones. Antigen selects those clones with high binding affinity, after which the B cell clones expand in number. Upon interaction with T cells, B cells undergo differentiation to plasma cells, the terminal antibody-secreting cells. We have also mentioned that the helper T cells are essential regulatory cells with the basic property of interacting with antigen bound to an antigen-presenting cell, while, at the same time, recognizing a self-protein, the Class II glycoproteins of the MHC. The cytolytic T cell recognizes antigen also in a presenting cell, but in their case, the interaction is usually restricted by Class I molecules. The general properties of the Class I and Class II molecules were outlined in Chapter 6. T helper cells secrete lymphokines that activate macrophages; T cytolytic cells can kill cells bearing antigen; both cells are essential components in resistance to a wide range of infectious agents. The present chapter describes, in depth, three essential regulatory interactions taking place among macrophages, T helper, and T suppressor cells: 1) the activation of T helper cells by antigen presented by phagocytes; 2) the differentiation of B cells to produce antibodies; and 3) the activation of suppresor mechanisms, many of which center around the generation of suppressor T cells.

MACROPHAGE-LYMPHOCYTE INTERACTIONS

Chapter 5 introduced the concept of macrophages as antigen-presenting cells. An essential step in the initiation of immunity to all polypeptide antigen is the activation of T helper cells, a process requiring the interaction of the helper T cells with the phagocytes. Our understanding of this interaction derives mostly from experiments using cell culture techniques in which the component cells of this response have been isolated and then recombined under defined conditions. The next series of experiments explain the basic interactions.

Experiment I: The recognition of antigen by the helper T cells requires macrophages and is restricted by the Class II polypeptides of the MHC. (The following protocol is taken from experiments by A. S. Rosenthal and E. M. Shevach, who discovered this important phenomenon.) (Figure 8.1)

Guinea pigs from two inbred lines, strain 2 and 13, and their F1 offsprings ([2 x 13]F1), are immunized with the protein ovalbumin (OVA). A few days later the animals are sacrificed, their lymphocytes are harvested, and the T cells are isolated free from any contamination with accessory cells. The T cells are placed in culture; to some cultures are added OVA, alone, or with macrophages of either strain 2 or from strain 13. It is important to note that strains 2 and 13 differ only at the I region of the MHC. After three to four days,

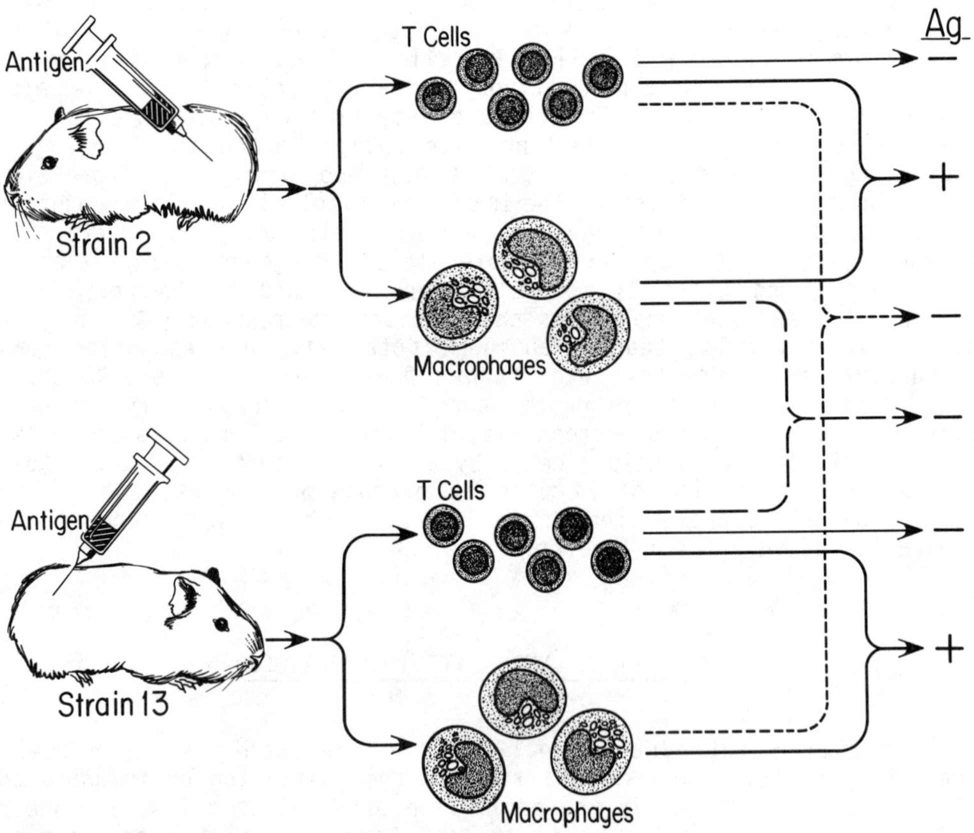

Figure 8.1. The explanation is in the text.

radiolabeled thymidine is added to the culture; and after several hours, the amount of label incorporated in the DNA of the lymphocytes is measured. (Normally, lymphocyes are in a resting state; but upon productive interaction with antigen, they will synthesize DNA and divide.) The following results are obtained:

Group	OVA-Primed T Cells (Strain)	Macrophages (Strain)	OVA	Proliferation
1	2	—	—	—
2	2	—	+	—
3	2	2	—	—
4	2	2	+	++++
5	2	13	—	+
6	2	13	+	+
7	13	—	—	—
8	13	—	+	—
9	13	13	—	—
10	13	13	+	++++
11	13	2	—	+
12	13	2	+	+
13	(2 x 13)	2	—	—
14	(2 x 13)	13	—	—
15	(2 x 13)	2	+	++++
16	(2 x 13)	13	+	++++

(— = no proliferation; + = proliferation)

The main findings, summarized in Figure 8.1, are that: 1) the T lymphocytes will not proliferate to antigen in the absence of macrophages (Groups 2 and 8); 2) the presence of macrophages is not sufficient; there has to be a match between the T cell and strain from which the macrophages are obtained (4 versus 6; 10 versus 12). You should note two other results, that T cells from the F1 responded to antigen on macrophages from either strain (15 and 16), and that an allogeneic interaction is taking place between the helper T cell and the macrophage from the opposite strain in the absence of antigen (5 and 11).

The basic results apply to all species and to all proteins, including natural proteins, synthetic polypeptides, and proteins of microorganisms.

Experiment II: The Class II polypeptides are the key modulatory molecules restricting the interactions between T helper cells and macrophages. The results of Experiment 1 using two strain combinations differing at the I region clearly indicate that this genetic segment is involved in the interaction between T cells and macrophages. A direct role for the I region products, the Class II molecules, can be demonstrated in the following experiment where two manipulations are done: 1) macrophages that bear Class II molecules are compared to those not bearing them; and 2) antibodies to Class II molecules are used to attempt to block the interaction.

The first manipulation consists of eliminating Ia-bearing macrophages by treatment with anti-Ia antibodies (a mixture of antibodies to all Class II polypeptides) and fresh serum as a complement source. Killing Ia-positive macrophages leaves Ia-negative macrophages which constitute approximately one-half the number of macrophages in the preparation. In the second manipulation, the anti-Ia antibodies are added in order to bind to the Ia on the macrophages and induce their internalization in vesicles, leaving the Ia-positive macrophages free of Ia on their membrane.

The OVA-specific T cells are placed in culture, plus OVA, and the following:

1. No macrophages = no proliferation

2. Mixture of Ia-positive and Ia-negative macrophages = proliferation

3. Ia-negative macrophages (treatment with anti-Ia plus complemement) = no proliferation

4. Mixtures of Ia-positive and Ia-negative macrophages together with anti-Ia antibodies = no proliferation

5. Ia-negative macrophages plus lymphokine = proliferation

The elimination of Ia-positive macrophages (Group 3) or capping off Ia from the membrane (Group 4) abrogates antigen presentation. In Group 5, the macrophages from Group 3 (i.e., containing only Ia-negative because of the treatment) were cultured with a preparation of T cell lymphokines that stimulate Ia biosynthesis. Antigen presentation is now reconstituted.

Experiment III. Antigen presentation requires physical contact between T lymphocytes and macrophages. A macrophage-secreted growth factor, interleukin 1, then promotes T cell growth. The role of phagocytes could be to actually present the antigen (plus Class II molecules), to secrete a growth-promoting molecule, or both. These possibilities are tested in the following experiments where two protocols are used—one involving the response of immune T cells to antigen; the second involving the response to the plant lectin Con A (Chapter 5) which stimulates growth of most T helper cells. The response to Con A requires accessory cells. A conditioned medium from macrophages, a medium from a forty-eight-hour culture of macrophages, is used to substitute for macrophages (macrophage supernatant, below).

OVA-primed T cells are cultured with the following additions:

	Stimulus	Macrophages	Macrophage Supernatant	Proliferation
1.	—	—	—	—
2.	—	+	—	—
3.	—	—	+	—
4.	OVA	—	—	—
5.	OVA	+	—	++++
6.	OVA	—	+	—
7.	Con A	—	—	—
8.	Con A	+	—	++++
9.	Con A	—	+	++

Figure 8.2 summarizes the results of this experiment. The response to OVA, which is restricted by the I region gene products, requires the physical presence of macrophages (compare No. 5 to No. 6). The response to Con A is macrophage dependent (No. 7 versus No. 8), but the physical presence of the macrophage is not required since a macrophage-conditioned supernatant partially replaces them (group No. 9). The growth factor acts only on Con A-stimulated cells (note Nos. 3 and 9). The growth factor is interleukin-1 (IL-1) described in Chapter 5.

Recent experiments suggest the following events: the T cell recognizes antigen and Class II molecules on the macrophage surface. Firm contact is established between the two cells. This produces two changes: 1) the macrophage increases its rate of secretion of IL-1, and 2) the T cell expresses receptors on its surfaces for the growth factor interleukin-2 (IL-2). IL-1 stimulates the release of IL-2 by the activated T cell; this IL-2 will now bind to the T cells having IL-2

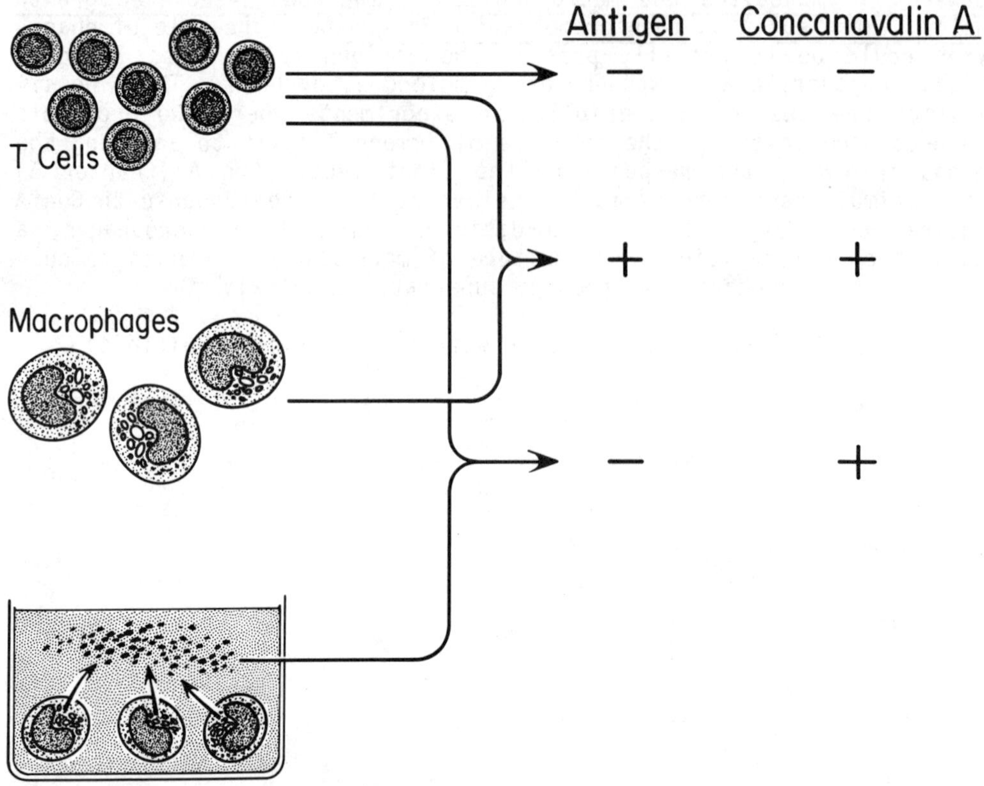

Figure 8.2 The explanation is in the text.

receptors and promote their growth. The growth of the T cells requires the continuous presence of IL-2.

In the case of the Con A response, the lectin promotes the development of the IL-2 receptor, while the IL-1 in the macrophage supernatant stimulates the secretion of IL-2 by the T cells.

What is happening to the antigen bound to the macrophage? The antigen molecules are bound to the macrophages and then internalized in vesicles where they go through processing stages involving partial catabolism. Antigen fragments are then transported to the membrane where they may contact the Class II polypeptides. Inhibition of the intracellular processing, inhibits the presentation. Biochemical studies trying to determine whether antigen complexes to Ia molecules are now being evaluated.

Experiment IV. Clonal response of T cells: T cells, like B cells, are also clonally restricted. In the case of T cells, the restriction applies not only to the recognition of antigen but also to the recognition of the combination of antigen and the Class II molecules. This important issue can be examined by testing the specificity of clones of antigen-reactive T cells. For example, T cells are harvested from F1 crosses of two inbred mouse strains, H-2b and H-2k, and placed in culture with macrophages of either strain plus antigen. The antigen-reactive T cells will proliferate, while the remaining cells not reacting with antigen will die within a few days. After a week, the helper T cells are obtained and restimulated on fresh macrophages and antigen; this cycle is repeated for one to two months. After these responses, clones of T cells are obtained, each clone derived from a single antigen-reactive lymphocyte. Each clone is now tested on the macrophages from either strain. Thus, a clone derived from (H-2b x H-2k)F1 strain of mice selected on H-2k responds to antigen presented on H-2k macrophages but not H-2b macrophages or vice versa. Clearly, the F1-immunized mice contains two sets of T cells: each set is reactive with the antigen plus one of the allelic form of the Class II molecules.

A point of crucial importance is whether there are clones of T cells that react with antigen in the context of an allogeneic Class II molecule. Clearly, these clones, if present, are not found after conventional immunization (Experiment 1), although T cells reactive with allogeneic Class II (without antigen) are easily detected. Clones of T cells reactive with antigen, in the context of allogeneic Class II molecules nevertheless can be found, but one must use several methods to select for them; the allogeneic T cells (those that proliferate upon recognition of foreign Ia and give rise to the mixed lymphocyte reaction) have to be eliminated first from the culture; the remaining cells are then cultured on a long-term basis, as in Experiment 4, with allogeneic macrophages and antigen. Eventually, clones of T cells will be selected out, reacting with antigen, presented only by macrophages bearing specific allogeneic Ia antigens.

The conclusion is that the thymus generates antigen-reactive clones that have specificity to many allelic forms of Class II molecules; however, the clones that are favored to expand in number are those that react with syngeneic Class II, because these are the molecules normally found in the antigen-presenting cells of the individual. Clones strongly reactive with self Ia alone are probably eliminated in the thymus, while, in contrast, those strongly reactive with allogeneic Ia (and responsible for the MLC) are maintained, leave the thymus, and will be responsible for the reactions of transplantation immunity.

At this point, two issues concerning T cell reactivity with antigens need to be addressed. First, the haplotype of a Class II molecule determines whether presentation of an antigenic determinant will take place. Thus, an important point to bear in mind is that not all antigenic determinants can be presented in the context of a given MHC Class

II haplotype. For each haplotype there are some antigenic determinants that will be presented, and others that will not. This determines, therefore, whether proteins will be immunogenic in a given individual. In fact, proteins with a restricted number of antigenic determinants may not evoke any response in individuals of selected haplotypes. We will consider this phenomenon in Chapter 10 when we discuss immunogenetics. In fact, the function of the Class II molecules was discovered following the observation that some strains of inbred animals responded to synthetic polypeptide antigens, while others did not. It was after these discoveries that the cellular interactions described in this chapter were studied.

The second issue concerns the strong reactivity of T lymphocytes for allogeneic MHC antigens. This issue has presented immunologists with a considerable puzzle, magnified by the finding that a relatively large fraction of all T lymphoyctes are specific for MHC alloantigens. Are there enough T cells to recognize foreign antigens and alloantigens or, alternatively, can the same T cell clones be capable of reacting to MHC alloantigens and foreign antigens plus self-MHC molecules? Recent studies with cloned T cell lines selected for their specificity for foreign antigens in the context of self-MHC molecules revealed that a small fraction of these clones show concomitant reactivity for MHC alloantigens, in the absence of the foreign antigens which induced their selection. Therefore, some of the same T cell clones can be specific for both antigen plus self-MHC and allo-MHC molecules.

B-T CELL COLLABORATION

The helper T cells can interact with B cells and promote their growth and differentiation. We will first describe the two basic systems in which B-T cell collaborations were discovered: the response to foreign red cells and to hapten-carrier conjugates.

Experiments Studying the Anti-Red Cell Response. The first studies on T and B cell interactions in immune responses were carried out in 1966 by Henry Claman and coworkers investigating the humoral response of mice to sheep red blood cells (SRBC). Lethally irradiated mice (650 to 750 R) were injected intravenously with varying numbers of either spleen, thymus, or bone marrow cells or with a mixture of thymus and bone marrow cells from normal or immune syngeneic donors. The cell transfer was followed by a challenge with SRBC. The spleens of the recipient were assayed for anti-SRBC antibody-forming cells at various times thereafter with the following results:

Group	Source of Cells	Anti-SRBC Response
I	Normal marrow	±
II	Normal or immune thymus	—
III	Thymus and marrow	3+ (synergy)
IV	Normal spleen	3+
V	Immune spleen	4+

The results showed synergy between thymus and bone marrow cells for antibody responses to SRBC. Neither the transplant of normal marrow nor of normal or SRBC-immune thymus cells permitted a hemolysin response (Groups I and II). However, a marked response was observed when thymus and marrow cells were transferred together in the same recipient (Group III). The bone marrow contained the antibody-producing cells which could function only in the presence of helper cells present in the thymus inoculum.

This interpretation was proven to be correct by subsequent experiments. A. J. S. Davies and associates immunized chimeric mice, which had bone marrow and thymus cells bearing distinct minor cell surface antigens. (Chimeric mice contain two different populations of cells varying at the major and/or minor transplantation loci; see Chapter 6). Following immunization, they separated the two cell types and determined that the bone marrow-derived cells were the source of the antibody-producing cells, whereas the thymus cells did not produce antibody but markedly increased the antibody production of the bone marrow-derived cells.

Particularly noteworthy were the experiments of J. F. A. P. Miller and associates. They analyzed the capacity of various lymphoid cell types to restore the IgM-anti-SRBC antibody response of irradiated mice. Lethally irradiated mice were injected with bone marrow (now known to be the source of B cells), thoracic duct cells (consisting of a majority of T cells), or both; and the number of antibody-forming cells was determined a week later by a plaque assay (PFC) (described in Chapter 4).

Donor Cells	Anti-SRBC PFC Response
Syngeneic bone marrow (BM)	73
Syngeneic thoracic duct lymphocytes (TDL)	97
Syngeneic BM plus TDL	877

Whereas transfer or either syngeneic bone marrow cells or thoracic duct lymphocytes alone failed to reconstitute immunocompetence, the anti-SRBC response was restored by concomitant transfer of the two donor cell types to the same recipient.

The origin of the antibody-producing cells was then determined. Adult thymectomized lethally irradiated CBA mice were injected with syngeneic CBA bone marrow and with thoracic duct lymphocytes (TDL) from (CBA x C57BL)F1 mice. The mice were then immunized with SRBC. The presence of distinct H-2 antigens on the bone marrow and TDL cells permitted Miller and associates to ask whether the antibody-secreting cells were derived from the bone marrow of the thymus, using specific alloantisera against the H-2 antigens of the CBA or C57BL strains. At the peak of the primary response, the spleen cells were removed and assayed for anti-SRBC antibody-producing cells by the Jerne plaque-forming assay before and after treatment with the alloantisera and complement. Under these experimental conditions, a cell which has been lysed by anti-H-2 antibody and complement cannot synthesize and release antibody to form a red cell plaque. The anti-CBA antiserum decreased the number of anti-SRBC-producing cells by 95%, whereas the anti-C57BL antiserum, specific for antigens expresssed only on the TDL cells, had no effect. This experiment established that the precursors of antibody-producing cells, now identified as the B cells, are derived from the bone marrow and not from the thymus, although B and T cells are required to interact specifically with antigen for the response to develop.

Since the initial studies demonstrating the requirement for cell interactions in the sheep erythrocyte system, analogous interactions have been demonstrated in the *in vivo* humoral response to all protein antigens and to hapten-carrier conjugates. The latter class of antigens has been the most effective tool to analyze the respective roles of T and B cells in antibody responses and the specificity of these cells for different determinants on hapten-carrier conjugates.

Experiments Studying the Anti-Hapten Response. The introduction of haptenic determinants into immunogenic carrier proteins by Landsteiner (see Chapter 2) provided a powerful tool for the analysis of specific interactions between antigen and B and T lymphocytes. Immunization with hapten conjugates elicits anti-hapten antibody responses only when the hapten is coupled to a carrier molecule which is "immunogenic". Particularly strong responses are elicited only by hapten conjugates of thymus-dependent antigen. Indeed, non-immunogenic molecules serve poorly or not at all as effective carriers for haptens. In the case of hapten conjugates of autologous molecules, the conjugation procedure often causes denaturation and results in the creation of an immunogenic carrier molecule. Moreover, optimal hapten-specific secondary responses require challenge with the hapten-carrier conjugate used for primary immunization (i.e., the "carrier" effect) (see Table 8.1). This concept of the "carrier effect" in antibody responses states that: immunization with a dinitrophenylated (DNP) conjugate of a protein carrier such as ovalbumin (DNP-OVA) enables the immunized animal to develop a secondary or anamnestic anti-DNP antibody response only to a challenge with DNP-OVA but not to a challenge with DNP conjugated to an unrelated protein carrier such as bovine gamma globulin (BGG). The anti-hapten antibodies produced by such immunization were highly specific for the haptenic determinant employed (e.g., little, if any, contribution to binding energy was attributable to determinants on the carrier). These observations indicated the existence of an additional recognition mechanism for the carrier molecule, involving the T cells. Indeed, helper T cells required for anti-hapten antibody responses of B cells are specific for determinants of the carrier molecules. The determinants which stimulate helper T cells and B cells have to be presented on the same molecule for effective T-B cell cooperative interaction.

Two *in vivo* experimental models have been used to establish these points:

1. The adoptive secondary anti-hapten response following transfer of hapten-primed and carrier-primed cells into irradiated recipient mice.

2. The use of preimmunization or supplemental immunization with free carrier to enhance primary and secondary anti-hapten antibody responses in guinea pigs and rabbits (Table 8.1, Groups 3 and 4).

Table 8.1

Helper Cells are Specific for Carrier Proteins in Antibody Response to Hapten-Protein Conjugates

Group	Primary Immunization	Supplemental Immunization	Secondary Challenge	Anti-Hapten Secondary Response
1	DNP-OVA	None	DNP-OVA	+++
2	DNP-OVA	None	DNP-BGG	No response
3	DNP-OVA	BGG	DNP-BGG	++++
4	DNP-OVA	BSA	DNP-BGG	No response

Table 8.1. Guinea pigs were immunized with 3 mg of DNP-OVA (dinitrophenylated ovalbumin) in saline and challenged three weeks later with 1 mg of DNP-OVA or DNP-BGG (bovine gamma globulin). Groups 3 and 4 were given supplemental immunization a week before primary immunization with 0.05 mg of BGG in complete Freund's adjuvant. Note that a secondary anti-hapten response was obtained only in Groups 1 and 3.

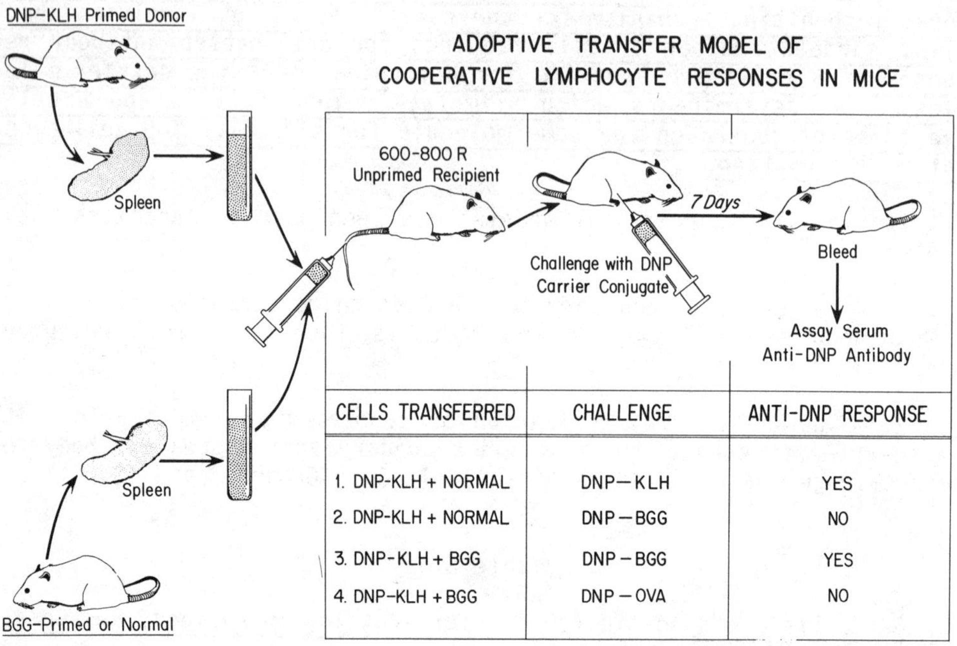

CELLS TRANSFERRED	CHALLENGE	ANTI-DNP RESPONSE
1. DNP-KLH + NORMAL	DNP—KLH	YES
2. DNP-KLH + NORMAL	DNP—BGG	NO
3. DNP-KLH + BGG	DNP—BGG	YES
4. DNP-KLH + BGG	DNP—OVA	NO

Figure 8.3. The explanation is in the text.

Figure 8.3 shows the protocol for studying collaboration between T and B cells in the response to hapten carrier. One group of mice are immunized with dinitrophenylated hemocyanin from giant keyhole limpet (DNP-KLH), a very strong immunogen, and a second set with bovine gamma-globulin (BGG). A third set of mice are not immunized. The cells are harvested and transplanted as indicated. There is no anti-DNP response when cells from DNP-KLH and from normal mice are transferred together and challenged with DNP-BGG (Group 2). Only challenge with DNP-KLH is effective. However, DNP-KLH cells and BGG cells synergize to induce the response to DNP-<u>BGG</u>. <u>The carrier effect is, therefore, reproduced by cell transfer</u>.

The cells from the BGG-immune mice interacting with DNP-BGG are the T cells. Their treatment with anti-Thy 1 (an antigen specific for T cells) and complement abrogates the response in Group 3 (i.e., T cells are killed selectively, leaving only B cells). In contrast, treatment of cells from DNP-KLH-immune mice with anti-Thy 1 (and complement) had no effect. Furthermore, depletion of B cells from the DNP-KLH-immune mice abrogates the response (B cells can be depleted by passing the spleen suspension through culture dishes to which anti-Ig are bound. The B cells become adherent, while the T cells remain free).

The carrier effect can be overcome if the animals, independently, receive supplemental immunization with a secondary carrier protein and are then challenged with the hapten on this second carrier. This experiment is illustrated in Table 8.1 by Groups 3 and 4.

Guinea pigs primed with DNP-OVA failed to respond to a secondary immunization with a heterologous conjugate, DNP-BGG (Group 2). However, if DNP-OVA-primed animals received an intervening supplemental immunization with unconjugated BGG, they not only developed secondary anti-DNP antibody responses to DNP-BGG, but the magnitude of such responses was greater than those elicited by secondary challenge with the original immunizing conjugate DNP-OVA. (This is because the DNP-OVA was first given in saline, while the supplemental antigen was given in Freund's adjuvant, a very strong immunizing vehicle. Moreover, this phenomenon was not restricted to secondary responses. Under appropriate conditions of dose and timing, guinea pigs or rabbits immunized with free carrier BGG manifest enhanced primary anti-DNP antibody responses following primary immunization with DNP-BGG. The kinetics as well as the magnitude of anti-DNP antibody production are sharply augmented under such conditions. (This is because the DNP-OVA was first given in saline, while the supplemental antigen was given in Freund's adjuvant, a very strong immunizing vehicle.)

These experiments establish the cooperative interaction of two distinct recognition processes for carrier and haptenic determinants. Furthermore, the carrier recognition is not mediated by serum antibody as shown by the inability of either small or large amounts of antiserum to the carrier to duplicate the effect of supplemental immunization with the second carrier protein. Contrasting with the inability of anti-carrier antibodies to do so, T cells from syngeneic animals immunized to the second heterologous carrier will transfer anti-hapten responsiveness to recipient animals which themselves have not been exposed to supplemental carrier immunization.

While the T-macrophage interaction is the main event resulting in clonal expansion of the T helper clone, the interaction of the T helper cells with B cells has a major effect on B cells. This interaction results in the growth of B cells and in their differentiation to antibody-secreting cells. During differentiation, the B cell switches its expression of heavy chain class from a cell that has IgM and IgD to a secretory cell that releases any one of the major Ig isotypes.

Many steps in the B-T cell interaction are similar to those taking place between the macrophage and the T cell. We envision the following three stages in the interaction of B cells and T cells: 1) recognition of antigen by the B cell by way of surface immunoglobulin; 2) B cells then present antigen to T cells—both cells interact in a process modulated by Class II polypeptides; 3) T cells secrete lymphokines that promote B cell growth and differentiation. (The T helper cells that collaborate with B cells result from the stimulation of clones that were selected and expanded by antigen presented by the phagocytes.)

In the first stage, The B cell will bind antigen by way of its Ig receptor and will cap and internalize it (Chapter 5). Following this process, an immunogenic determinant appears on the cell surface, and now, in Stage 2, the T helper cell recognizes and binds to the B cell. Thus, B cells first serve as antigen-presenting cells, presenting a determinant similar to that initially presented by the macrophage.

The collaboration between the T cells and the macrophage is also restricted by Class II molecules of the MHC. The phenomenon is identical in most respects with that described earlier for macrophages and T cells and will not be detailed. An experiment showing this collaboration is shown in Table 8.2.

In the third and final stage of the interaction between the T-B cell, the T cell will secrete lymphokines. Such lymphokines will have the potential to act on any B cell undergoing cell division, inducing them to maintain growth while also differentiating them, i.e., the lymphokines will act in a polyclonal manner. For example, B cells that have been stimulated briefly with the polyclonal mitogen LPS will keep proliferating under the influence of lymphokines from activted T helper cells. Differentiation to plasma cells also takes place. In the case of resting B cells, the lymphokines stimulating only terminal differentiation without enlarging the clones. The effects of lymphokines is not restricted by MHC, i.e., for example, mixtures of T helper cells with syngeneic macrophages may stimulate the growth of B cell blasts from an allogeneic strain.

There are a number of issues currently studied which have not been resolved. The molecular nature of the lymphokines that acts on B cells is not known, nor is their relationship to other lymphokines, such as those described in Chapter 7. We do know that lymphokines that act on B cells (called thymus-replacing factor by some) are certainly different from IL-2. Other unsettled issues are whether all B cells respond in the manner described above and whether there are families of T helper cells which direct the isotype switch. There are some indications that some sets of T helper cells may even recognize the isotype or idiotype on surface Ig. The regulation of B cell differentiation is obviously a complex issue, probably involving multiple steps.

Thymic-independent antigens. Antibody responses can be initiated by some antigens in the apparent absence of T helper cells, thus the term thymic-independent antigens. Thymic-independent antigens are usually bacterial products, including lipopolysaccharides (LPS) from Gram-negative organisms, or polysaccharides with repeating antigenic

Table 8.2

I-Region Genes Restrict T-B Cell Cooperative Interactions

Strain of Hapten-Primed B Cells	Strain of Carrier-Primed T Cells	Secondary Responses in (a x b)F1 Irradiated Recipients
a	a	++++
b	b	++++
a	b	—
b	a	—
b	(a x b)F1	++++
a	(a x b)F1	++++
(a x b)F1	a	++++
(a x b)F1	b	++++

Table 8.2. Carrier-primed T cells were adoptively transferred to (a x b)F1 recipients which were irradiated; then anti-Thy-1 and C-treated, hapten-primated spleen cells (B cells) were adoptively transferred to the same (a x b)F1 recipients. The animals were challenged with the hapten-protein conjugates and the secondary secondary anti-hapten response measured as an indication of T-B cell cooperative interactions.

determinants. Many of the thymic-independent antigens—but in particular LPS—induce polyclonal stimulation of B cells, i.e., every B cell is stimulated to grow and differentiate. The LPS molecules get incorporated into the B cell membrane and stimulate the cell. The same type of polyclonal stimulation may develop with repeated binding of B cell receptors to antigen with multiple identical determinants.

The response of thymic-independent antigens is characterized by its moderate to low intensity, its restriction to the production of antibodies of the IgM class, and its limited immunological memory.

INTERACTIONS WITH SUPPRESSOR T CELLS

The suppressor T cells (Ts), originally discovered by R. Gershon, are a distinct class of lymphocytes whose function is to inhibit specifically the immune response. Ts are normally found within the thymus, the lymphoid organs, and the blood. They are highly radiosensitive to X-irradiation and to radiomimetic drugs like cyclophosphamide. Ts slowly disappear after thymectomy, even in the adult individual (such a procedure in the adult does not affect T helper cells). It follows that the Ts decrease with aging when the thymus involutes. All these characteristics indicate that Ts are relatively short-lived cells.

Ts bear distinctive surface proteins that distinguish them from T helpers and cytolytic T cells. In the mouse, the species where they were first identified and studied best, the effector Ts bear low levels of Ly1 and moderate levels of Ly2; conventionally, we call them Ly1-Ly2+ inasmuch as they are not killed with antibodies to Ly1 (with complement). Ts also express I-J-controlled antigenic specificities (Chapter 7), which distinguishes them from cytolytic T cells which are also Ly1-Ly2+ but I-J negative. In humans, Ts bear the T8 marker. The ratio in blood for positive cells for T4, a marker for helper cells, and positive for T8, the marker for both cytolytic T cells and Ts, is about 2. Inversion in this ratio is taken as an index of an increase in relative Ts activity over T helpers.

Historical Analysis. Specific unresponsiveness has been known for some time, although it was not realized to be the result of suppressor T cells until the findings of Gershon. Suppressive phenomena and tolerance are, in fact, deeply interrelated. One of the early experimental observations now attributed to Ts suppression were studies on the inhibition of contact sensitivity to simple chemicals by C. Sulzeberger and extended by M. Chase, J. Battisto, and their colleagues. Intravenous or oral administration of a contact-sensitizing chemical—such as dinitrofluorobenzene which binds to epsilon amino groups of lysine of proteins—produced a state of unresponsiveness to the same chemical when later applied to the skin. In untreated individuals, the direct application of the same chemical to the skin induces a typical delayed sensitivity state (Chapter 7). This contact sensitivity state results from the activation of the T helper cells by Langerhans cells containing the sensitizer bound to epidermal proteins. We know that, in the case of the treated individual, the first intravenous administration of the chemical resulted in its conjugation to autologous proteins in blood and to the preferential stimulation of Ts, which then inhibited the development of cellular immunity.

Ts were originally identified by the adoptive transfer of lymphocytes from antigen-unresponsive mice. Gershon and Kondo injected mice with high doses of sheep red cells (SRBC). This high dose of antigen was found to induce a very poor response. They then harvested the splenic lymphocytes from the treated mice and co-transferred them together with normal thymocytes into thymectomized, X-irradiated mice previously reconstituted with bone marrow cells. Such recipient mice contained B cells but were T cell deprived. The mice were then injected with a standard amount of SRBC capable of inducing a strong antibody response in normal mice:

Group 1 Received no thymocytes: antibody titer of less than 1.

Group 2 Received thymocytes from untreated mice: antibody titer of 6.

Group 3 Received thymocytes from untreated mice plus lymphocytes from mice given high doses of SRBC: antibody titer of 1.

(Antibody titer is log 2 of the reciprocal of highest serum dilution inducing hemagglutination.) Group 1 made no antibody response because of an absence of helper T cells; therefore, their B cells could not get help for the anti-SRBC response. The mice in Group 2, in contrast, made an anti-SRBC response since they had been reconstituted with T cells. The comparison between Groups 1 and 2, then, clearly shows the need for the T-B cell interactions analyzed previously. Group 3 shows the new finding—the addition of lymphocytes from the hyporesponsive mice inhibited the T-B interaction.

This experiment indicated that T lymphocytes, which heretofore had always been responsible for inducing immunity, were also capable of inhibiting an immune response. Later studies, of E. Boyse and H. Cantor, established that lymphocytes that transferred positive immunity, and those that suppressed it had different sensitivities to treatment with anti-Ly antibodies. This indicated the existence of two distinct T cell subsets responsible, respectively, for help and suppression. Following these results, it became apparent that suppressor T cells were important cellular elements that were responsible for many of the various phenomena of immunological tolerance (Chapter 9). Ts were later recognized as participating also in the normal response to protein antigens. Thus, the response to proteins results from the critical balance of two opposing T cells—the T helpers and the Ts.

Suppressor T cells have been shown to be capable of suppressing specifically a large variety of T and B cell responses. Accordingly, Ts can be induced that specifically suppress T cells responses such as delayed-type sensitivity, contact sensitivity, or target cell killing by cytolytic T cells. Similarly, suppressor T cells have been identified that can suppress B cell immunity either through their effects on helper T cells or even directly by suppressing antibody synthesis by plasma cells.

Generation of Ts. Ts are now known to be activated in two general conditions: 1) during a physiological immune response, and 2) under a variety of situations that favor the development of Ts over T helper cells.

Concurrent with the appearance of T helper cells and the development of the response to antigen, Ts are stimulated. The physiological development of Ts can be viewed as a cellular mechanism that inhibits and controls the expansion and continuation of the immunological process. The Ts contribute, therefore, to the decay with time of the immune response (together with other factors to be considered in the next section). The generation of the Ts has been studied in selected systems and has been found to be a highly complex process involving various cells in what is termed the suppressor circuit. These interactions include a first step in which an Ly1+2- Ts inducer cell, also termed Ts1, is generated following the interaction with antigen and an antigen-presenting cell. The details of this interaction are now being studied and are largely unknown. The Ts1-inducer cell appears to be distinct from the conventional Ly1+ helper T cell discussed in the previous section. The nature of the antigen-presenting cell which activates Ts1 cells is not clear, although it bears on its surface antigenic determinants encoded in the I-J locus of the MHC and it may be a distinct antigen-presenting cell from the one which activates helper T cells. Perhaps, the antigen-presenting cell is a macrophage at some stage in its maturation or perhaps is it represented by a different accessory cell. Ts1-inducer cells in the suppressor circuit then trigger the development of Ts2 effector cells. Depending upon the system, some Ts2 cells are specific for antigen and others display specificity for the idiotypes on the Ts1 cell and the B cell. The Ts2 cell, in turn, interacts specifically with a third suppressor T cell in the circuit, Ts3, which is an antigen-specific effector cell induced as the result of the original immunization. These Ts3 cells, also termed effector suppressors, are responsible for the suppression phenomena observed. They are activated by a specific factor produced by the Ts2 cells.

Such suppressor T cell circuits involving the activation of a Ts1 cell inducing a Ts2 suppressor, which, in turn, activates a Ts3 effector cell, have been documented in the specific suppression of both cellular immunity and antibody production. In several systems, the induction of Ts1 and Ts3 cells, as well as the interactions between Ts2 factor and Ts3 cells, are restricted by genes in the I region of the MHC.

As stated above, the Ts interact with each other by way of soluble mediators. These mediators are proteins that are presently being characterized. One of the best studied molecules is the Ts3 factor. It is a two-chain molecule in which one chain displays antigen specificity and the other chain bears determinants with anti-I-J alloantisera.

In those systems where suppression of the response is achieved, the final effector cell appears to regulate the system by inhibiting the helper cells. However, as was mentioned previously, suppresor T cells are also able to suppress the reactions of delayed and contact sensitivities in *immune* animals and the synthesis and secretion of immunoglobulins by *plasma* cells. The issue remains where the cells responsible for these various activities are the same or are distinct subclasses of suppressor T cells.

Conditions which favor the generation of suppressor T cells:

1. *A high or very low dose of antigen*—for every protein antigen, there is an amount that gives rise to an optimal response. This amount varies from protein to protein. Increasing the amount may result in a decreased response. Too little antigen will not induce immunity. Under both extreme circumstances, Ts will be preferentially activated.

2. *The kind of antigen*—proteins that remain in circulation or extracellular fluids without being taken by phagocytes will tend to induce Ts in contrast to proteins that are immediately trapped by the phagocyte system.

3. *Repeated administration of antigen*—most situations in which antigen is continuously administered can give rise to strong Ts activity. In chronic infectious diseases, there is always a strong Ts component, because of the persistence of small amounts of antigen released into the blood, i.e., tuberculosis, parasite infections. The same situation applies to tumors, in which the growth of the tissues is favored by the presence of Ts.

4. *The route of administration*—the intravenous route favors the development of Ts. Ts are preferentially induced when antigen circulates for long periods of time before being taken up by phagocytes in lymphoid tissue. Also, administration of some antigen by the oral route may favor Ts activity.

5. *Age*—very young individuals have a clear tendency to develop strong Ts activity in contrast to older individuals. Aged individuals have low Ts activity.

6. *Deficit in Ir gene function* (Chapter 10).

As one can note from this list, three closely interrelated conditions favor the development of Ts: the lack of development of helper T cells, the bypassing of accessory cell function, and the presence of free antigen for long periods of time. It is possible that, in these situations, some of the Ts might have interacted with antigen *directly* without the help of macrophages. This conclusion is based on two findings: 1) in culture, Ts can be generated in situations where conventional macrophages are decreased or eliminated; and 2) Ts can be enriched by their attachment to antigen bound to insoluble matrices. However, it is also possible, in light of recent evidence indicating the need of antigen-presenting cells for the induction of Ts, that a distinct class of antigen-presenting cells is involved in this process, as discussed earlier.

An important issue is whether Ts may be specific for an Ig class. There is scattered experimental evidence in favor of Ts directed to Ig of a given class or allotype. The best evidence so far comes from the IgE antibody response. The IgE response must be carefully controlled since high titers of IgE antibody can be extremely dangerous because of their ability to release vasoactive amines of mast cells (Chapter 14). In experimental systems, it has been found that the IgE antibodies can be induced in high titers, but rapidly decreases, followed by an IgG response. This disappearance appears to be caused by Ts that selectively inhibits the IgE antibody response.

A final consideration is whether polysaccharides can trigger Ts. All the systems studied so far indicate that Ts are best stimulated by protein antigens. In one thymus-independent response, to the pneumococcal polysaccharide, it has been found that elimination of circulating lymphocytes enhances the response implying a level of Ts under normal conditions.

Specificity of Suppression. The generation of Ts is highly specific, as specific as the generation of helper T cells. There is, however, a clear element of non-specificity once the effector Ts are activated. The end result of such activation of effector Ts is to inhibit the specific response while, at the same time, affecting to some extent the response to unrelated antigens. The phenomenon of antigenic competition consists of the inhibition of the response to one antigen when administered at a critical time after immunization with an immunogenic protein.

The non-specific component can be identified in adoptive transfer experiments using the hapten-protein systems discussed before. For example, take three sets of cells—B cells enriched for anti-DNP memory cells, T helper cells from ovalbumin (OVA)-immune mice, and Ts to bovine gamma globulin (BGG)—and then carry out adoptive transfer into X-irradiated mice:

	Transfer	Challenge	Anti-DNP Antibodies
1.	B (anti-DNP) + Th (vs. OVA)	DNP-OVA	+++
2.	As above plus Ts (vs. BGG)	DNP-OVA	+++
3.	As No. 2	DNA-OVA and BGG	+

The Ts cells activated by BGG could induce suppression of the response to an unrelated protein (DNP-OVA). However, they could be triggered only by its specific antigen, BGG.

Target of Ts. In many systems, the inactivation of T helper cells appears to be the target of Ts, but exactly how this is done is not clear. One recent report claims that Ts inhibit helper T cells from secreting IL-2, thus stopping T helper and cytolytic clones from expanding in number. It is possible that Ts directed to idiotypic determinants could also inhibit B cell function.

Brief Comment on Helper and Suppressor T Cell Function. Many of the interactions resulting in the generation of helper and suppressor T cells are reasonably well understood and have been outlined in this chapter. It is clear, however, that the crucial balance between helper and suppressor T cell function is extremely complex, and many of its features remain to be settled. The complexity of the suppressor circuit has been recently magnified by studies from Gershon's laboratory, indicating that there are countersuppressive influences. The conditions that favor the development of countersuppression, thus favoring helper function, are now being studied.

COMMENTS ON THE TERMINATION OF THE IMMUNE RESPONSE

We have considered a number of important phenomenona concerned with the induction of an immune response. The response is obviously extremely complex since it involves a number of critical interactions among at least four major types of cells: macrophages, helper T cells, suppressor T cells, and B lymphocytes; each of these cells interacts with antigen by way of receptor molecules, some of which are different from each other. Also crucial in the response are the various gene products of the MHC which determine all responses involving T lymphocytes. Each cell studied in an isolated way, as it is now possible to do, shows a multifaceted pattern of response and a clear capacity to regulate the others. Macrophages process antigen, can stimulate induction of helper T cells, and can secrete modulatory factors that influence lymphocytes. Helper T cells obviously help B cells, as well as other T cells, and are also involved in delayed sensitivity and antimicrobial immunity. This last example is one of the best, showing a complete circle of stimulation, i.e., macrophages ——> T cells ——> macrophages (Chapter 7). Suppressor T cells control immune response. Finally, B cells respond in positive or negative ways, depending on the structure of the antigen and on the other regulatory cells (Chapters 5 and 9).

Finally, what causes the termination of the immune response? Many factors have been discussed and analyzed, some quite extensively. Those considered important are:

a. The elimination of the antigen. The duration of antigen in an immunogenic form in macrophages is relatively short-lived. Once the antigen disappears from the macrophage, the response dwindles.

b. The presence of antibody. Antibody molecules can bind available antigen and stop it from interacting efficiently with lymphocytes. It is thought that physiologically antibody plays a homeostatic role in shutting off the reponse. For example, experiments have been done in which animals are subject to plasmapheresis a few days after an immune response is initiated (i.e., the blood is withdrawn, and the red cells are then separated from the plasma and reinfused back). The removal of the antibody in the plasma is accompanied by a new burst of antibody in blood, suggesting that the level of serum antibody was controlling the production of antibody. In other experiments, antibody administered with antigen can be found to decrease an ongoing immune process. An appropriate example is the prevention of erythroblastosis fetalis by giving Rh-negative pregnant mothers antibodies to Rh-positive red cells (Chapter 2).

c. The emergence of suppressor T cells. We have discussed these. We emphasize here that Ts are normally activated during a conventional immune response, and these contribute very significantly to its termination.

d. The anti-idiotype response. There is evidence in favor of an antibody response to the idiotypes expressed on B and T cells. This anti-idiotype response may also serve to stop the stimulation of the idiotype-bearing clones.

REFERENCES

Gershon, R. K. A disquisition on suppressor T cells. Transplant. Rev., 26:170, 1975.

Katz, D. H. Lymphocyte Differentiation, Recognition, and Regulation. Academic Press, Inc., New York, 1977.

Katz, D. H., and Benacerraf, B. (eds). The Role of Products of the Histocompatibility Gene Complex in Immune Response. Academic Press, New York, 1976.

Moller, G. (ed). Immunol. Rev., Volume 26, 1975 (contains nine articles dealing with the early studies on suppression).

Moller, G. (ed). Immunol. Rev., Volume 50, 1980 (contains nine articles dealing with suppression and tolerance to haptens).

Paul, W. E., and Benacerraf, B. Functional specificity of thymus-dependent lymphocytes. Science, 195:1293, 1977.

Rosenthal, A. S. Determinant selection and macrophage function in genetic control of the immune response. Immunol. Rev., 40:136, 1978.

Singer, A., and Hodes, R. Mechanisms of T cell-B cell interaction. Ann. Rev. Immunol., 1:211, 1983.

Unanue, E. R. The regulatory role of macrophages in antigenic stimulation. Part Two: Symbiotic relationship between lymphocytes and macrophages. Adv. Immunol., 31:1, 1981.

CHAPTER 9

Immunological Tolerance

Immunological tolerance, also referred to as specific immunological unresponsiveness, is the acquired inability of an individual to express specific cell-mediated or humoral immunity to a molecule or antigenic determinant to which it would otherwise respond. Such an individual tolerant to an antigen preserves his capacity to respond to other antigens. Immunological tolerance is as specific in this respect as immunity. The phenomenon of immunological tolerance is the basis for our inability to mount immune responses against our own tissue antigens. Tolerance to self, however, does break down with resulting autoimmune diseases of severe life-threatening consequences. The statement that the presence of an antigen since birth is responsible for our inability to recognize it as antigen has been substantiated. Thus, individuals lacking an autologous component as a result of genetic mutation form strong responses against the missing molecule if immunized with it. For example, guinea pigs genetically deficient in the C4 component of complement develop high levels of antibodies to C4 when immunized with normal guinea pig serum containing C4 protein. Under the same conditions of immunization, normal guinea pigs do not make anti-C4 antibodies.

The selective inability to develop immune responses to an antigen requires contact with this antigen under conditions that lead to specific tolerance rather than immunity. The antigens that have been used to study tolerance include cells bearing allogeneic histocompatibility antigens, proteins, synthetic polypeptides, haptens, polysaccharides, and live microorganisms. In very few instances have autologous antigens been tested.

Tolerance can be induced in the newborn or in the adult. The newborn is by far most sensitive to tolerance induction. We first describe examples of tolerance in newborn and adults and then consider its cellular basis.

Neonatal tolerance: Antigens which normally stimulate immune responses in adults can induce immunological unresponsiveness in newborn animals who have not yet developed immunological competence. This high susceptibility to tolerance of immunologically immature individuals is believed to be the explanation for self-tolerance. Tolerance to cellular antigens, such as the histocompatibility antigens, can be elicited in newborn animals. Such tolerance results in the acceptance of allografts and in the maintenance of the chimeric state (i.e., the individual will have circulating allogeneic cells).

The first example of tolerance to cellular antigens was discovered by R. Owen in 1945 in dizygotic cattle twins. These are non-identical twins (i.e., derived from two different ova) that share a common placental blood supply resulting in the exchange of blood cells during fetal life. After birth, it was found that each calf was a chimera having a mixture of its own hematopoietic cells plus that of its twin. The dizygotic calves were unable to mount an immune response to the other's foreign alloantigens. Inspired by this observation, Sir Peter Medawar and his associates in Britain showed that such dizygotic cattle twins were mutually tolerant of skin grafts from one another, regardless of differences in sex and color. Previous to these studies, analysis of infection with the non-pathogenic virus, the lymphocyte choriomeningitis virus (LCM), had disclosed a curious phenomenon: the virus given at birth was not eliminated by the host and persisted throughout the life of the mouse; in contrast, inoculation of the virus into adults resulted in its elimination. These two observations led M. Burnet and F. Fenner to postulate that contact with antigen during early life could lead to a specific state of unresponsiveness.

Medawar and his group proceeded actively to produce immunological tolerance to histocompatibility antigens by injecting embryos of inbred CBA mice *in utero* with live spleen cells of histoincompatible A strain mice. When such CBA mice grew to adulthood, they were found to be specifically tolerant of skin grafts from histoincompatible A strain donors; the CBA mice tolerant to A skin were able to reject allografts of other strains bearing different histocompatibility antigens. Such a state of tolerance could be abolished by injecting lymphoid cells from an adult syngeneic CBA donor, for example:

	A Graft	BL/6 Graft
CBA mouse—not treated	Rejection	Rejection
CBA mouse—inoculated with A cells during embryonic or neonatal life	No rejection	Rejection

The studies of transplantation tolerance were rapidly reproduced in other species, most notably in chickens by Hasek. Hasek induced tolerance by fusing the chorioallantoic membranes of two embryos and thus interconnecting their blood vessels. He thus produced artificially what was found naturally in cattle by Owen, i.e., the mixing of blood cells during embryonic life.

(It is clear that the history of tolerance centers around the studies discussed above in the young. The results were dramatic and called attention to the possibility that the lack of responsiveness to self had the same basis, i.e., contact with antigen during an immature stage of the immunological system. Other observations, however, called attention to manipulations that could produce a state of immunoresponsiveness in adults. We refer in particular to the studies of contact sensitivity discussed in Chapter 8. Another classical study of unresponsivenesss was produced by Felton by injecting high doses of pneumococcal polysaccharide into mice.)

Tolerance to histocompatibility antigens have now been extensively analyzed using protocols akin to those used by Medawar, i.e., injecting cells immediately after birth. The induction of the tolerant state requires the inoculation of a critical number of live hematopoietic cells right after birth (cells from other organs or dead cells do not induce tolerance). The state of tolerance can be tested by skin grafting or in a mixed lymphocyte culture by examining for proliferation of T helper cells or for the development of cytolytic T cells (i.e., lymphoid cells from the inoculated host are cultured with lymphoid cells from the donor). The induction of tolerance also depends on the degree of antigenic disparity between the host and the tolerogen. In the mouse, it is difficult to induce a tolerant state with certain combinations of alloantigens differing strongly at H-2. The induction of tolerance has been examined using recombinant inbred strains where the tolerogen (i.e., the lymphoid cells inoculated at birth) differ selectively at Class I or Class II loci, or at both, with the host (the newborn mouse). Differences only at Class I induce a state of tolerance but less efficiently than differences in Class II. Differences through the whole H-2 appears to be the most effective. The cellular basis of this phenomenon is discussed later.

Tolerance to protein antigens can also be induced at birth. Tolerance induction requires giving the protein antigen very soon after birth, before the individual acquires immunocompetence, as was the case for alloantigens. Species where the immune system is well developed at birth are, in general, very difficult to tolerize. The induction of tolerance depends greatly upon the antigen; with strongly immunogenic proteins, it is more difficult to induce tolerance. In contrast, weakly immunogenic proteins, particularly if injected for several times, will induce a prolonged state of unresponsiveness. These proteins circulate for long periods of time, a factor that helps maintain the tolerant state. The length of tolerance induction depends, again, upon the amounts of antigen given as well as their immunogenicity. Finally, tolerance to microorganisms is difficult, if not impossible, to induce except in the case of some viruses. We mentioned before the results with LCM which, inoculated at birth, stays in the host tissues without inducing cytopathic effect.

<u>Tolerance in the Adult:</u> Tolerance can also be induced in the adult, although it is much more difficult than in neonates. Adult individuals have a fully mature immune system that is ready to respond to antigen presented under suitable conditions. Critical conditions have to be met for induction of tolerance in adults:

1. In all cases, the ease of tolerance induction in adults is inversely related to the inherent immunogenicity of the antigen. For example, a weak immunogen, albumins, which circulate for long periods and are poorly trapped in lymphoid organs, require a less stringent regiment for tolerance than a strong immunogen, like foreign erythrocytes. These are rapidly eliminated and taken up by accessory cells of the lymph nodes or spleen. Haptens attached to non-immunogenic proteins can induce tolerance in contrast to those bound to strong immunogens (Table 9.1).

2. The dose of antigen: the use of very low doses of antigen, such as bovine albumin, below the threshhold dose which is immunogenic; or the use of very high doses. This experiment gives rise to the concept of two zones of tolerance induction—low- and high-zone tolerance.

3. The metabolizability of the antigen: proteins that are not degraded will induce tolerance. The best example is to use a hapten like DNP bound to two synthetic polypeptides, one made up of L-amino acids, the other of d-amino acids. The latter are poorly degraded by the host and remain in tissues for long times and do not stimulate T cell immunity. Such polypeptides are highly tolerogenic (Table 9.1). A second example is tolerance to polysaccharides. Administration of polysaccharides in ten- to one-hundredfold higher amount than the immunizing dose is effective. Polysaccharides also remain in tissues for long times and do not stimulate T cells. In these two examples, tolerance is usually at the level of the B cell.

4. The injection of antigen in a form that is free of large polymers: in this way, the uptake by macrophages is bypassed or decreased. This applies particularly to proteins like albumins or immunoglobulins which can be made to polymerize and will then be readily taken up by macrophages of tissues and lymphoid organs.

5. The route of administration: the intravenous route is the preferred route for tolerance induction. The oral administration of some proteins or small chemicals is also an effective way to induce tolerance.

6. The interaction with Fc receptors: immunoglobulins can be highly tolerogenic, a finding that has been used to induce tolerance by attaching small chemicals to them. For example, DNP bound to autologous Ig is a very efficient tolerogen, much more than bound to its $F(ab')_2$ fragment or to other autologous proteins like albumin. It is thought that this tolerogenic effect is, in fact, caused by binding of the Ig to the Fc receptor of B cells, inducing a negative signal.

7. The use of immunosuppressive agents: given together with antigen, it favors the development of tolerance by reducing the number of active immunocompetent lymphocytes. Immunosuppression has been induced with X-irradiation or with drugs that interfere with cell division such as methotrexate, cyclophosphamide, and 6-mercaptopurine.

Table 9.1

Tolerance to DNP Induced in Adult Mice

Immunizing Molecule			Results	
	Half-Life	Uptake	Immunity	Tolerance
DNP-KLH	Minutes	++++	++++	—
DNP-deagg HGG	Days	+	±	+++
DNP-agg HGG	Minutes	+++	+++	—
DNP-autologous IgG	Days	+	—	+++
DNP-autologous albumin	Days	±	—	+
DNP-L-GL	Minutes	++	—	±
DNP-D-GL	Minutes	++	—	+++
DNP-SIII	Minutes	++	±	++

Table 9.1 DNP-KLH = DNP on hemocyanin; DNP-deagg HGG or DNP-agg HGG = DNP on monomer or polymer human IgG, respectively; DNP-L-GL or -D-GL = DNP on the synthetic polymer made of glutamic acid and lysine either with L- or D-amino acids; DNP-SIII = DNP on pneumococcal polysaccharide. Immunity is defined as the capacity of the molecule to induce an immune response. Tolerance is tested by injecting the mice with DNP-agg HGG, an obligate immunogen.

Table 9.1 summarizes some of these points in an experiment studying the response to the DNP hapten in mice. In all these examples we are examining the anti-DNP antibody response. Immunity in the Table means that the antigen was capable of inducing anti-DNP antibodies. Tolerance is tested by challenging the mice for a second time, with an obligatory immunogen as carrier, one that always induces a primary immune response—in our example with aggregated or polymerized Human Gamma Globulin. Referring to Table 9.1, DNP-KLH is a strong immunogen taken up avidly by phagocytes and readily induces T helper cells. Clearly, tolerance is not induced with such a strong antigen which readily stimulates a response and generates immunological memory. DNP-deaggregated human IgG (HGG) is a poor immunogen that can effectively induce tolerance, while aggregated HGG, as mentioned, is a strong immunogen. The examples with DNP-autologous IgG or albumin show the importance of a non-immunogenic protein as carrier of the hapten. The fact that DNP-autologous IgG is a better tolerogen than DNP on mouse albumin indicates the importance of Ig as carriers for induction of B cell tolerance. The polymer made of glutamic acid and lysine (GL) illustrates the need for metabolizing the protein. The compound made of L-amino acids is degraded, while that made of d-amino acids resists proteolysis and remains for long periods in the tissues of the individual. The use of DNP conjugated to pneumococcal polysaccharide also illustrates the effects of molecules that are retained in tissues without much degradation. The pneumococcal polysaccharide is very slowly eliminated.

The lack of responsiveness of anti-DNP B cells in these examples could be as: 1) a direct result of functional inactivation of the T helper cells, therefore, stopping their collaboration with B cells; or 2) a direct inactivation of the B cells by the tolerogen. In all the examples except for those using deaggregated or aggregated HGG, we are measuring effects on B cells since the carriers used for tolerance induction differs from those used in the challenge. Operationally, we are, therefore, examining only the effect of the tolerogen on the DNP-B cells. In the example with HGG, the effect could be at either carrier or hapten recognition.

CELLULAR BASIS OF TOLERANCE

Immunological tolerance can affect the T lymphocyte or the B cells, or both. At the T cell level, tolerance may result from the functional disappearance of the T helper clones and/or the development of T suppressor cells (Ts). As can be noted, many examples discussed in the induction of tolerance were also mentioned in Chapter 8 in the context of the induction of Ts.

Crucial for understanding the cellular basis of tolerance were experiments first performed by J. Chiller and W. O. Weigle in the mouse. The Chiller-Weigle experiment was performed in the following manner: as illustrated in Figure 9.1, inbred mice are tolerized with one injection of a suitable dose of deaggregated human gamma globulin (HGG); such mice can be shown to be tolerant to HGG as manifested by their incapacity to develop anti-HGG responses to subsequent challenge with aggregated HGG. We have mentioned that aggregated HGG is an Ig preparation polymerized by heat; the aggregated HGG is rapidly taken up by macrophages and is strongly immunogenic. In contrast, deaggregated HGG is a soluble preparation where polymers have been removed by ultracentrifugation; deaggregated HGG bypasses uptake and is tolerogenic. Chapter 5 discussed this experiment using albumin instead of gamma globulins.

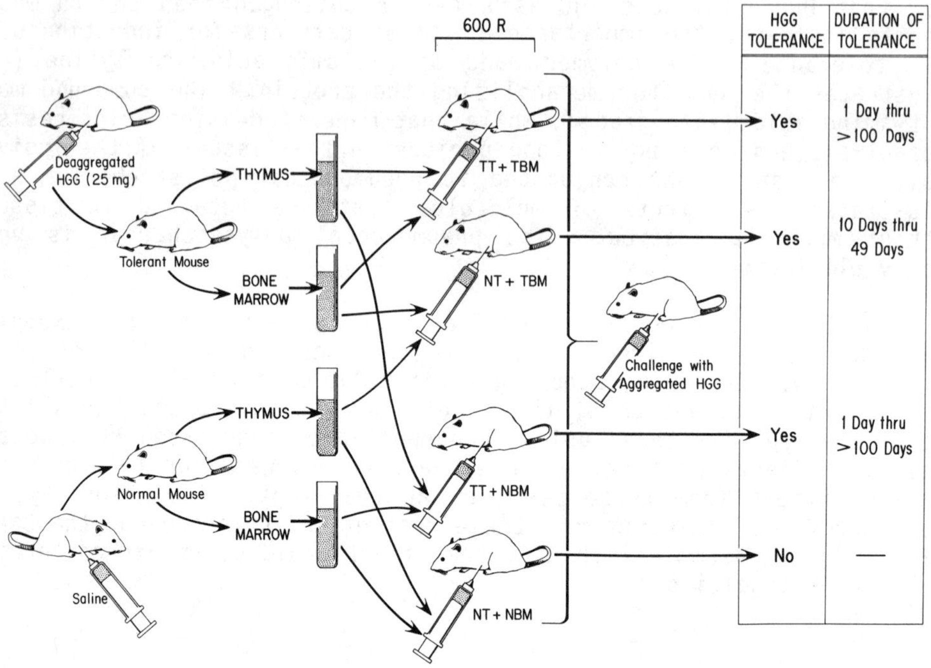

Figure 9.1. The protocol of Weigle and Chiller to study tolerance at the cellular level: NT = thymus cells from normal; TT = thymus cells from tolerant; NBM = bone marrow cells from normal; TBM = bone marrow cells from tolerant. The explanation of the experiment is in the text.

At various times after administration of the deaggregated, tolerogenic HGG, the mice are sacrificed and used as donors of thymus and bone marrow cells for transfer to irradiated syngeneic mice. Also, the tolerant bone marrow or thymus cells were transferred in combination with thymus or bone marrow cells from normal mice.

The transfer follows the protocol described in Chapter 8. HGG, as most proteins, is a thymus-dependent antigen. The immune response to it requires collaboration between specific B and T cells. The bone marrow cell inoculum provides the B cells, while the thymocytes provide the progenitors of helper T cells. The recipients are then immunized with a suitable dose of aggregated HGG and then sacrificed after an appropriate interval for analysis of their spleens for HGG-specific PFC responses.

Figure 9.1 shows the different kinds of combinations. Transfer of bone marrow and thymus cells from normal mice results in an anti-HGG response (note NT + NBM). In contrast, the transfer of bone marrow and thymus cells from tolerant mice (TT + TBM) did not produce a response. Mixing thymus or bone marrow cells from tolerant with normal counterparts induced different patterns of response. At some time the bone marrow cells, though derived from a tolerant mouse, made antibodies when combined with normal thymocytes. This indicated that the tolerant lesion was in the T cell. This point was confirmed when the T cells from this same mouse would not collaborate with normal bone marrow cells.

Using this system, it was shown that T cells were tolerant very rapidly after induction (within twenty-four hours). The tolerant state was maintained in T cells for around one hundred days. The bone marrow population also became tolerant, but not until Day 10 to 11. Recovery in this population occurred by Day 50. By comparison, intact tolerant mice manifested tolerance in parallel with that of the T cell population, i.e., an animal whose bone marrow population had recovered by Day 60 would nevertheless be functionally unresponsive due to absence of immunocompetent HGG-specific T cells.

The experiments demonstrated that: 1) <u>both T and B lymphocytes are susceptible to tolerance induction</u>; 2) <u>that the susceptibilities of these two lymphocyte classes differ considerably in both the dose of tolerogen and the time required for tolerance induction</u>; 3) <u>that the duration of tolerance is shorter in B cells than in T cells</u>; 4) <u>finally, that the immunological status of the whole animal reflects more generally that of the T cell population, in the case of a thymus-dependent antigen</u>.

We will first discuss the tolerant lesion at the level of T cells. What is the problem in the tolerant T cells in this model of HGG tolerance? Although there is no complete agreement among cellular immunologists on this regard, it is apparent, however, that tolerance has a strong component of suppression caused by the generation of antigen-specific Ts. In Chapter 8, we have discussed the situations that induce Ts, one of which is the bypass of classical macrophage-T helper cell induction. Using deaggregated HGG, there is poor uptake by macrophages and limited antigen presentation at the same time that the antigen circulates for long periods. How can Ts be shown in the model of HGG tolerance? Simply by co-transferring the tolerant cells together with known sets of T helpers and B cells into X-irradiated hosts. Under these circumstances, the tolerant cells will inhibit the collaboration between the helper T cells and the B cell (although this is not always easy to demonstrate).

Whether or not clones of T helper cells are inactivated by the tolerogen is not a settled question. The difficulty lies in that helper T cells cannot be measured directly (nor can Ts). Helper T cells are always measured in functional bioassays. The lack of helper

T cells could mean that the clone is not there (i.e., that the tolerogen eliminated it); that the clone is there but in an inactive form; or that is has never been expanded, i.e., never stimulated. These issues remain to be settled.

Suppressor T cells have also been found to be a major component in tolerance to very low doses or very high doses of protein antigen. Also, the inhibition of contact sensitivity by administration of a sensitizer intravenously (discussed in Chapter 8) is caused by Ts. This is the example where the reactive chemical dinitrofluorobenzene is injected intravenously, binding to innumerable self-proteins in the circulation and on cells. This creates the activation of Ts. Later, the chemical is applied to the skin, also binding to self-proteins at high density. In normal circumstances, the application to the skin induces a state of delayed sensitivity by activation of T helper cells. However, in the individual given the DNFB intravenously, the Ts inhibit the development of T helper cells.

Ts have a major role in tolerance to protein during the neonatal period of life. It has recently been found that, in the mouse, a species in which neonates are born very immature, there is a paucity of Ia-bearing macrophages in lymphoid organs and in tissues as well as of Langerhans cells. Thus, the neonate cannot activate helper T cells and the entrance of antigen during this period will, therefore, lead to stimulation of Ts. The lack of expression of Ia in the neonate could be due to the high levels of prostaglandin E and to alpha-fetoprotein, both of which inhibit Ia synthesis.

What happens to the T cells in the case of tolerance to cellular alloantigens administered during neonatal life? There is agreement that many instances of tolerance to alloantigens are caused by Ts. However, in some situations, no Ts are found, implying a functional deletion of T helper cells. In examples where tolerance has been induced selectively to Class I alloantigens, no Ts are found but only absence of T helper cells (these are the examples mentioned in the section on neonatal tolerance where neonatal mice are injected with allogeneic cells from recombinant mice differing only at K or D, the Class I loci of the mouse H-2). In contrast, tolerance to Class II molecules or to Class I and II, in combination, result in stimulation of Ts as well as having a functional absence of T helper cells.

In summary, although the basis for T cell tolerance is not entirely settled, there is good evidence arguing in favor of a major involvement of Ts. Ts are induced, resulting in tolerance, in situations that do not favor classical antigen presentation and T helper cell induction. Future research should establish the possible defect of T helper cells in tolerance.

What is happening with B cells in the examples of tolerance described previously? As noted in the experiment of aggregated HGG, B cell tolerance in adults can be induced using large amounts of antigen at a time when there is no activation of helper T cells. In the examples in Table 9.1 using haptens, tolerance at the B cell level could be induced using carriers which were either poorly immunogenic or non-immunogenic for T cells. Particularly effective were the use of: 1) synthetic polypeptides made of d-amino acids; 2) polysaccharides; and 3) non-immunogenic gamma globulins.

These observations indicate that, in circumstances where little or no helper T cell function normally exists, then direct interaction of the antigen with the B cell receptors at the appropriate concentration preferentially generates a tolerogenic signal to such cells. Conversely, in the presence of helper T cell function, an immunogenic signal to B cells results. What events determine this difference have to be settled.

In culture the interaction of the Fc receptor of B cells with an immunoglobulin generates a powerful inhibitory signal that makes the cell unresponsive to further stimulation. The nature of this signal is not known, but it could explain the ease of induction of B cell tolerance with haptens bound to non-immunogenic IgG (Table 9.1) or with deaggregated HGG (Figure 9.1). The incubation of B cells with non-metabolizable antigen appears to result in capping, followed by a limited reexpression of surface Ig in some B cells.

Finally, tolerance in B cells from young, neonatal animals is different from tolerance in B cells from adults. Again, these studies need to be done with cells from animals born very immaturely (like the mouse) or, otherwise, with cells obtained from early fetal life. We mentioned in Chapter 5 that B cells from newborns are immature and display only IgM in their membranes and no C3 receptors. When such B cells are manipulated in tissue culture, it becomes readily apparent that a brief interaction with a number of antigens, in the absence of T cell stimuli, readily induces tolerance. Recent studies have indicated that the B cell from newborn mice, after binding and capping its receptors, cannot regenerate new Ig. This implies that somehow these cells are at a particularly sensitive stage where interactions of membrane Ig with antigen result in powerful tolerogenic effects. It implies that perhaps B cell tolerance induced early in life may be accounted for by deletion of the clone of B cells, at least for a period of time.

The following experimental protocol illustrates the high susceptibility of B cell from neonates to tolerance induction:

1. Harvest B lymphocytes from newborn or adult mice.

2. Portion each set into tubes and incubate with 0.1 to 100 ug per ml of DNP-HGG (dinitrophenylated human gamma globulin) for twenty-four hours.

3. Remove the DNP-HGG by washing. Then, add DNP-LPS, culture for four days, and assay for number of antibody-forming cells by a

plaque method. DNP-LPS is *E. coli* lipopolysaccharide to which DNP groups are attached. DNP-LPS is a polyclonal activator for B cells and induces differentiation of all B cells.

Results: B cells from newborn mice were inactivated by the brief exposure to DNP-HGG (0.1 to 1.0 ug) and were unable to respond to the polyclonal stimuli. B cells from adult mice were partially unresponsive at the high concentration of 100 ug per ml. At 1 and 10 ug per ml, B cells from adult mice responded strongly with numerous anti-DNP, plaque-forming cells.

Finally, the question can be raised whether there are changes in macrophages responsible for tolerance induction. In all examples of tolerance, the cellular lesion is at the level of the T cell or the B cell. However, defects in macrophages could possibly favor induction of a tolerant state. We referred before to the situation in mouse neonates where the macrophages cannot express Ia because of suppressive influences in the environment. This lack of Ia may well be a crucial element favoring the lack of response in the neonate. These studies have not been done in humans, although initial reports do indicate a significant decrease in Ia-bearing monocytes immediately after birth.

Another example of tolerance induction resulting from a defect in antigen presentation can be found in studies using ultraviolet irradiation. UV light selectively damages the skin Langerhans cells. This damage results in failure to develop contact sensitivity upon percutaneous sensitization and in development of T suppressor cells.

Recovery from Experimentally Induced Tolerance: The tolerant state induced by various means in adult animals differs, in general, from natural tolerance to self-antigens in that the acquired tolerant state exists for a finite time and then subsides. The length of the tolerant state will vary depending on the animal model, type of tolerance, and mode of induction. Recovery from the tolerant state can either be spontaneous or induced.

The rate of spontaneous recovery generally reflects the generation time of stem cell precursors of the immunocompetent lymphocytes rendered specifically tolerant. This will, of course, also be governed by the presence of residual tolerogen in the animal which may be capable of tolerizing new cells as they emerge from the stem cell pool.

Several factors regulate the rate of spontaneous recovery. For example, recovery of responsiveness to T-dependent antigens will be delayed if the tolerant animal has been thymectomized or if it is very old. On the other hand, recovery is enhanced by factors which favor the rate of replacement of immunocompetent cells such as moderate doses of X-irradiation (which stimulates regeneration of bone marrow stem cells) or by transfusion of syngeneic lymphoid cells from a non-tolerant donor.

The state of acquired tolerance can be terminated or "broken" by certain experimental manipulations. There are three basic models for breaking tolerance: 1) the tolerant state induced to a protein (No. 1) can be broken by immunizing the animal, at an appropriate time, with a related protein (No. 2), provided there is suitable cross-reactivity between both (actually, the best situation is when protein 2 cross-reacts moderately, about 15%, but not too much, less than 75%). However, if protein 1 is administered at the same time of immunization with protein 2, the tolerance will not be broken.

The explanation is as follows: the animal is immunized with protein 2 at a time when the tolerance to protein 1 is found only in the T cells, for example, two months after immunization in the cases of Figure 9.1. The helper T cells will recognize only the determinants of protein No. 2 not shared with protein 1. The animal is still tolerant to protein 1 at the T cell level and, therefore, will not have helper T cell activity against those carrier determinants in common between 1 and 2. (These helper T cells collaborate with B cells reactive with various determinants in protein 2, including the shared determinants between 1 and 2.) Administration of protein 1, together with 2, stops the breaking of tolerance because B cells are again tolerized by protein 1. Table 9.2 summarizes these points.

2. Tolerance induced to a hapten conjugated to a protein carrier (i.e., DNP-OVA) can be broken by immunizing the animal with a DNP conjugate of an unrelated carrier such as DNP-BGG. In the second example, tolerance to DNP-OVA exists only at the level of OVA-reactive T cells. Immunizing with a different carrier like BGG permits collaboration with the anti-DNP B cells.

3. Tolerance to certain self-antigens, such as thyroglobulin, the main protein of the thyroid acini, can be broken by immunizing the animal with either denatured or hapten-conjugated thyroglobulin. We explain the third example by the fact that altering the native protein creates new antigens to which normal T cells are reactive, and which can then provide help to the B cells.

The case of autologous proteins: The issue of reactivity to self-antigens is discussed at length in Chapter 13, in the section on Autoimmunity. The question of whether B cells, helper T cells, or Ts are responsible for tolerance to self has been addressed in part by trying to immunize with self-antigens. Such immunization is indeed effective under special conditions and depending on the nature of the antigen. Here we want to stress the fact that maintenance of self-tolerance requires the continuous presence of the antigen—the example of the congenital absence of C components that we cited in the introductory paragraph to this chapter. A dramatic experiment which addresses this issue is that reported E. L. Triplett in frogs. During the embryonic stage of development, the pituitary gland was removed. When the embryos matured, the pituitary was implanted back into its original donor, which proceeded to react against it, rejecting the gland. A

Table 9.2

Breakdown of Tolerance by Cross-Reactive Immunization

Experimental Animal	Antigenic Determinants Recognized by Lymphocyte Clones when Challenged with:	
	Protein 1	Protein 2
Normal		
T cells	a,b,c	a,d,e
B cells	x,y,z	x,w,v
Tolerant to Protein 1		
T cells	_ _ _	_,d,e
B cells	x,y,z	x,w,v
Tolerant to Protein 1 Plus Excess of Protein 1		
T cells	_ _ _	_,d,e
B cells	_ _ _	_,w,v

Table 9.2. In this experiment, proteins 1 and 2 are deliberately chosen to have different antigenic determinants for T and B cells. Protein 1 contains determinants a, b, and c, each of which is recognized by different T cells clones (anti-a, anti-b, etc.), and determinants x,y,z, recognized by distinct B cell clones. Protein 2 contains determinants a,d, and e for T cells and x,w,v for B cells. Note that a and x are common to both proteins. The second and third columns show the available clones found in the T and B populations of the three different groups and to which the immune response is directed. Tolerant to Protein 1 animal immunized with Protein 2 will make an anti-x response because of T cell help through determinants d and e; this means that the antibodies will bind to protein 1 (to the common x determinant). Tolerant to Protein 1 Plus Excess of Protein 1 shows B cell tolerance to the common determinant x shared between Proteins 1 and 2. Hence, no anti-x antibodies are made capable of binding to Protein 1.

control in which only half of the pituitary was removed during the embryonic stage accepted the graft. Clearly, these experiments indicate the presence of self-reactive lymphocytes which remain inactive physiologically when exposed to the antigen which persists since early life. In our view, such lympocytes most likely remain inoperant in great part by maintenance of an active Ts.

REFERENCES

Billingham, R. E., Brent, L., and Medawar, P. B. Actively acquired tolerance of foreign cells. Nature, 172:203, 1953.

Gershon, R. K. A disquisition on suppressor T cells. Transplant. Rev., 26:170, 1975.

Howard, T. G., and Mitchison, N. A. Immunological tolerance. Prog. Allergy, 18:43, 1975.

Katz, D. H., and Benacerraf, B. Immunological Tolerance: Mechanisms and Potential Therapeutic Applications. Academic Press, Inc., New York, 1974.

Moller, G. E. (ed.) Transplantation Tolerance. Six papers in Immunol. Rev., Volume 46, 1979.

Nossal, G. J. V. Cellular mechanisms of immunologic tolerance. Ann. Rev. Immunol., 1:33, 1983.

Owen, R. D. Immunogenetic consequences of vascular anastomeses between bovine twins. Science, 102:400, 1945.

Triplett, E. L. On the mechanisms of immunogenic self-recognition. J. Immunol., 89:505, 1962.

Weigle, W. O. Immunological unresponsiveness. Adv. Immunol., 16:61, 1973.

CHAPTER 10

Immunogenetics

This chapter considers two genetic systems that control all immunological phenomena: the genes for Immunoglobulins and for the Class II MHC molecules. The structure of antibodies was described in Chapter 3. This chapter describes the organization of the Ig genes and their expression on B cells. The MHC, including its gene organization, was described in Chapter 6. The role of MHC products in cellular interactions was considered in Chapters 7 and 8. We describe here the effect of the MHC genes in controlling responses to proteins (Ir genes).

GENETICS OF THE IMMUNOGLOBULIN MOLECULES

Many of the studies on Ig gene expression have utilized techniques of molecular genetics, including recombinant DNA methods. This approach has revealed that, during the process of differentiation of a stem cell to a B cell and ultimately to an antibody-producing cell, there are a number of changes taking place in the organization and expression of various Ig genes. These changes or rearrangements of the Ig genes are essential for: a) the development of a specific antibody-combining site; and b) for the expression of different heavy chain isotypes—the class switch. The gene rearrangements that create the antibody-combining site take place during the non-antigen-driven differentiation of the B cell, i.e., the change from the stem cell to the immature B cell bearing an IgM molecule on its membrane. These gene rearrangements are responsible for the diversity of specificities of antibody molecules. The gene rearrangements that follow antigen stimulation of a B cell result in the switch in heavy chain classes while conserving the specificity of the antibody-combining site. Thus, it is by changes in gene organization that the two functions of Ig molecules—the specific one of antigen binding and the non-specific or effector one—are largely modulated.

Other genetic decisions are made by the B cell during its differentiation. The expression of heavy chain and light chain genes follows in sequence. Thus, a very early B cell—the pre-B cell—expresses only heavy chain in its cytoplasm but not on its membrane. At a subsequent stage, the light chains are synthesized, and the entire IgM molecule is assembled (immature B cell). Subsequently, IgM, and later IgD, are expressed and placed on the cell surface. The B cell also expresses the genetic information of only one chromosome, either the maternal or paternal allele. This phenomenon of allelic exclusion is the only example found in eukaryotic autosomal genes. Isotype exclusion is another phenomenon in which a B cell decides to express the genes for either kappa or lambda light chains. The antibody molecules made by a single plasma cell bear either kappa or lambda chains but not both (Chapter 3).

Organization of Ig Genes: There are three unlinked families of Ig genes, those for the kappa L chain, lambda L chain, and the H chain. In the mouse, these are located in chromosomes 6, 16, and 22, respectively; in humans, in chromosomes 2, 22, and 14. Each chromosome contains the genes coding for the variable and constant parts of the chain. In the germ line, the genes are organized as segments (exons) made up of a continuous sequence of nucleotides (about 330) that code for each of the domains of the Ig molecule. These gene segments (or simply genes) are separated from each other by sequences of DNA that are silent and are never expressed in the final translated protein—the non-coding or the intervening sequences or introns.

The first molecule in biology where it became apparent that more than one gene coded for a single polypeptide chain was the Ig molecule. The studies that first led to this finding were made before the advent of gene cloning. The early studies were based on the inheritance characteristics of allotypes and idiotypes (Chapter 3). Of particular importance were the studies on rabbit allotypes. The rabbit Ig allotypes were first described by J. Oudin at the Pasteur Institute, in Paris, who coined the name for intraspecies antigenic determinants of Ig molecules. Oudin immunized a rabbit with a rabbit antibody-antigen complex. He found antibodies that reacted with rabbit Ig from some but not all rabbits. The antibodies were reacting with unique determinants that were inherited as autosomal traits. Different allotypic systems, each with several allelic forms, were identified for the constant region of the gamma, alpha, and mu H chains and the kappa and lambda L chain. Most importantly, the rabbit is unique in having an allotypic marker in the variable region of the H chain. These a allotypes are accounted for by several amino acid substitutions localized to the framework region of the VH chain. C. W. Todd made the very important observation that a given a allotype could be found in IgG or IgM (for example, Ig molecules could be found that were gamma-positive, a1-positive, or mu-positive, a1-positive; a1 is an allele of the a locus). From these results, one could gather that two genes were involved, i.e., one gene coding for the variable region, where the allotype was localized, and the second gene for the constant region. In other studies, the allotypes of Groups e and d (in the H chain constant regions) were shown to be linked to those of Group a (V region allotypes). Crossover between C and V region allotypes were documented for rabbit families, providing further support for the conclusion that at least two separate genes were involved in the synthesis of an antibody H chain. The crossover frequency for CH and VH genes of the rabbit was estimated at 0.3%. Other studies on the sequence analysis of several light chains showed portions of great variability, at the N terminus, with portions of similar sequence at the C terminal half of the molecule. These results led W. J. Dreyer and J. Bennet to postulate that a single polypeptide chain of the Ig molecules must be encoded by two genes, one encoding the variable, the other the constant regions.

This postulate of Dreyer and Bennet was found to be correct when molecular analysis of the Ig genes was carried out, starting with the studies of S. Tonegawa at the Basel Institute in Switzerland. The description of Ig genes that follows is based on studies on mouse Ig which have been the most extensive to date. The Ig genes of the three unlinked families are organized as follows: For the kappa L chain, there are three sets of genes: V, J, and C genes. The V genes, about 290 nucleotides long, code for about ninety-five amino acids of the variable region (up to the third CDR, i.e., complementary determining region or hypervariable region). There are about three hundred V genes organized in tandem and separated by non-coding sequences. (Each V gene is preceded by a small gene segment coding for the signal peptide). The J genes include four to five different gene segments (also separated by introns) of about forty nucleotides long that code mainly for the fourth framework region of the variable chain. The C gene is a single gene segment that codes for the entire constant domain of the kappa L chain. The C gene is separated from the J gene by a long intron of about 1,100 nucleotide pairs. As noted, the variable domain is coded by two different genes, V and J, that are separated from each other by non-intervening sequences in the germ-line or in non-Ig-producing cells.

The genes coding for the lambda chain in the mouse are represented by two V genes (termed V1 and V2) and three pairs of J and C genes, J1C1, J2C2, J3C3 (corresponding to the subtypes of lambda chains in the mouse). A fourth pair, J4C4, is defective and not expressed. The V1 gene is joined usually with J1 or J3, and the V2 with J2. Lambda light chains in the mouse are of limited heterogeneity and comprise only 5% of the total Ig.

In the heavy chain there are four groups of gene segments: V, D, J, and C. The VH genes comprise a cluster of about one-hundred to two-hundred different segments, each about 295 base pairs coding for about ninety amino acids, including the third framework region. The D genes are represented by small segments of variable length that code for part of the third CDR (from six to seventeen residues). There are twelve different D genes. The J segment codes for the last ten to fifteen amino acids of the fourth framework region and comprises four different genes.

The complex of genes coding for the H chain constant region are organized as eight different sets of genes, in the mouse in the order mu, delta, gamma-3, gamma-1, gamma-2b, gamma-2a, alpha, and epsilon (Figure 10.1). (In the human, the CH gene sets contain nine genes: for mu, delta, gamma-1, gamma-2, gamma-3, gamma-4, epsilon, alpha-1, and alpha-2.) The CH genes are organized into exons, each coding for one of the domains of the molecules; some Ig (the genes for gamma, for example) contain a separate segment coding for the hinge region located between the exons coding for the first and second domains). The delta gene complex is peculiar in having only two exons coding for the constant regions and, in between them, an exon for the hinge. The delta gene is close to the mu segments. All the genes for a particular class or subclass are accompanied by two small exons coding for the intramembranous protein of the Ig molecule. The two exons are situated about two thousand nucleotide pairs 3' to the exon coding for the last domain of the secreted Ig.

<u>Generation of Diversity</u>. The great number of antibody-combining sites are created, to a great extent, as a result of rearrangements of the different gene segments encoding for the variable region; the V and J segments for L chains; and the V, D, and J for the H chain. For the L chains, each V gene associates at random with any of the J genes (<u>V-J joining</u>). In the case of the H chains, the V genes rearrange, first with any of the D genes, and then with any of the J genes (<u>V-D-J joining</u>). <u>This random rearrangement, therefore, creates a number of V-J and V-D-J combinations, depending upon the number of genes encoded in the germ line</u>. In the germ line and in non-antibody-producing cells, the various gene segments are not joined, maintaining their organization as was described above. During the differentiation of the B cell, the joining process then takes place. In the early stage of the pre-B cell, the genes for the H chains are first expressed and rearranged, followed by a similar process for the L chain genes. Once the H and L polypeptides are transcribed and translated, they assemble in the endoplasmic reticulum to form the molecule with a unique combining site.

The manner in which V-J and V-D-J joining occurs is not firmly established. There are many who agree that the rearrangements take place within each chromosome, although arguments have been raised for an unequal crossing over. Some clues on how the joining may take place come from the analysis of the intervening sequences between the various gene segments. All the V and D genes are followed by short, highly conserved sequences of seven and nine nucleotides separated by a space of unconserved nucleotides of either twelve or twenty-three nucleotide pairs in length. The D and J segments at their 3' side also contain a nonamer and heptamer (also separated by a space of twenty or twenty-three nucleotide pairs). The nonamer and heptamer that follow the V (or D genes) are inversely complementary to those that precede it (in the D or J segments). One hypothesis is that, during recombination, these conserved sequences come together or join with a specific enzyme looping out and deleting the intervening sequence.

There are two other mechanisms that increase the diversity of the variable region and which result from the joining of the different segments. One of the mechanisms occurs at the site of the joining (functional site diversity). The joining ends of V with J, V with D, or D with J are not precise and can vary by several nucleotides, giving rise to different amino acids from those encoded in the germ-line genes. (For example, particularly prominent is a "hot spot" at position 96 of kappa L chain in the mouse.) Another mechanism—functional insertion diversity—occurs with V-D and D-J joining and consists of the insertion of one to four nucleotides. These nucleotides are thought to be added in a template-independent way perhaps by the action of a terminal deoxynucleotidyl-transferase.

A final mechanism that increases the diversity is somatic mutation. A high rate of mutation was first documented among murine myelomas of the lambda type. This observation was later extended by nucleotide analysis. The rate of mutation of the Ig genes is high, occurring selectively at the V, D, or J segments but not at the C gene segments. Among the V chains, the mutations are also found in the intervening sequences although less frequently than in the gene segments. The mutations can be accounted for by changes in a single nucleotide pair. It is thought that the mutational event follows the V-J or V-D-J joining. The actual molecular mechanism responsible for the mutation is not known. It is possible that mutations appear to be frequent in the Ig gene because it is a system that selects for them through the antigen molecule.

In summary, then, antibody diversity arises from:

1. the number of genes in the germ line

2. the rearrangement of the different germ-line segments that code for the variable region

3. the process of functional site diversity

4. the process of functional insertion diversity

5. somatic mutations

6. combination of H and L chain

Concerning the number of antibody-combining sites capable of being generated, we can consider the information available on kappa and heavy chain genes in the mouse. The kappa gene with three hundred V genes and four J genes can give rise to 1.2×10^3 different combinations; the H chain genes with two hundred V genes, twelve D genes, and four J genes can give rise to 9.6×10^3; thus, the combination of H and L will give rise to about 10^7 antibody-combining sites. (This does not take into account points No. 3, 4, and 5 above; however, many of the genes so identified may not be expressed.)

Allelic and Isotype Exclusion. Allelic exclusion refers to the random expression by B cells or plasma cells of the maternal or paternal allele for each H or L chain. The other example of allelic exclusion in biology is at the level of X chromosome where one of the alleles remains nonfunctional. It was postulated by Lyon that one or the other X chromosome in somatic cells of females is rendered inactive at some early embryonic stage. Isotype exclusion refers to the phenomenon whereby a B cell expresses the genes for either kappa or lambda L chains, but not for both.

Allelic exclusion of the Ig genes can best be studied using the allotype markers. In Table 10.1 we describe an example using the B cells of a heterozygous rabbit and three different allotype markers. Two of the markers are localized in the H chain: the a marker, to the V region, linked with the d marker in the C region. The third, the b marker, is in the kappa L chain. Note that, while the individual antibody-producing cells exhibit only one allele of each group, any combination of paternal or maternal allotypes may be observed. Allelic exclusion takes place in all three families of Ig genes, for kappa L chain, lambda L chain, and heavy chains.

The molecular basis of allelic and isotypic exlcusion needs to be established. Definitely, the allelic- or isotypic-excluded protein is not synthesized by the B cell. The examination of L chain genes from B cell tumors has indicated that only one allele is functionally rearranged, while the other remains as in the germ line. In a significant number, however, one of the genes is defectively rearranged (joining the V gene with a non-J segment or vice versa). These aberrantly rearranged genes may be transcribed and even translated but do not encode functional L chains. With regard to the H chain genes, a high number of them are rearranged but aberrantly, and some can be transcribed and translated. The same phenomenon appears to hold for isotype exclusion where the rearrangement of the kappa or lambda gene is accompanied by aberrant rearrangements or no rearrangements at all of the other chain. The hypothesis has been made that allotypic exclusion develops by some mechanism in which the genes that are rearranged inhibit the subsequent rearrangement of the other allele. The same mechanism would apply for the exclusion of kappa-chain or lambda-chain genes.

Changes in Heavy-Chain Genes. The changes in expression of H-chain genes by the B cell is an important phenomenon that still requires elucidation at the molecular level. The small, immature B has exclusively membrane IgM; later the cell acquires membrane IgD to become a double producer. Following cellular interactions with T helper cells, there is a class switch with cells producing and secreting Ig of a different isotype. Such cells showing class switch will have on their membrane IgM plus the new Ig. The new Ig will also be secreted. The consensus is that the switch in isotypes follows the order of the heavy chain genes (i.e., that a mouse B cell will first switch to gamma-3 and then to gamma-1, to gamma-2b, to gamma-2a, etc.). Such orderly class switching has not been proven. It is very possible

Table 10.1

Phenotypes of Ig-Producing Cells in a Rabbit with Genotype

a1a2/b4b5/d11d12

	Mother	Father	Offspring
Genotypes	a1, d11/a1, d11	a2, d12/a2, d12	a1, d11/a2, d12
	b4 /b4	b5 /b5	b4 /b5
Phenotype in Plasma Cells	a1, d11, b4	a2, d12, b5	a1, d11, b4
			a1, d11, b5
			a2, d12, b4
			a2, d12, b5

(The parents were chosen to be homozygous at all three loci; note that the offspring plasma cell show allelic exclusion. The explanation is in the text.)

---

that a cell will switch to one isotype without having to express the intermediate ones. The switch in H chain genes could occur by two possible mechanisms: a) by rearrangements of the C genes in the germline configuration so that exons coding for some genes would be deleted and the remaining one brought into closer approximation with the rearranged V-D-J genes; or b) by the formation of a long primary RNA transcript which is later processed, resulting in the expression of multiple-messenger RNA. Evidence for these two processes have been brought forth. Clearly, the transcription of the H chain genes is a complex process regulated by biochemical events still not clearly understood (Figure 10.1).

The small B cell produces only membrane IgM. Apparently, a short-lived primary RNA transcript is made and from this derive two messenger RNA, one for membrane mu, the other for secreted mu. Both mRNA have been identified. As expected, the mRNA for membrane mu is longer than that for secreted mu and codes for the membrane and cytoplasmic portions of the molecule. Furthermore, the B cell translates both mRNA but expresses only the membrane IgM. The secreted mu chain contains core carbohydrates but lacks some terminal sugars. The reasons for a lack of assembly of the secreted mu are not known. Following activation, however, the secreted IgM is assembled and released.

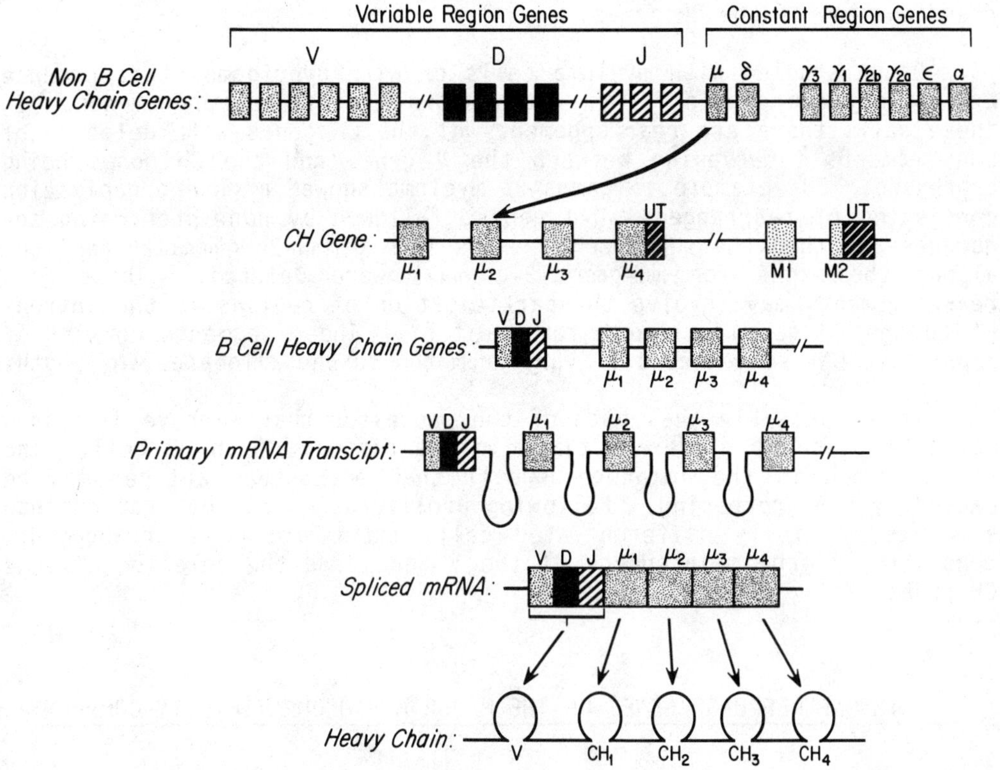

Figure 10.1. Organization of Heavy Chain genes. In non-B cells, the varous gene segments (depicted as boxes) are organized as shown in the graph; the V, D, and J segments are separated from each other. Each segment coding for the constant region is organized into exons and introns, as depicted, for the mu constant region genes (second line). Each box represents an exon coding for a constant domain. In the B cell (third line), the VDJ segments are now rearranged and joined, presumably, from a long primary messanger RNA, the mature mRNA for the Heavy Chain is generated.

At a later stage, the B cell co-expresses IgM and IgD on its cell surface. Such double producers have the same organization of mu and delta genes and bear mRNA for membrane and secreted mu and delta chains. Thus, it appears that the same VH sequences are spliced from a long primary RNA transcript and joined to the sequences for mu or delta. The same process has been thought to take place for the class switching of some immature B cells in culture. For example, in a B cell line that switched from IgM to IgG2b production, there was no rearrangement of the CH genes.

Other studies with myeloma cells or with hybridomas that produce exclusively one single isotype have shown a different phenomenon. In these cells there are rearrangements of the CH genes with deletion of DNA segments intervening between the V genes and the CH genes being expressed. For example, a gamma-2b myeloma showed a gene organization consisting of rearranged V-D-J genes, followed by non-intervening sequences and then the sequence of exons from gamma-2b-gamma-2a-epsilon-alpha; the exons for mu-gamma-3-gamma-1 were deleted. These gene rearrangements may involve the participation of regions in the introns 5' to the CH genes called S for "switch". These segments consist of repetitive DNA sequences that vary from ten to one kilobases in length.

It is possible that both of the processes that we have discussed may take place at different times in the history of the B cell. The class switch in the immature B cell that encounters antigen may be caused by RNA processing. Following proliferation and maturation into a secretory, fully differentiated cell, there are gene arrangements consisting of the maintenance of the V genes and the deletion of some CH genes.

THE IMMUNE RESPONSE GENES OF THE MAJOR HISTOCOMPATIBILITY COMPLEX

The MHC of the species was described in Chapters 6, 7, and 8. Chapter 6 described the organization of the genes, the characteristics of the two major gene products, the Class I and II molecules, and their role in cellular interactions and transplantation reactions. Chapters 7 and 8 described the role of Class I and II molecules in regulating the interactions of helper or cytolytic T cells. The purpose of this section is to review an aspect of Class II MHC genes not described earlier, which is their control of *in vivo* responses to selected protein antigens.

The studies described before established that the T lymphocytes are selected to recognize foreign antigens only when presented in the context of autologous MHC molecules. They also illustrated how Class II A and E polypeptides, the Ia antigens, determine the critical interactions that T cells undergo with macrophages and B cells, resulting in the generation of an immune response. Because the Class II molecules are extensively polymorphic, one should expect that individuals of different haplotypes may differ in their ability to develop T cell responses to selected antigens. After all, the Class II molecules play an essential contribution to the specificity of T cells. Indeed, *it* was found that low responsiveness or non-responsiveness to certain antigens was associated with selected MHC haplotypes. It is not surprising, therefore, that historically the MHC-linked Ir genes, and in fact the I region and its products, were discovered and defined in studies concerned with the genetic analysis of inbred strains of animals to respond to distinct protein antigens.

Three types of antigens have been most useful in the identification of the MHC-linked Ir genes:

1. Synthetic polypeptides with limited structural heterogeneity;
2. Alloantigens differing slightly from their autologous counterparts, i.e., minor histocompatibility antigens; and
3. Complex multideterminant antigens administered in limited immunizing doses, in conditions where only the most immunogenic determinants are recognized.

The discovery of specific MHC-linked Ir genes depended upon experiments where the immunological system is presented with a challenge of highly restricted heterogeneity and specificity. These conditions tend to limit the possibility of specific interaction between the antigens and clones of immunocompetent cells. The experiments revealed that the response of experimental animals to a wide variety of antigens is under the control of dominant MHC-linked Ir genes. All the antigens under Ir gene control share an important characteristic: they are thymus-dependent antigens. No MHC-linked Ir gene control has been observed to date for thymus-independent responses.

The first experiments that revealed differences in the immune responsiveness of individual animals to a selected antigen were carried out in random-bred guinea pigs with a DNP conjugate of the homopolymer of L-lysine, DNP-PLL. Breeding studies revealed that the ability to respond to DNP-PLL was controlled by a single dominant autosomal gene that determined both the ability to develop specific cellular immunity to DNP-PLL and anti-DNP antibodies. The DNP-PLL responder animals were able to produce specific antibodies to any haptens to which the PLL carrier was conjugated. Thus, the genetic control of the response to DNP-PLL could be attributed to the ability of the responder animals to recognize the PLL carrier as an immunogen. The defect in "non-responder" guinea pigs, unable to respond to DNP-PLL, was not due to their inability to synthesize anti-DNP antibodies. Accordingly, the immune defect in DNP-PLL non-responder animals could by bypassed if the animals were immunized with DNP-PLL coupled to an immunogenic T-dependent carrier such as ovalbumin (OVA), i.e.:

DNP-PLL:	No anti-DNP response
DNP-OVA:	Anti-DNP antibodies made
DNP-PLL-OVA:	Anti-DNP antibodies made

(The guinea pigs are unresponsive to PLL because of some defect at the level of the generation of helper T cells. In the case of immunization with DNP-PLL-OVA complex, the DNP-PLL behaves operationally as a hapten, the OVA being the carrier [Chapters 2 and 8]. Since the non-responder guinea pigs can respond to OVA, it will be able to generate helper T cells that collaborate in the anti-DNP antibody response.)

These experiments led to the conclusion that the specific process controlled by Ir genes did not concern the capacity to form antibodies but rather the ability to generate helper T cell activity. These studies were then extended to the two inbred strains of guinea pig strains 2 and 13. (These strains were later shown to differ primarily at the I region of the MHC of the guinea pig.) Similar studies on the genetic control of specific immune responsiveness were done with other synthetic antigens, the copolymers of L-glutamic acid and L-alanine (GA) and of L-glutamic acid and L-tyrosine (GT). These experiments are illustrated in Table 10.2, where responsivesness is shown to be linked to MHC loci.

Table 10.2

Inheritance of Specific Ir Genes and of the Major Histocompatibility Loci of Guinea Pigs of Strain 2, Strain 13, (2 x 13)F1, and Backcrosses

	Strains				
Antigens	2	13	(2 x 13)F1	(2 x 13)F1 x 13	(2 x 13)F1 x 2
DNP-PLL	+	—	+	+ (50%) - (50%)	+ (100%)
Glutamyl alanine copolymer (GA)	+	—	+	+ (50%) - (50%)	+ (100%)
Glutamyl tyrosine copolymer (GT)	—	+	+	+ (100%)	+ (50%) - (50%)

Table 10.2. Plus indicates responsiveness and presence of major histocompatibility specificities associated with the responsive status.

Similar observations were made in the mouse by H. McDevitt, M. Sela, and collaborators when studying the response to the (T-G)A-L polypeptide described in Chapter 2. They found strains of mice that responded immunologically but others that did not. By breeding experiments and using genetic strains that differed only at the MHC, they established that there was a very close linkage between the capacity of a strain of mice to make an immune response and its MHC haplotype (Chapter 6). The immune response genes were mapped using recombinant inbred strains of mice. The genes mapped in a new region of the H-2 complex between the K and D regions. This region was defined as the I region (Chapter 6). Similar I regions to which Ir genes map and which also code for the major antigens capable of stimulating mixed leukocyte reactions were later detected in other mammalian species.

The identification of Ir genes in the I region motivated an attempt to prepare antibodies against determinants coded for by the I region genes. Mice and guinea pigs which differ genetically only at the I region were immunized reciprocally with each other's lymphoid cells; the alloantisera obtained detected a new class of antigens expressed on most B cells, a large fraction of macrophages, and also on a small percentage of T cells. These antigens were given the generic name of Ia antigens and corresponded to the Class II molecules discussed in Chapter 6. The anti-Ia antibodies were later used to characterize the nature of the molecules (Chapter 6).

The development of anti-Ia alloantisera detecting specificities on lymphocytes and macrophages provided another approach to the characterization of I region gene products. Loci coding for serologically distinct I specificities were mapped to the I-A and I-E subregion, defined by Ir genetics as indicated above. These Ia antigens of the I-A and I-E subregions are found primarily on B cells and marophages (Chapter 7). Another subregion defined by serological techniques and designated I-J codes for determinants on suppressor T cells and suppressor T cell factors.

The discovery that some I region loci that code for the Ir genes also code for the Ia antigens with distinct specificities raised the question whether the Ia molecules are themselves the Ir gene products. There is general agreement that this is the case. Ir genes equal Ia antigens, the Class II molecules of the MHC. Studies in mice and guinea pigs, in particular, indicated a close association between Ia specificities and Ir gene-controlled responses. Also, monoclonal antibodies to Ia antigens blocked the *in vitro* response to antigen controlled by Ir genes. Two other findings on responses to selected antigens are of particular significance. The response to selected antigens, exemplified by the GLPhe (composed of glutamic acid, lysine, and phenylalanine) synthetic polypeptides required two complementing Ir genes, one encoded in I-E, the other in I-A: the F1 mice from two appropriate non-responders could make a response. Later biochemical studies established that the E polypeptides were coded in two loci, the alpha chain in I-E and the beta chain in I-A (Chapter 7). Finally, a mutation in the beta chain of A polypeptide has been found to correlate with distinct changes in the response to protein antigens.

The analysis of the cellular interactions (Chapters 7 and 8) and the Ir gene studies described here led to the conclusion that all antigenic determinants are recognized in the context of the A or E Class II molecules of a given specificity (haplotype). Take, for example, six antigenic determinants, numbered 1 through 6, and four haplotypes of the A molecules labeled a, b, d, and k. A pattern of response could be:

	1	2	3	4	5	6
a:	+	+	—	+	+	—
b:	+	+	+	—	+	+
d:	—	—	+	+	—	+
k:	+	+	—	+	+	+

Individuals of a given haplotype, say a, will be able to respond to a selected series of determinants 1, 2, 4, and 5 but not 3 and 6. A protein containing a single determinant, say number 3, will be immunogenic on individuals bearing haplotypes b and d but not in those bearing a and k. A protein that contains multiple determinants—say 1 to 5—will evoke responses in individuals of most haplotypes—in our case, all of them. To see "Ir gene effects", one would then have to give this protein in such small amounts so that only dominant determinants are recognized. In our example, if the dominant determinant (i.e., the strongest) is 4, we would find that haplotype b would be a nonresponder to the protein when given in limiting amounts. However, administering high doses would allow the response now by way of the minor determinants 1, 2, 3, or 5. A diagram with the actual data of responder and non-responder status of various strains of mice to a number of proteins is shown in Figure 10.2.

The Cellular Locus of Ir Gene Effects. Since the Class II molecules are the Ir genes, it follows that these genes are operating at the level of the cells that carry them—normally the macrophage or the B cell. The question remains whether the defect in non-responders to a given antigenic determinant lies at the level of interaction of Class II molecules with the antigenic determinant in the presenting cell or with the recognition by T cells of the Class II molecules plus antigens. In the first case, one needs to postulate that Class II molecules and a specific determinant enter into some complex or close interaction and that the T cell receptor interacts with the complex. With some alleles, simply, this combination will not take place (determinant selection hypothesis). The second hypothesis requires that the

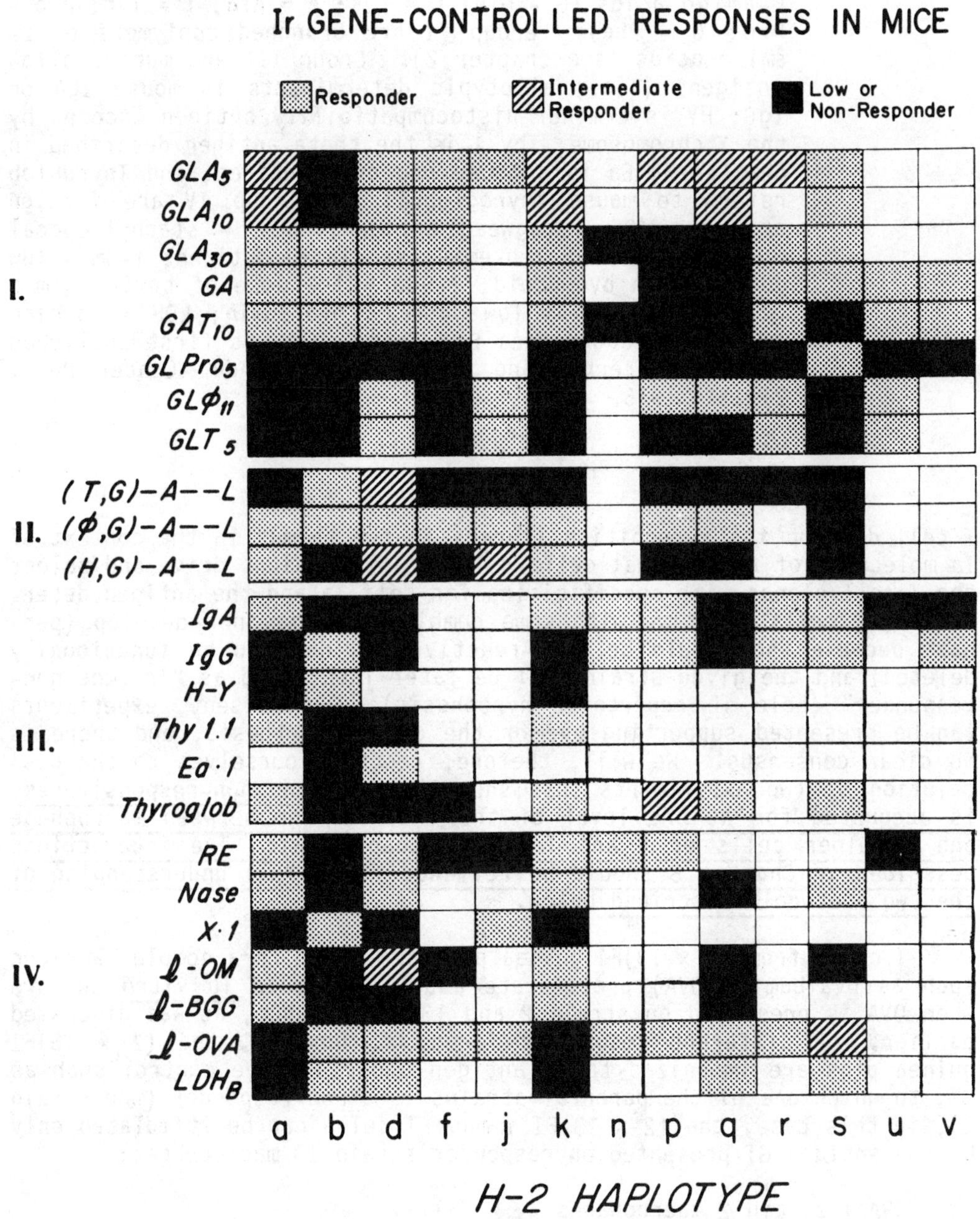

Figure 10.2. The explanation for this figure is on the next page.

Figure 10.2. This diagram shows the response of various inbred strains of mice of the indicated H-2 haplotypes to four sets of antigens. Group I refers to random linear copolymers of L-amino acids (G - Glu; L = Lys; A = Ala; T = Tyr; Pro = Pro; Ø = Phe). Group II are branched coplymers of L-amino acids (see Chapter 2). Group III are murine allo-antigens (i.e., allotypic determinants in mouse IgA or IgG; HY is a minor histocompatibility antigen encoded by the Y chromosome; Thy 1 is the theta antigen described in Chapter 5; Ea is a mouse red cell antigen; and Thyroglob refers to mouse thyroglobulin). Group IV are foreign antigens (RE = ragweed antigen; NASE = staphylococcal nuclease; X1 = a leukemia-associated antigen; 1-OM = low dose of hen ovomucoid; 1-BGG = low dose of bovine gamma globulin; 1-OVA = low dose of ovalbumin; LDH = porcine lactic dehydrogenases B. This table was first published by D. Benacerraf and D. H. Katz in Adv. Cancer Res., 21:121, 1975.

T cell develop its recognition library in the thymus in the context of Ia molecules of the stromal cells. These interactions drive and select the T cell clones with specificities for self-Ia and the antigen determinant; T cells reactive with some combinations may not develop (perhaps because they would be self-reactive and need to be functionally deleted) and the given strain will be later identified as "Ir gene non-responder" (hole in repertoire hypothesis). At present, experiments can be presented supporting one or the other hypothesis, and there is no clear consensus. We will, thefore, restrict ourselves to the description of two experiments that show that Ir gene non-responsiveness is accounted for at the level of the interactions between macrophage and T helper cells or B and T cells (Chapter 8). The interactions described in Chapter 8 should be reviewed for a full understanding of the two protocols described below.

T cells from (2 x 13)F1 guinea pigs immunized to a complex antigen such as ovalbumin (OVA) proliferate equally well in *in vitro* culture when OVA is presented on strain 2 and 13 macrophages, as was discussed earlier. A different result is found if, however, the (2 x 13)F1 guinea pigs are immunized to an antigen under Ir gene control such as GT, to which one of the parental strains is a non-responder (the strain 2); in this case, the (2 x 13)F1 immune T cells can be stimulated only by the antigen GT presented on responder strain 13 macrophages:

OVA + strain 2 macrophages:	++++
OVA + strain 13 macrophages:	++++
GT + strain 2 macrophages:	No response
GT + strain 13 macrophages:	++++

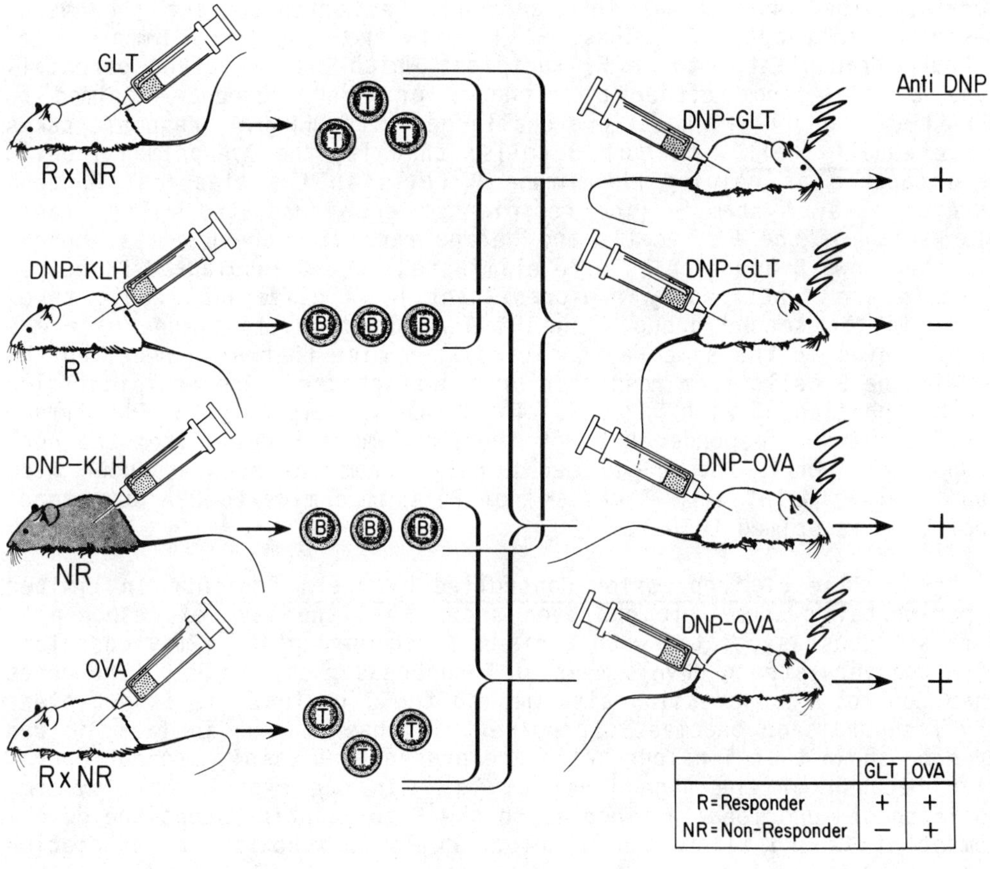

Figure 10.3. The explanation is in the text.

The same approach can be used to study Ir gene function in B cells. A typical experiment is shown in Figure 10.3. This is a complex but very important experiment that follows the experimental protocol designed to demonstrate I region control of T-B cell cooperation analyzed in Chapter 8. Some inbred strains of mice respond to the synthetic random copolymer glutamyl-lysyl-tyrosine (GLT), while others do not. The response to a complex, multideterminant antibody as OVA, however, was found to be similar among the various inbred strains at the usual doses of immunization. Thus, mice from a strain unresponsive to GLT respond perfectly well to OVA. The experiment is done as follows: F1 mice, crosses between a responder strain and non-responder strain to GLT, are divided into two groups: one group is immunized with OVA, another with GLT. Both groups will respond to both antigens. Subsequently, the T cells are isolated from each and assayed for the capacity to help B cells from the responder or non-responder parental strain. The assay takes into account the hapten-carrier phenomenon described in Chapter 8. Thus, F1 T cells from the group immunized to OVA are transplanted to an F1 recipient which also received parental-type B cells from either a responder or a non-responder primed to DNP-KLH. When the F1 hosts are challenged with DNP-OVA, response takes place equally well with both B cells; that is, the OVA-primed T cells were capable of helping DNP-immune B cells in the classical hapten-carrier assay system. (The recipients were irradiated after transplantation of the F1 T cells and before receiving the B cells, hence, all their own B and T cells were eliminated; the transplanted F1 helper T cells are functionally radioresistant.) A different result takes place in the second group. The F1 T cells from GLT-immune mice are transplanted in the same way to irradiated mice that also received the DNP-immune B cells from responder or non-responder. The recipient mice are now challenged with DNP-GLT. The F1 cells help only the DNP-immune B cells from a responder but not the DNP-immune B cells from the non-responder! Thus, the DNP-primed B cells from the non-responder mice can receive "help" from T cells from F1 primed mice to OVA but cannot from T cells primed to GLT.

The Case of Suppression Controlled by the I Region. In limited experimental systems, it has been shown that the lack of response to some antigens associated with a given I region haplotype may correlate with the very strong development of T suppressor cells (Ts). The genes that control T suppression also map to the I region. It is not clear why T suppression becomes so prominent in these cases; in fact, it can even be shown that T helper cells are present but simply are not operative because of the high level of Ts. In one experimental system, addition of monoclonal antibodies to the E polypeptide stops the development of Ts and allows for T helper cells to function in association with the A molecules. Perhaps this system operates by the recruitment of Ts by helper T cells that recognize antigen and the E molecules. The involvement of the I region in suppression also involves the I-J molecules. These determinants are found in factors that regulate suppression (Chapter 8). At present, it is not clear whether I-J maps to the I region, nor do we know the structure of its gene products.

REFERENCES

Benacerraf, B. Role of MHC gene products in immune regulation. Science, 212:1229, 1981.

Germain, R. N., and Benacerraf, B. A single major pathway of T lymphocyte interactions in antigen-specific immune suppression. Scand. J. Immunol., 13:1, 1981.

McDevitt, H. O., and Chinitz, A. Genetic control of the antibody response: relationship between immune response and histocompatibility (H-2). Science, 163:1207, 1969.

Moller, G. (ed). Ir Genes and T Lymphocytes. Immunol. Rev., 38, 1978.

Tonegawa, S. Somatic generation of antibody diversity. Nature, 302: 575, 1983.

Wall, R., and Kuehl, M. Biosynthesis and regulation of immunoglobulins. Ann. Rev. Immunol., 1:393, 1983.

CHAPTER 11

Tumor Immunology

A vast literature supports the concept that tumors bear antigens different from those of the normal host tissue and to which the immune system of the animal can respond. In recent years, a great deal of effort has been directed to determining the nature of such immune responses to tumor-associated antigens (TAA's), to exploring the manner in which these responses affect tumor growth, and to finding methods able to regulate the anti-tumor response to the host's benefit.

Attempts to demonstrate immunity to malignant tissue were made in the early 1900's. Tumor cells from one mouse grew only for a limited time when transplanted to another and then were rejected. We discussed in Chapter 6 that these experiments used outbred mice and that the rejection was due to responses to normal tissue alloantigens. The first clear-cut reports of syngeneic tumor immunity involved chemically induced tumors. Using inbred mice, small pieces of a sarcoma were transplanted from one mouse to another. After allowing the tumor to grow for a short while, the blood supply to the tumor was interrupted by tightly tying a suture around the base of the tumor. This ligation technique caused the malignant cells to die. The animals, thus cured of their tumors, were then able to reject a second implant of the same sarcoma, but not of other unrelated cancers. Mice not immunized by the ligation technique were unable to stop the growth of the sarcoma (Figure 11.1). Later, it was established that differences in normal tissue antigens were not responsible for the tumor rejection. Immunization, either with skin grafts or by injection of tissue cells, did not protect mice from tumor grafts coming from the donors of the normal tissue. The tumors possessed unique antigens distinct from those present on non-malignant cells.

Chemically Induced Tumors. Three important concepts in tumor immunology came from studies on chemically induced tumors:

1. Non-dividing (heavily irradiated) tumor cells can be used to immunize animals. This provides a way of examining immunity to tumors that disseminate early after transplant and thus cannot be candidates for treatment by ligation/excision.

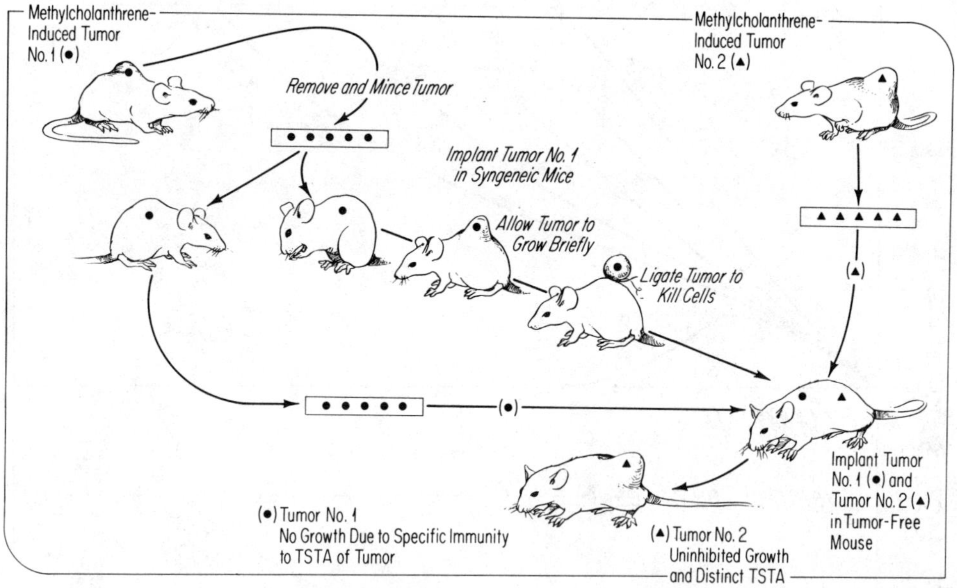

Figure 11.1. Active immunization by the growth and ligation method. Viable cells from a chemically induced tumor are transferred to a syngeneic recipient. After a brief period of tumor growth, the site of the tumor is ligated (or tied) to prevent blood flow and to kill the tumor. Alternatively, the area containing the malignant tissue can be surgically removed. The tumor-free animal is then rechallanged with cells from the original tumor. The first tumor is rejected due to the prior immunization of the animal with the same tumor, while the antigenically unrelated tumor grows in the same manner as it would in a completely untreated animal. This demonstrates that 1) tumor immunity exists and 2) it is highly specific.

---

2. <u>The resistance of animals immunized to syngeneic tumors is quantitative.</u> Non-immune animals permit growth of smaller inocula than immunized animals. Progressive tumor growth occurs in immune animals when larger numbers of tumor cells are transferred (Figure 11.2).

3. <u>Each tumor induced by carcinogenic chemicals is antigenically distinct from all others, as assessed by cross-immunization-transplant experiments.</u> Thus, two tumors induced in different animals by the same chemical, in one animal by the same chemical, or even different parts

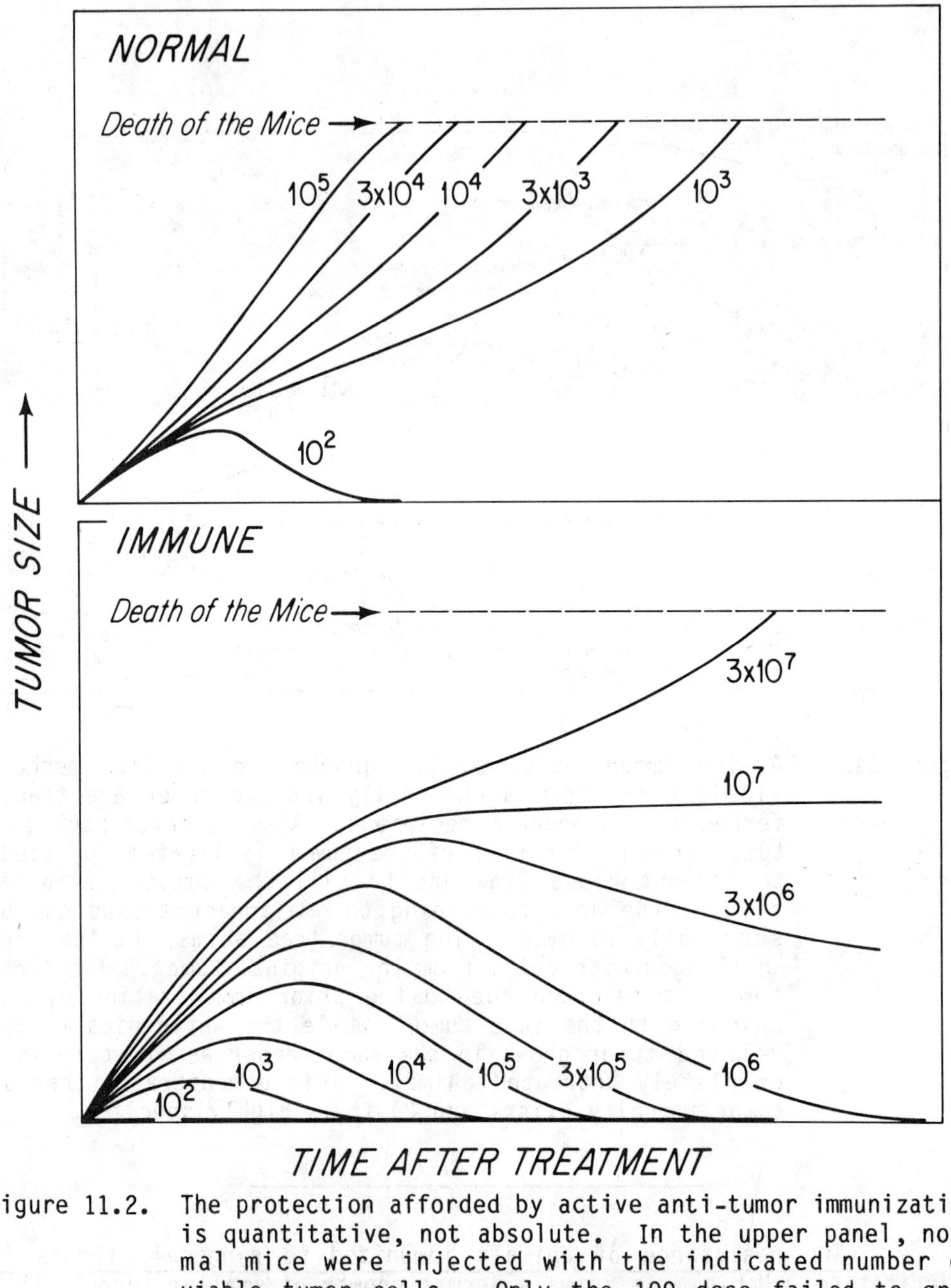

Figure 11.2. The protection afforded by active anti-tumor immunization is quantitative, not absolute. In the upper panel, normal mice were injected with the indicated number of viable tumor cells. Only the 100 dose failed to grow progressively. Higher numbers of tumor cells grow until the animal dies, with the rate of growth dependent on the initial tumor load. In the lower panel, the growth of the same tumor in actively immunized mice is illustrated.

of one large tumor induced by one chemical, are immunologically distinct from one another in transplantation tests. Recent studies have confirmed that the immunodominant tumor-specific transplantation antigens (TSTA's) of chemically induced tumors are distinct (Figure 11.3) but have also provided some evidence suggesting a sharing of weaker tumor-associated antigens (TAA). Some of these shared TSTA's may be associated with endogeneous RNA viruses found to be present in certain chemically induced sarcomas.

Virus-Induced Tumors. Virus-induced tumors also bear TAA's capable of inducing rejection responses. However, in contrast to chemically induced tumors, different tumors induced by the same virus, or family of viruses, share TSTA's (Figure 11.3). This is true even for tumors arising from different tissues. In certain systems, such as tumors induced by DNA viruses, such as SV40 and polyoma, the common TSTA's are distinct from antigens of the virus itself, since cells transformed by these viruses do not produce virus. Immune responses to tumors induced by viruses are often very strong in comparison to those generated to chemically induced tumors.

Tumor-Associated Antigens. The precise nature of most tumor antigens is unknown. It is clear that the tumor-specific transplantation-type of antigens (TSTA) are located at the cell surface where they are accessible to the receptors of effector cells and antibody. In carcinogen-induced tumors, the uniqueness of TSTA's suggests that they arise from mutational events affecting some previously normal cell product. In virally induced tumors, the sharing of TSTA's is apparently due to the fact that viral products, such as capsid proteins for the RNA tumor viruses which bud continuously from transformed cells, or non-virion products controlled by the viral genome of DNA tumor viruses, serve as the target antigens. These virally induced TSTA's are common in all cell types transformed by the virus. Recent evidence suggests that the recognition of virally induced TSTA's by cytolytic T cells is restricted by the H-2 complex in mouse model systems. This indicates that H-2 products and TSTA's may interact on the cell surface to form the actual antigen seen by the particular effector cell (see Chapter 7).

In addition to transplantation-type antigens, tumors also possess several other types of tumor-associated antigens. Many tumors have so-called "oncofetal" antigens, which are actually embryonic or fetal cell products re-expressed in the transformed (malignant) adult tumor cell because of depression of the fetal genes. Examples of such antigens in man include alpha-fetoprotein, secreted in large amounts primarily by hepatocarcinoma cells, and CEA (carcino-embryonic antigen), produced by tumors of the gastrointestinal tract, especially colonic adenocarcinomas. These oncofetal antigens are not involved in the host anti-tumor response; when secreted in large quantity (such as alpha-fetoprotein), they can serve a clinically useful purpose as a marker for tumor load and recurrence or metastases after therapy.

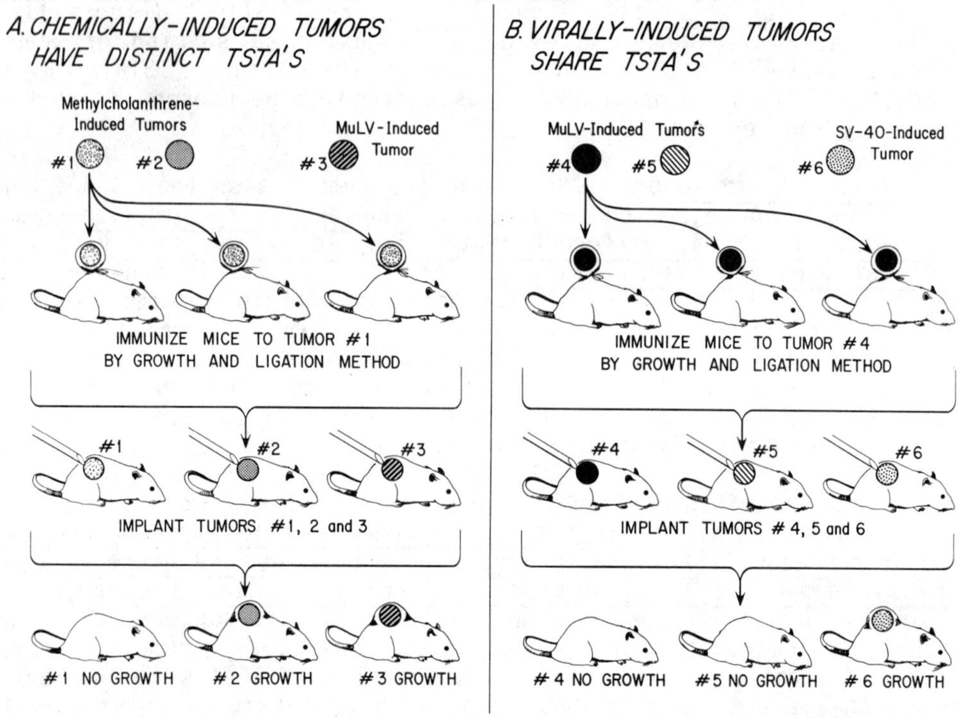

Figure 11.3. Chemically induced tumors have distinct TSTA's, while virally induced tumors share TSTA'a. This is illustrated diagrammatically in this figure. In panel A, mice are immunized by growth-ligation to the chemically induced methylcholanthrene fibrosarcoma #1. Different immune mice are then challenged with an appropriate number of viable cells from tumor #1, a distinct methylcholanthrene tumor #2, or a murine leukemia virus (MuLV)-induced tumor #3. All tumors are syngeneic to the recipient. As can be seen, only tumor #1 is rejected by the mice immune to tumor #1. Even though it was induced by the same chemical in the same inbred strain, tumor #2 is not rejected, nor is the unrelated virally induced tumor #3. This contrasts with panel B. In this case, immunization to MuLV-induced tumor #4 protects against both tumor #4 and MuLV-induced tumor #5, but not the unreleated SV-40-induced tumor #6. Thus, tumors induced by the same virus in animals with the same MHC antigens clearly share TSTA's.

A third type of antigen is found in tumors caused by DNA tumor viruses. This antigen, called the T antigen, is specific for the inducing virus but is not a structural protein of the virus. It stimulates antibody production in the tumor-bearing host. The use of such antibody in the immunofluorescence test reveals high concentration of T antigen in the nuclei of tumor cells. The T antigen probably represents a viral protein produced early after infection and necessary for viral reproduction and cell transformation. The appearance of this antigen serves as a useful marker for infection and/or transformation of cells by DNA tumor viruses. Because of its internal location, however, it is not an important antigen in tumor rejection phenomena and is thus distinct from TSTA's.

IMMUNE SURVEILLANCE

The demonstration of specific immunity to tumor-associated antigens provided the experimental basis for the theory of immune surveillance. This theory states that the immunological mechanisms underlying rejection of allografts actually evolved as a means of distinguishing self from non-self, the latter being malignantly transformed cells bearing TAA's. The immune system maintains "surveillance" over the body, rejecting small clones of malignant cells, as they arise, if they are sufficiently distinct antigenically from normal tissue. Though widely accepted for its simplicity and logical appeal, this concept is by no means established as true by hard data. Whether such a "surveillance" mechanism functions at all has been widely debated. Attempts to test the prediction of this theory have yielded both supporting and non-supporting data. Cells transforming spontaneously *in vitro* in the absence of immunoselection have very little *in vivo* immunogenicity, yet, the theory would predict that lack of immune selection would yield highly immunogenic tumors. The frequency of spontaneous or chemically induced tumors in mice immunosuppressed by anti-lymphocyte serum (ALS) or due to congenital lack of a functional thymus (nude mice) is no different than in immunologically intact animals, though the loss of the surveillance mechanism should result in increases in tumor frequency in the former group. Very small tumor inocula, approaching in cell number the early stages of clonal tumor development, rather than being efficiently rejected, often "sneak through" the immune defenses of the host, while larger inocula are rejected. On the other hand, immunosuppressed animals are much more susceptible to tumor development by oncogenic viruses such as polyoma than are immunologically intact controls. In man, clinical immunosuppression results in increased tumor frequency, as the theory predicts. In mice, progressive tumor growth after murine sarcoma virus inoculation is inversely related to immune response to the tumor. Finally, "natural" immunity to certain virally induced tumors exists and appears to correlate with tumor resistance.

It is likely that immune surveillance does operate to prevent development of some malignancies. Immunoregulatory events, ill-defined, non-specific mechanisms of defense and local anatomic and physiologic conditions may play important roles in the surveillance process. Attention has been focused on Natural Killer (NK) cells as the possible cellular mediators of immune surveillance (see below).

CELLULAR IMMUNITY AGAINST TUMORS

The basis for resistance to tumors resides in the cellular, rather than humoral, immune compartment. This was established in early experiments using two methods. In one, "neutralization" of tumor cells by admixture with immune, but not normal, lymphoid cells was observed when such mixtures were inoculated into syngeneic recipients unable themselves to reject the tumor (Figure 11.4). The second method was adoptive transfer of immunity by cells transplanted to normal syngeneic recipients. Cells from tumor-immune animals protected the new host against subsequent challenge with the appropriate tumor, using either chemically or virally induced tumors.

The ability of antisera to affect tumor growth has also been tested. In only a few cases *in vivo* has antisera from tumor-immune animals been able to passively protect non-immune animals from tumor growth. This protection can be seen mainly against leukemias. In most other cases, such sera had no effect or enhanced tumor growth for reasons discussed below.

At least four different cell types have been found to play a role in tumor immunity: 1) T lymphocytes; 2) B lymphocytes; 3) NK cells; and 4) macrophages. The basic properties of these cells were reviewed in Chapter 5.

Helper and Cytolytic T Lymphocytes (CTL). The importance of T lymphocytes in the adoptive transfer of tumor immunity and in mediating *in vitro* tumor cell destruction is well documented. Helper T cells play a role by regulating the expansion of CTL (Chapter 7) and by secreting mediators. Prominent among the lymphokines is interferon-gamma which can 1) activate macrophages, and 2) increase NK cell activity. The CTL are thought to function not only by directly killing tumor cells but also by secreting interferon-gamma. Except for the antigenic determinants to which they are directed, no significant differences are known between CTL directed to tumors or to cells bearing alloantigens. Thus, information derived from studies of the latter apply to the former.

Demonstration of the role of CTL in immunity to syngeneic tumors comes largely from experiments employing virally induced tumors of rats and mice. In many experiments, adoptive transfer of immunity to tumors depended upon T lymphocytes from the immune donors. These same T cell

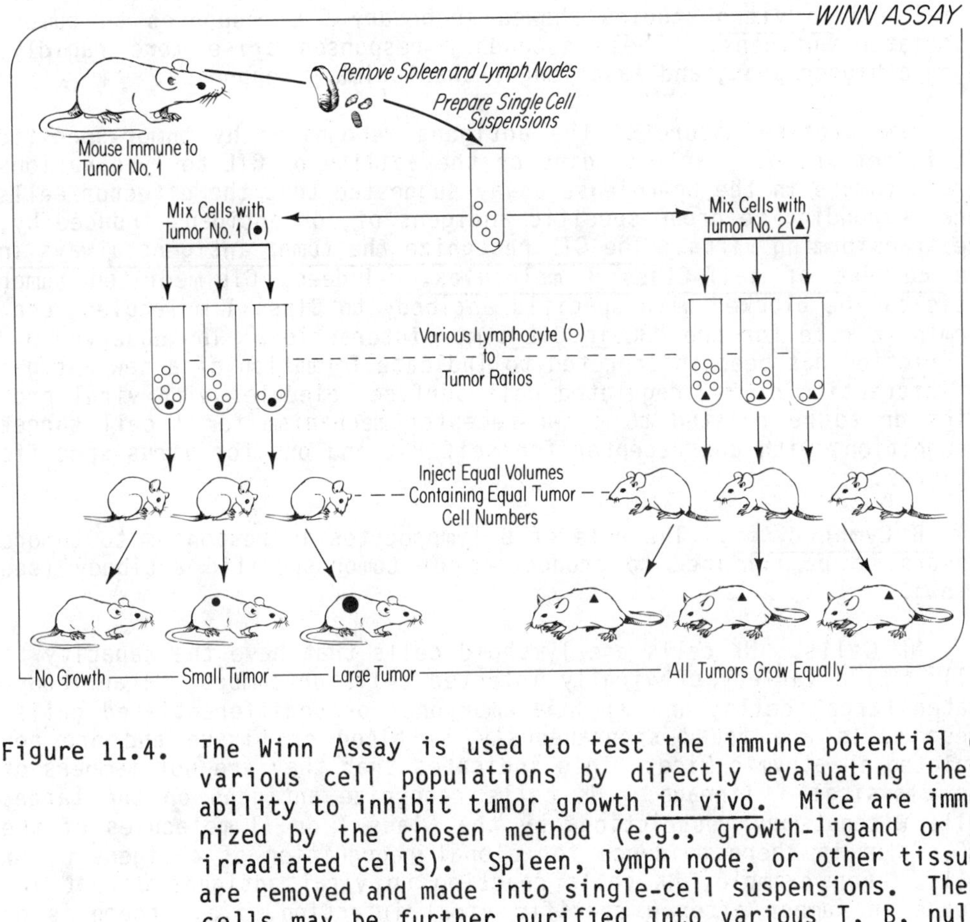

Figure 11.4. The Winn Assay is used to test the immune potential of various cell populations by directly evaluating their ability to inhibit tumor growth in vivo. Mice are immunized by the chosen method (e.g., growth-ligand or X-irradiated cells). Spleen, lymph node, or other tissues are removed and made into single-cell suspensions. These cells may be further purified into various T, B, null, macrophage, or other subpopulations. Differing numbers of the immune cells are then mixed with constant tumor cell numbers and the mixtures injected subcutaneously into normal or immunologically incompetent syngeneic mice. If the chosen immune cell source has anti-tumor activity, this will be seen as a decreased rate of tumor growth compared to control mice receiving normal cells mixed with the same number of tumor cells. Furthermore, the specificity of this anti-tumor activity can be tested using mixtures with a second tumor not used for the immunization of the effector cell donor.

---

populations mediated in vitro lysis of tumor cells labeled with chromium-51, indicating the presence of CTL (Chapter 7). Furthermore, in vitro restimulation of lymphoid cells bearing anti-tumor CTL, with the original tumor, resulted in the selected growth of the CTL and in increased tumor destruction by the cultured cells. Clearly, both animal and *in vitro* studies showed secondary CTL responses to tumor-associated antigens. These secondary responses arise more rapidly, reach a higher peak, and last longer than primary responses.

The precise nature of the antigens recognized by tumor-specific CTL is not known. Early studies on the ability of CTL to lyse various target tumors in the Cr-release assay suggested that the effector cells were responding to group-specific antigens of, or antigens induced by, the transforming virus. The CTL recognize the tumor antigens always in the context of self-Class I molecules. Indeed, CTL-mediated tumor lysis can be blocked with specific antibody to Class I molecules, confirming a role for the MHC in CTL-tumor interaction. The observed H-2 restriction has been interpreted to indicate formation of a new antigen by interaction of H-2-regulated cell surface molecules with viral proteins or to be related to a two-receptor mechanism for T cell target recognition, with one receptor for self H-2 and one for virus-specific antigens.

B Lymphocytes. The role of B lymphocytes in responses to tumors appears to be confined to production of tumor-specific antibody (see below).

NK Cells. NK cells are lymphoid cells that have the capacity to kill: 1) a variety of virally infected cells or tumors, 2) antibody-coated target cells, and 3) some embryonal or undifferentiated cells. These cells are found spontaneously in blood or tissue and are not depleted in athymic mice. This indicates that they are not members of the classical T lineage. NK cells recognize antigens on the target cells without any restrictions by the Class I or II molecules of the MHC. Nor is there evidence for clonal recognition of antigens by NK cells. For example, NK cells reacting to viral antigens do not increase in number after a specific viral infection, i.e., there is no immunological memory insofar as NK activity is concerned. The activity of NK, however, can be regulated, in two ways: 1) interferons increase the number and activity of NK cells. In fact, interferon causes multiple effects: dormant NK cells readily become active, an active NK can bind more target cells, NK cells can repeat cycles of binding and killing targets several times. The effect of interferon can be produced with as little as a ten-minute incubation followed by a one-hour period of time in which new protein synthesis is necessary. 2) Prostaglandins of the E class inhibit NK activity.

The precise role of NK cells in anti-tumor defense needs to be established. In the mouse, different inbred strains display different levels of NK, and this level correlates well with the capacity of the mice to develop anti-tumor defense. Mice with high levels of NK have a lower incidence of spontaneous or induced tumors. In an experimental system involving mice, transplantation of NK cells from high-level inbred strains results in protection against some tumors. In contrast, cells from low-level inbred strains did not protect. In humans, there is some relationship between levels of NK cells found in peripheral blood mononuclear cells and the extent of tumor growth. Thus, there is a great interest at present on whether the concept of immune surveillance can be accounted by the NK cell. The spontaneously high level of NK in normal blood, their capacity to recognize many antigens, and the relationship between NK level and tumor growth discussed above are all persuasive arguments for these cells having a critical role.

Whether NK cells have a protective effect in conjunction with antibody is not established. NK cells have Fc receptors and *in vitro* can kill target cells coated with antibody by the mechanism known as antibody-dependent cellular cytotoxicity (ADCC). There is no firm evidence on whether this mechanism operates in anti-tumor defense.

Macrophages. We discussed in Chapter 7 that macrophages, activated by T cell-derived lymphokines, can kill tumor cells. It is believed that such activated macrophages may play a role in anti-tumor immunity. Indeed, macrophages have been found to infiltrate tumors. The tumor-bearing macrophages can be shown at some stages of the tumor growth to be activated and to destroy the tumor cells. However, as the tumor grows, the macrophages are less activated and inhibited in their response to lymphokines. This indicates that the process of macrophage activation can be suppressed in the actively growing tumor. Since macrophage activation is dependent on T cell activity, it follows that processes that modulate T cell function can affect the degree of macrophage activation.

In vivo evidence for the participation of macrophages in tumor rejection is limited. Some investigators have claimed that injections of agents which affect macrophages may promote tumor growth. Since these agents (silica, for example) may affect other cells, the interpretation of the result must be made with reservation. Microscopic observations have revealed a lack of tumor cell multiplication in viral-induced sarcomas, at sites of heavy monocyte infiltrates. We do not know if this is a primary antitumor effect of macrophages or a scavenging response to already damaged and dead cells. Finally, irradiated mice have been shown to be unable to reject tumor allografts when provided with immune lymphoid cells fully capable of transferring adoptive tumor immunity to non-irradiated recipients, suggesting a necessary role for a radiation-sensitive, non-lymphoid cell, presumably a monocyte, in tumor rejection. It is apparent that clearcut data on this point is not yet at hand.

Other Immune Anti-Tumor Mechanisms. Antibody: Antibodies to tumors can produce several possible effects: 1) kill tumors, by fixation of complement; 2) kill tumors by way of an ADCC mechanism; or 3) produce antigen-antibody complexes involving soluble tumor antigens, resulting in inhibition of various cellular effectors. Overall, the role of antibodies in anti-tumor defense has been highly controversial. The best evidence indicates some degree of protection against leukemias. In solid tumors, the evidence points to a negative effect that will be further analyzed below.

MECHANISMS OF ESCAPE FROM ANTI-TUMOR DEFENSES

In the face of these myriad potential means at an animal's disposal for destroying tumor cells, the ability of small numbers of tumor cells to escape destruction and grow until causing the death of the host requires some mechanism(s) by which the tumor cells circumvent or blunt the immune response. Several such mechanisms have been documented to date (Table 11.1).

The simplest mechanism possible for a tumor to escape destruction by an immune response is simply to bear no antigens that the immune system recognizes as foreign. Although a few examples of tumors appear to meet this criterion, these negative results may simply indicate that such tumors engender weak responses that cannot be measured by standard assays. The vast majority of tumors tested for active immunization elicit some, albeit often weak, immunity; animals bearing tumors almost invariably demonstrate some immune reactivity to their tumors. Hence, absence of a response because of lack of antigenicity cannot explain successful tumor growth in most cases. Under certain circumstances,

Table 11.1

MECHANISMS OF ESCAPE FROM ANTI-TUMOR DEFENSES

1. Lack of recognizable TAA's	Weak. Essentially all tumors tested can be shown to be immunogenic to some degree.
2. Maximal immune response quantitatively insufficient to compete with tumor growth rate	Fair. Consistent with quantitative nature of protection after active immunization with tumor.
3. Inhibition of response by "blocking factor" (antibody or antigen-antibody complexes)	Fair. Experimental data exist in several species both at *in vitro* assay level and *in whole* animal.
4. Inhibition of response by suppressor T cells and factors	Good. Directly demonstrated in several model systems both *in vivo* and *in vitro*.
5. Protection due to tumor architecture or tumor cell secretion of inhibitory materials	Good. Based on morphologic observations and some *in vitro* and *in vivo* experiments.

however, particular animals may be incapable of responding to certain TAA's by virtue of a lack of the appropriate immune response (Ir) gene(s).

A second possibility is that the response elicited is simply too weak to cope with the tumor burden. Since in most, but not all cases, tumors can be shown to be highly susceptible to immune destruction in vitro, it is commonly assumed that weakly immunogenic tumors escape destruction by producing new cells faster than the limited number of immune effectors i.e., a simple quantitative failure of the immune system. Some support for this hypothesis comes from studies on the ability of actively or adoptively immunized animals to resist graded doses of tumor. With continuing immunization or with transfer of greater numbers of preimmunized cells, the minimum number of tumor cells needed to get a "take" also increases, as if each immune effector could kill a fixed number of tumor cells. Any tumor in excess would escape to kill the host.

It appears, however, that more complex mechanisms than these are responsible for the failure of the immune system to contain tumor growth. The most widely studied and documented mechanism is that involving soluble blocking factors, present in the serum of tumor-bearing hosts. Such factors can be demonstrated to interfere with in vitro cytotoxicity assays, as well as to enhance tumor growth in vivo. They have been found in studies involving chemically induced, virally induced, and spontaneous tumors in several species. Because such material could block immune function in an antigen-specific manner, they were presumed initially to be antibodies. Subsequent isolation of active serum fractions showed that efficient blocking was mediated by antigen-antibody complexes. Blocking complexes can be eluted from the surface of lymphoid cells from tumor-bearing animals; these cells, freed of blocking complexes, will demonstrate a previously undetectable cytotoxicity in vitro.

Most of the studies looking at blocking factors employ the microcytoxicity assay which detects largely ADCC effector function. Since such cells require free Fc receptors to mediate ADCC, antigen-antibody complexes should inhibit cytotoxic function. Because of the blocking properties of immune complexes, B cell stimulation by tumors is a two-edged sword.

Another example of the immune system acting against itself and favoring tumor growth, involves specific suppressor T lymphocytes. These cells, which play important roles in the regulation of immune responses other than to tumors, have been found to be present and active in animals with growing tumors. Such suppressor T cells inhibit the development of effector anti-tumor responses, including the development of cytolytic T cells. Transfer of spleen or thymic cells from mice bearing an actively growing tumor into normal mice results in promotion of growth of freshly implanted tumors.

Experiments have been done attempting to selectively eliminate T cells from mice bearing an actively growing tumor using critical doses of anti-lymphocyte serum (ALS). ALS is an antiserum obtained from rabbits immunized with murine lymphocytes. Injected into mice, it affects primarily circulating T cells. Furthermore, small amounts of ALS appear to selectively deplete the suppressor T cell population. More recent studies have reproduced the effect of ALS by injecting tumor-bearing mice with antisera to the I-J region of the MHC. These antibodies affect the suppressor T cells.

How do the suppressors enhance tumor growth? It has been demonstrated that the T suppressor pathway involved in regulating tumor immunity is complex and involves several sets of Ts. Thus, tumor antigen triggers can stimulate a first set, termed Ts-1 (inducer) cells, which produce a specific suppressor factor that activates a second population of Ts. These Ts-2, in turn, produce another soluble specific factor which acts in concert with a third, antigen-primed Ts population (Ts-3). The result of this latter interaction is the release of a suppressive molecule that inhibits helper T cells, thus preventing effective CTL or antibody production.

Finally, it is possible that the tumor cells may produce molecules that have a negative effect on the immune system. Tumor cells release soluble membrane proteins and are, therefore, a continuous source of antigens which may stimulate the Ts pathway rather than the helper T cells. Aside from these, there is some indication of as yet uncharacterized molecules released by the tumor that directly inhibit macrophage activation and NK cell activity. The role of these molecules is now being studied.

SOME COMMENTS ON IMMUNOTHERAPY

Because the immune system, left alone, is often unable to cope with tumor growth, many attempts to augment its effectiveness have been made. Two general approaches have been employed to this end: 1) prophylactic or therapeutic immunization with normal or treated tumor cells identical or sharing antigens with the tumor against which an augmented specific immune responses is desired; and 2) treatment with a variety of non-tumor-related adjuvant materials to increase specific or non-specific resistance to tumors.

As outlined above, inoculation of animals with viable tumor cells at a dose which causes temporary growth, then regression, or surgical removal or destruction of a progressively growing tumor, usually results in relatively strong specific resistance to rechallenge with the original tumor. Similar results can be achieved with some, but not all, tumors if cells are heavily irradiated and given repeatedly as prophylactic immunizations to the host, prior to tumor transplant. Chemical treatment of the surface of tumor cells used for preimmunization has been reported to increase the ability of such cells to immunize. The techniques used include conjugation to protein or DNP and treatment with iodoacetate or *Vibrio cholerae* neuraminidase. In the last case, some success at therapy of established tumors, rather than prophylaxis, has been claimed. Cell-free vaccines, consisting of cell membranes or partially purified soluble extracts, have also shown ability to preimmunize against certain tumors. Finally, inoculation of oncogenic virus can protect against subsequent challenge with tumors caused by the same or related virus. In all these examples, the resistance is specific for the immunizing agent (tumor), and there is no increase in immunity to unrelated tumors. It is, therefore, believed that these methods act as any antigen does, by priming and boosting the animal to expand the number and perhaps activity of the relevant immune cells (i.e., induce memory) before suppressive or blocking mechanisms can interfere.

The second group of treatments involve several agents, almost all possessing the common ability to potently stimulate macrophages. An attenuated strain of mycobacterium, the Bacillus Calmette-Guerin or BCG, is the best studied of these materials. Pre-immunization with BCG leads to generally increased resistance to a whole range of tumors. Intralesional, but not systemic, administration of BCG can lead to partial or complete regression of growing tumors. These properties are also possessed by certain BCG components, including specially prepared cell walls, a methanol extract, and even certain purified cell wall components. A similar ability to cause a generally increased resistance to tumors and to cause local tumor regression when given intralesionally is possessed by *Corynebacterium parvum* and double-stranded RNA (poly I:C). When these agents are used prophylactically, animals having resisted growth of a given tumor, better than control animals, may show no increase in resistance to a second challenge of the same tumor. When these agents are used therapeutically, the cured animals usually exhibit increased immunity to rechallenge with the same, but not with an unrelated, tumor. These divergent results have been interpreted to indicate that the prophylactic treatments increase some non-specific (macrophage?) mechanism that prevents the tumor from growing upon transplant, thus resulting in rejection without sufficient antigenic stimulation to induce a specific response. In the therapeutic protocol, it is unclear whether non-specific rejection occurs and the specific immunity merely is increased or whether the function of the stimulated phagocytes is to act as an adjuvant to boost specific immunity, which then leads to tumor rejection.

Human Immunotherapy. There have been numerous attempts at human immunotherapy using some of these approaches. In France, physicians have treated patients with leukemia with cell vaccines prepared from allogeneic leukemia cells, with some small measure of success. In many countries, BCG or *C. parvum* is being tried in protocol studies on several solid tumors. Most work to date has been with malignant melanoma patients. BCG injected directly into melanoma skin lesions does lead to tumor regression locally in many cases. However, systemic regressions are rare. Use of widespread scarification immunization with BCG has led to very marginal improvement in the treatment of melanoma patients with metastatic disease. The complications of such therapy, consisting mainly of "BCG'osis", a systemic active BCG infection, or severe allergic responses, are becoming more frequent. C. parvum, used as a killed vaccine, may avoid the first type of complication but not the second. Some workers feel, however, that it may be more active than BCG. Treatment with interferon, which may act against tumors via augmentation of immune destruction of malignant cells, is currently being evaluated.

There is intense on-going research in development of monoclonal antibodies directed to specific tumor antigens (Chapter 4). These monoclonal antibodies would have the advantage of their exquisite purity and specificity and could be used not only to trace tumor deposits but to destroy them. The idea is eventually to attach a toxic molecule to the monoclonal and, in this way, selectively destroy the target cell.

REFERENCES

Fidler, I. J., and Poste, J. Macrophages and cancer metastasis. Adv. Exptl. Med. Biol., 155:65, 1982.

Hellstrom, K.E., Brown, J. P., and Hellstrom, I. Monoclonal antibodies to tumor antigens. Contemp. Top. Immunobiol., 11:117, 1980.

Herberman, R. B., and Ortaldo, J. R. Natural killer cells: their role in defenses against disease. Science, 214:24, 1981.

Kamo, I., and Freidman, H. Immunosuppression and the role of suppressive factors in cancer. Adv. Cancer Res., 25:271, 1977.

Moller, G. (ed). Antibody carriers of drug and toxins in tumor therapy. Immunol. Rev., 62:1982 (contains eight articles reviewing this form of immunotherapy).

CHAPTER 12

The Classical and Alternative Complement Sequence

The discovery of complement emerged from observations made just before the turn of the century, that normal serum exerts a destructive effect upon bacteria. This action of normal serum was lost when the serum was heated to 56 degrees C. The heightened bactericidal activity of serum from an immunized host was also lost when the serum was heated to 56 degrees C but could be restored by the addition of serum from a non-immune host, thereby indicating the involvement of at least two activities. The heat-labile element was termed complement by Bordet and the heat-stable factor, earlier termed sensitizing substance or amboceptor, is now known to be antibody. The antibody is of the IgM class when present in normal serum as natural antibody arising by subclinical and cross-reacting immunogenic exposure, and of the IgG class in the specifically immunized host.

The ease with which lysis of erythrocytes could be observed with complement and antibody directed to erythrocyte surface antigens led modern workers to use this target cell to develop intermediates bearing specific antibody and various complement components. These cellular intermediates were then used to define the order in which various complement components reacted, examine the stability of various steps in the sequence, delineate the effective one-hit nature of a productive interaction, and establish assays of exquisite sensitivity. With the application of modern techniques of protein chemistry to the purification of components assayed by the hemolytic cellular intermediates, the classical system was defined as being composed of nine sequentially acting proteins.

One of the most unusual aspects of the complement story relates to the discovery and rediscovery of the alternative complement pathway. During the early 1950's, Pillemer and associates observed that the incubation of normal human serum with certain microbial polysaccharides, such as the polysaccharide zymosan derived from yeast, in the presence of the appropriate cation, magnesium, led to the inactivation of the classical late acting complement components without apparent participation of the classical early acting components. When such a serum was activated with an immune complex, the utilization of the early acting classical components was profound and generally more marked than the inactivation of the late components. The discoverers of the zymosan effect noted that a non-complement protein was bound to the particle, and that the presence of this protein, termed properdin, was essential for the reaction sequence which led to late acting component utilization. Their observation attracted widespread interest because serum depleted of properdin, by adsorption with zymosan and removal of the particles by centrifugation, lost its capacity for lytic reactions against a diverse variety of microbial agents. The critique of the concept focused upon the alternative interpretation that the effect was due to the action of classical complement and a vast pool of natural antibodies of low affinity. Although Pillermer's original collaborators purified properdin in subsequent years and thereby established that it was not an immunoglobulin or complement component, it remained for others to rediscover the properdin system by approaches from several different directions.

The evidence for an alternative pathway to activation of the classical late acting components included: 1) the anti-complementary activity of immune complexes composed of 5S rabbit IgG (i.e., pepsin digested) and, therefore, lacking the classical complement component activating site; 2) the complement-activating or anti-complementary activity of a guinea pig immunoglobulin class (IgG1) naturally lacking the classical pathway activating site; 3) the immunochemical evidence that the enzymatically active components of the classical and alternative activating pathways were distinct; and 4) the finding that an anti-complementary protein in cobra venom acted without the involvement of the classical early reacting proteins.

The importance of the initial recognition of the properdin-dependent serum system is that it represented the first substantial approach to the definition of a non-specific human defense system. This postulate has recently been validated in molecular terms with the demonstration that the alternative or properdin pathway is composed of an alternative activating and amplification phase. The direction of the amplification step to the microbial surface affords the host a mechanism of augmented resistance with the capacity to distinguish non-self from self despite the lack of an antibody requirement.

The entire complement system, as currently understood, consists of nineteen plasma proteins (Table 12.1) whose designations conform to two conventions. The classical components, which are the plasma proteins responsible for the lysis of cells bearing antibody directed to cell surface antigens, are symbolized with a capital C and a number designating the component, eg., C1, C4, C2, C3 and C5 through C9. The alternative pathway factors, which lead into a lytic terminal sequence without a requirement for antibody, are denoted with a capital letter, eg., B, D and P (properdin) in recognition of their distinct nature and discovery after the classical components. A bar over a letter or number, as in $\overline{C1}$, indicates the enzymatically active form of the protein, and cleavage fragments are suffixed with lower case letters, eg., C3a and C3b, with the suffix "b" generally noting the larger of the two

Table 12.1

Physiochemical Characteristics of Proteins of the Complement System

	Approximate Molecular Weight (Daltons)	Serum Concentration (ug per ml)	Cleavage Fragments
Clq	390,000	70	
Clr	95,000	35	
Cls	85,000	35	
C4	180,000	430	C4a, C4b, C4c, C4d
C2	117,000	30	C2a, C2b
C3	190,000	1,300	C3a, C3b, C3c, C3d
C5	190,000	75	C5a, C5b
C6	128,000	60	
C7	120,000	55	
C8	163,000	55	
C9	79,000	200	
P (Properdin)	220,000	25	
D	25,000	2	
B	95,000	240	Ba, Bb
C$\bar{1}$INH	105,000	180	
C4bp (C4-binding protein)	1,100,000	250	
I (C3bINA)	93,000	50	
H (beta-1-H)	150,000	400	
S-protein	80,000	500	

fragments. The loss of defined activity by a protein, when not associated with alterations in the primary structure, is noted by the placement of the letter "i" after the protein as in C2i and Bi, which are major fragments whose binding sites have decayed so that they can no longer form a complex with another complement protein and express the peptide hydrolase activity of their respective active sites. When a protein loses a defined activity, as a consequence of peptide hydrolysis unaccompanied by fragmentation, it is denoted by a preceding "i" as in iC3b, the form of C3b with alpha chain cleavage and loss of hemolytic functions. The most critical step in the elaboration of the biologic functions of the complement system is generation of C3b, the major cleavage fragment of C3. All complement proteins may be grouped into functional divisions according to their interactions with C3 (Figure 12.1). There are two pathways for <u>initial cleavage of C3</u>, the classical and the alternative; <u>a single amplification mechanism</u> comprised of alternative pathway proteins which augment C3 cleavage once initial C3b has been generated; and a <u>final common effector sequence</u> which the initiation and amplifying pathways activate after C3b has been generated.

The activation of the complement system, by either the antigen-antibody-dependent classical pathway or the cell-surface-mediated alternative pathway, results in the elaboration of the cardinal factors of a host inflammatory response. This has directed attention from the original emphasis on the cytolytic potential to a more broadly based role in the amplification of specific and non-specific host defense.

THE CLASSICAL PATHWAY OF COMPLEMENT COMPONENT ACTIVATION FOR C3 CLEAVAGE (FIGURE 12.2)

If antibody-antigen aggregates are added to serum, the first component (C1) is bound and converted into an active protease that catalyzes the activation of the fourth (C4) and second (C2) components. Activated components in the form of major fragments C4b and C2a form a complex, C4b,2a, that has proteolytic activity and catalyzes the activation of the third component (C3).

<u>First Component (C1)</u>. C1 is formed from three subcomponents, C1q, C1r and C1s. In serum, which contains 5 mM Ca, C1r and C1s are in a tight equimolar complex but their interaction with C1q is weak. C1q binds weakly to monomer IgG but strongly to aggregated IgG (i.e., IgG bound to antigen, forming an immune complex). Electron microscopy shows C1q to have a hexamer structure. A variety of evidence suggests that interaction between C1q and aggregated antibody occurs through the second constant domain of the antibody and the non-collagenous heads of the C1q hexamer structure. C1q consists of six subunits, each containing a globular head connected to a collagen-like stem. This was

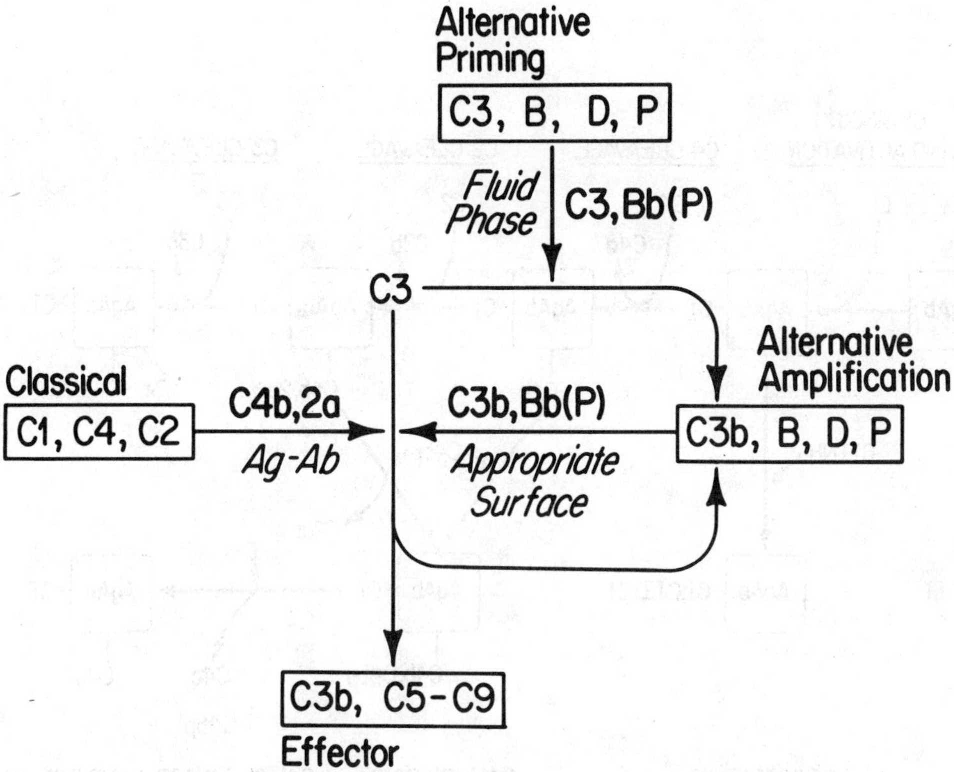

Figure 12.1. Relation of the classical and alternative pathways of complement activation to C3 and the effector sequence of complement. Antigen-antibody complexes (Ag-Ab) initiate formation of the classical pathway C3 convertase, which can cleave C3 to generate C3b and activate C5 to C9. The alternative pathway amplification C3 convertase, C3b,Bb, is assembled when C3b that was initially generated by the priming C3 convertase, C3,Bb, or by C4b,2a, is deposited on a surface with appropriate biochemical characteristics. Properdin (P) is shown in parentheses to indicate that it serves an augmenting but not always essential role in the function of alternative pathway C3 convertases. (From Fearon, D. T., and Austen, K. F., New Engl. J. Med., 303:259, 1980).

---

surmised from a combination of electron microscopy and selective degradation of "head" and "stems" with protease and collagenase, respectively. The globular portions carry the binding regions for the CH2

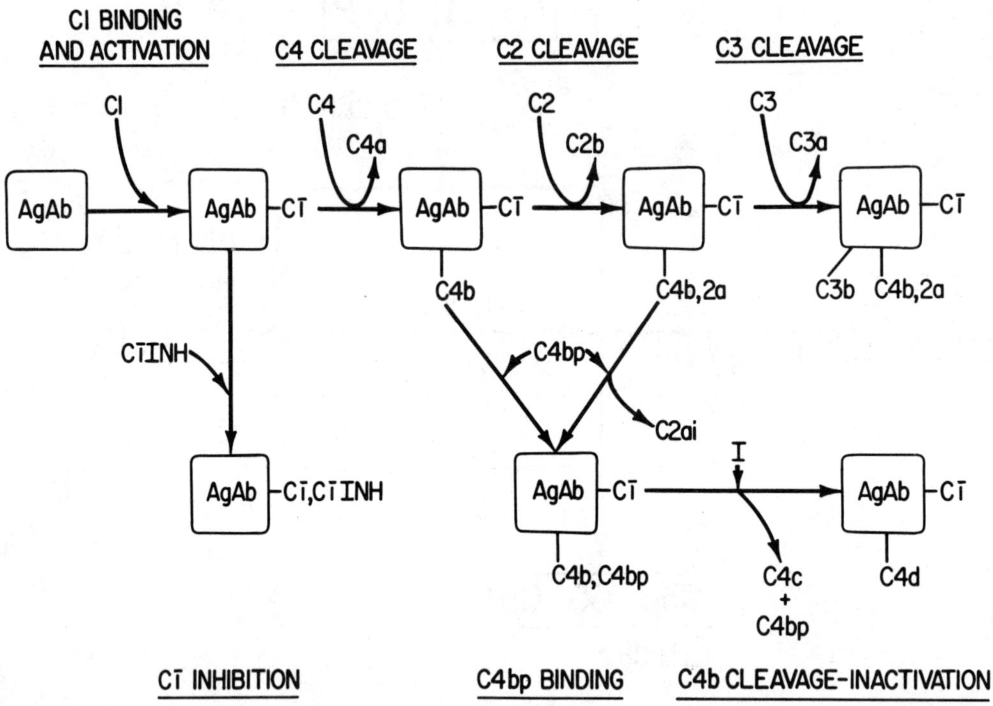

Figure 12.2. <u>The classical pathway of complement activation.</u> An antigen-antibody complex (Ag-Ab) initiates the reaction by binding C1 which then self-activates. The C1 cleaves C4 and C2 whose major fragments form a bimolecular complex, C4b,2a, the classical pathway C3 convertase. Formation of the C3 convertase is regulated by the control proteins, C1INH, C4pb, and I. (From Glass, D. N., Fearon, D. T., and Austen, K. F. In: The Metabolic Basis of Inherited Disease, Fifth Edition. Edited by J. B. Stanbury, J. Wyngaarden, D. Frederickson, M. Brown, and J. Goldstein. New York, McGraw-Hill, in press.)

---

domain of IgG with a valency of 3 to 5 Clq per IgG and the composite stem presents the binding region for the calcium ion-linked tetramer containing Clr and Cls. Crosslinking of Clq to an immune complex then induces a conformational change in Clr that catalyzes self-hydrolysis to generate C1r. The active site on the smaller of the disulfide linked chains of C1r then hydrolyzes C1s to yield C1s. C1s and C1r are both single chain polypeptides that form two chains of approximately 60,000 and 30,000 upon cleavage activation. The C1s subunit C1 is then involved in the cleavage of C4 and C2 to form the classical C3 convertase, C4b,2a.

<u>Fourth Component (C4)</u>. This component, a glycoprotein with a molecular weight of 180,000 and a beta electrophoretic mobility, is composed of three polypeptide chains linked by strong non-covalent interaction as well as by disulfide bonds; an alpha chain of 90,000; a beta chain of 70,000; and a smaller gamma chain of 33,000 molecular weight. Cleavage of C4 by C1s releases a 7,000 to 11,000 molecular weight fragment, designated C4a, from the N-terminus of the alpha chain; the residual major fragment is C4b. C4b serves five functions: 1) irreversible binding to immune complexes and cell membranes via a nascent site that otherwise undergoes rapid decay to fluid phase C4i, which is not capable of binding; 2) binding to immune adherence receptors present on a variety of cells via a stable binding site on C4b; 3) interaction with C1 to allow more efficient cleavage of C2; 4) continued binding to activated C2 to form C4b,2a, the classical pathway C3 convertase; and, 5) in the state of C4b,2a, interaction with C3b to form C4b,2a,3b, a protein complex called the classical pathway C5 convertase. Fluid phase C4i retains all the capacities of C4b except the binding to membranes by the nascent site. Several proposals have been advanced for the effect of C4b/C4i on C2 cleavage by C1. These include an allosteric modification of the active site of C1 to uncover the specificity for C2, an allosteric modification of the substrate C2 to expose the site vulnerable to proteolytic attack by C1s, and the provision of a site for deposition of the products, C2a, to allow interaction of C1s with additional C2.

<u>Second Component (C2)</u>. C2 is a single chain glycoprotein of 117,000 molecular weight which is cleaved by C1s into C2a and C2b. The C2a of 85,000 molecular weight bears the catalytic site, whereas the C2b of 35,000 molecular weight serves as an activation peptide with a linkage function. Thus, C2 has two interdependent sites uncovered by the action of C1s: an enzymatic site on C2a and a binding site for C4b on the smaller C2b fragment. C2a must be associated with C4b or C4bi in a magnesium ion-dependent binding in order to express C3 cleaving activity. The complex undergoes termperature-dependent decay due to release of C2i and attendant loss of C3 convertase function. The residual C4b is capable of reforming new C3 convertase upon cleavage of additional C2 by C1s. This indicates that the decay of the convertase is secondary to the loss of C2a and that native C2 displaces any residual C2b on the C4b site. C4b,2a is designated <u>classical C3 convertase</u> since it is derived from the interaction of the classical early components and may activate the effector sequence of complement, C3 to C9.

THE ALTERNATIVE ACTIVATION AND AMPLIFYING PATHWAYS FOR C3 CLEAVAGE

Although the alternative pathway was originally separated from the classical on the basis of an independent protein sequence leading to utilization of C3 (Figure 12.1), it is now clear that the alternative pathway proteins amplify both antibody-dependent and non-antibody-dependent C3 cleavage. The amplifying function is essential to any regulated expression of alternative pathway activation and augments antibody-dependent classical complement activation; thus, it serves both the non-immune and immune host. The proteins of the amplification pathway are the same as those of the alternative initiating pathway, namely, P, B, D and C3 with the only distinction being the requirement for the C3b state to shift their interaction to the amplified state. Their sequential interaction in the amplification phase (Figure 12.3), will be used to examine their structural and functional relationships. It will then be feasible to describe the likely molecular events in alternative pathway initiation.

Third Component (C3). C3, the substrate for classical C3 convertase, is historically factor A of the original properdin pathway. C3 is a beta globulin of 190,000 molecular weight; it is composed of two polypeptide chains, alpha of 120,000 molecular weight and beta of 70,000 molecular weight, linked by disulfide bonds. Cleavage of C3, during the initiation and amplification of the alternative pathway or by the classical C3 convertase yields a 6,000 to 8,000 molecular weight fragment, C3a, from the N-terminus of the alpha chain and a residual C3b fragment. The C3b fragment, like C4b of the classical C3 convertase, serves as the receptor for another protein that, in turn, provides the C3-cleaving site of the amplification C3 convertase.

B. B, designated in the original description of the properdin system, is now known to be a 100,000 molecular weight beta globulin consisting of a single polypeptide chain. B expresses some C3-cleaving activity when in a magnesium ion-dependent reversible association with C3b. C3 convertase activity is markedly increased upon cleavage by D to yield C3b,Bb. The 20,000 molecular weight activation fragment Ba, has alpha electrophoretic mobility. The 80,000 molecular weight active-site bearing fragment, Bb, decays from the bimolecular complex of C3b,Bb to yield Bi, a fragment with gamma mobility that cannot bind and thus is functionally inactive. The residual C3b is capable of reforming new C3b,Bb convertase upon association with additional B, with attendant D cleavage.

D. D, not recognized in the original description of the properdin pathway, is an alpha globulin, a single polypeptide chain, with serine esterase activity, of about 25,000 molecular weight. As noted, it cleaves B in the presence of C3b to uncover fully the C3 convertase activity of the bimolecular complex, C3b,Bb.

The analogies of the amplification pathway (Figure 12.3), to the classical initiating pathway (Figure 12.2), include 1) formation of a

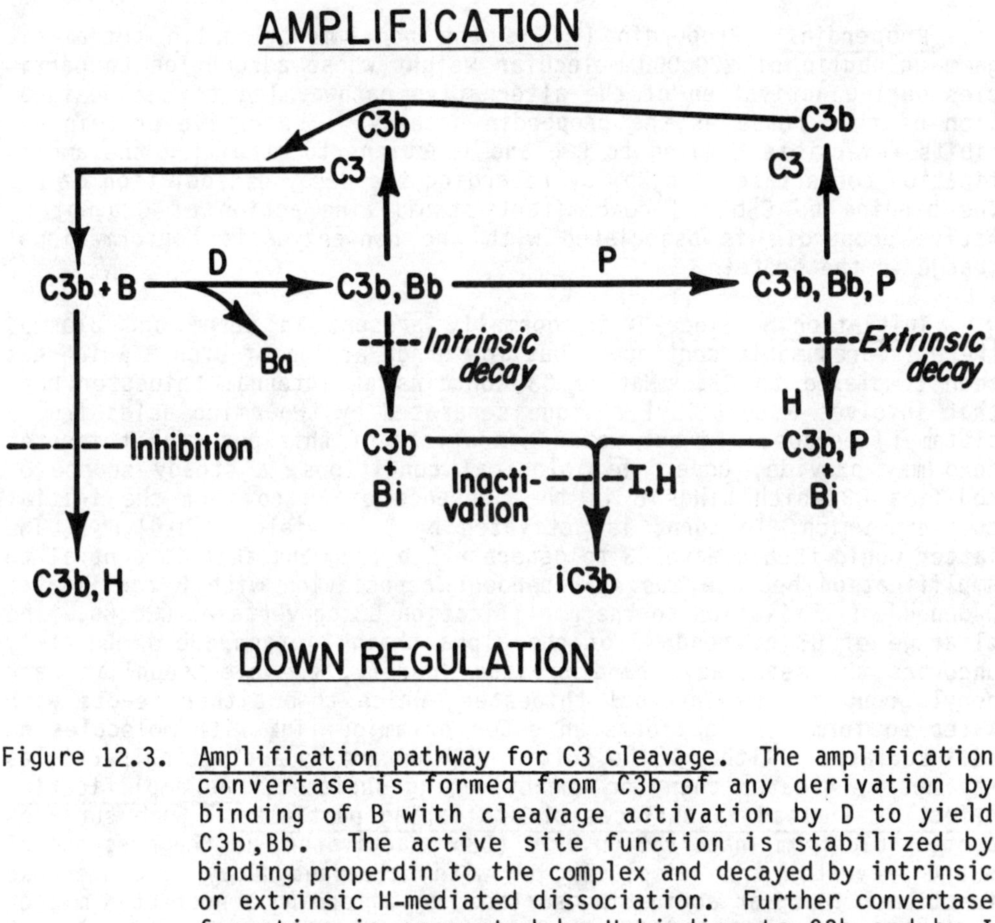

Figure 12.3. Amplification pathway for C3 cleavage. The amplification convertase is formed from C3b of any derivation by binding of B with cleavage activation by D to yield C3b,Bb. The active site function is stabilized by binding properdin to the complex and decayed by intrinsic or extrinsic H-mediated dissociation. Further convertase formation is prevented by H binding to C3b and by I cleavage of C3b to iC3b in the presence of H.

---

magnesium ion-dependent, bimolecular complex, C4b,2 and C3b,B; 2) the action of a serine esterase, C1 and D, to uncover the full C3 convertase function of the fragments 2a and Bb in the respective complex, C4a,2a and C3b,Bb; and 3) the decay of convertase function through release with loss of their binding sites of C2i and Bi. The differences are in the order of the molecular events. In the classical sequence, the fixation of antibody to antigen determines the site of C1 activation to C1 and the focus of deposition of the classical C3 convertase, C4b,2a. In the amplification pathway, the C3b deposition directs the focus of D dependent generation of the amplification C3 convertase, C3b,Bb, to that site. Since the substrate specificity of D for B is not expressed until the formation of the bimolecular complex, C3b,Bb, there is control of this capability without invoking a zymogen for D.

Properdin. Properdin (P) is the non-immunoglobulin tetrameric gamma globulin of 220,000 molecular weight whose adsorption to particles during activation of the alternative pathway led to the designation of this route as the properdin pathway. The native protein exhibits reversible binding to C3b and functions to stabilize the amplification convertase, C3b,Bb, by retarding the decay-dissociation of Bi. The binding to C3b and concomitant stabilizing action of C3b,Bb, by native properdin is associated with the non-enzymatic conformational change in the protein.

Initiation. Since D is normally present in serum and plasma, there is presumably continuous but low grade action of D on B which has been complexed to C3. Native C3 contains an internal thioester bond that involves a cysteinyl residue separated by two amino acids from a glutamyl residue. Direct water hydrolysis of this putative thioester bond may provide, under physiological conditions, a steady source of modified C3 which binds B in the presence of Mg to form the initial complex, which, in turn, is activated by D to yield C3(H2O),Bb. The latter would then cleave C3 to generate C3b fragment that is central to amplification because its Mg-dependent association with B facilitates D-dependent activation to the amplification C3 convertase, C3b,Bb. The cleavage of C3 at bond 77 of the alpha chain to form C3b immediately uncovers the metastable binding site, namely, the electrophilic carbonyl group of the internal thioester, which then either reacts with water to form C3bi or forms an ester or amide link with molecules on cell surfaces. Although the initial C3b uptake by activating particles may not be greater than for nonactivating surfaces, the amplification effect is limited to surfaces of activating particles. Such surfaces protect C3b from inactivation by I (C3b inactivator) in the presence of H and prevent H from displacing Bb with attendant decay of convertase function. Thus, an activating surface, by affording a protected microenvironment for C3b and C3b,Bb,P, advances the alternative complement pathway from slow fluid phase turnover, to intense particle-directed amplified C3 cleavage. The amplified deposition of C3b would alter the fate of the particle by facilitating phagocytosis or cytolysis. As the human host would normally clear C3b from self surfaces, there would be a biochemical basis for non-immune host resistance residing in the surface requirements for the action of the host regulatory proteins. If specific antibody were present to permit classical complement pathway initiation, the benefits of amplification would be further rewarded. Thus, the alternative pathway may be viewed as a two phase system: continuous, lowgrade C3 cleavage with complete regulation of the putative actions of C3b; and amplified cleavage of C3 by a C3b-dependent convertase protected from the regulatory mechanisms, generally by the nature of the surface taking up C3b from the fluid phase (Figure 12.4).

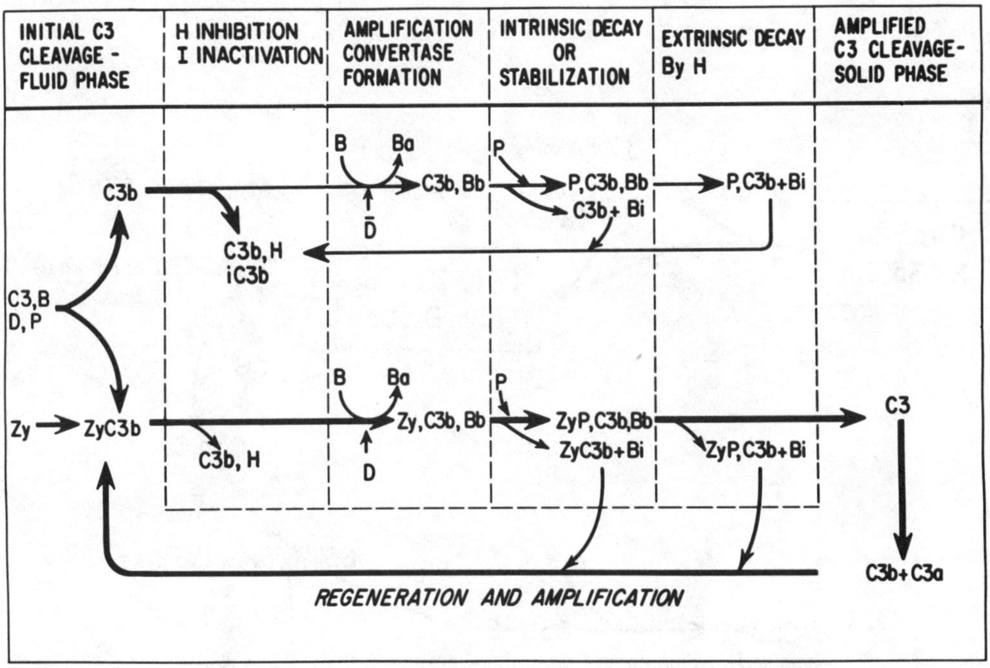

Figure 12.4. Activation of the alternative complement pathway. The continuous low-grade interaction of C3, B, D and P in the fluid phase generates C3b, which is inactivated in the fluid phase or after binding via its metastable binding site to a non-activating particle. Physiologic activation of the alternative pathway follows binding of C3b to an activating paticle, such as zymosan (Zy), that permits B association and P stabilization while impairing H binding. Inactivation of C3b by I in the presence of H produces iC3b, which is then cleaved to C3c and C3d by non-specific proteases. (Modified from Fearon, D. T., and Austen, K. F. In: Arthritis and Allied Conditions, Ninth Edition. Edited by D. J. McCarthy, and J. L. Hollander. Philadelphia, Lea and Febiger, 1979).

THE EFFECTOR COMPLEMENT SEQUENCE

The classical and amplifying C3 convertases recruit the effector proteins of the complement system, C3, C5, C6, C7, C8 and C9 (Figure 12.5).

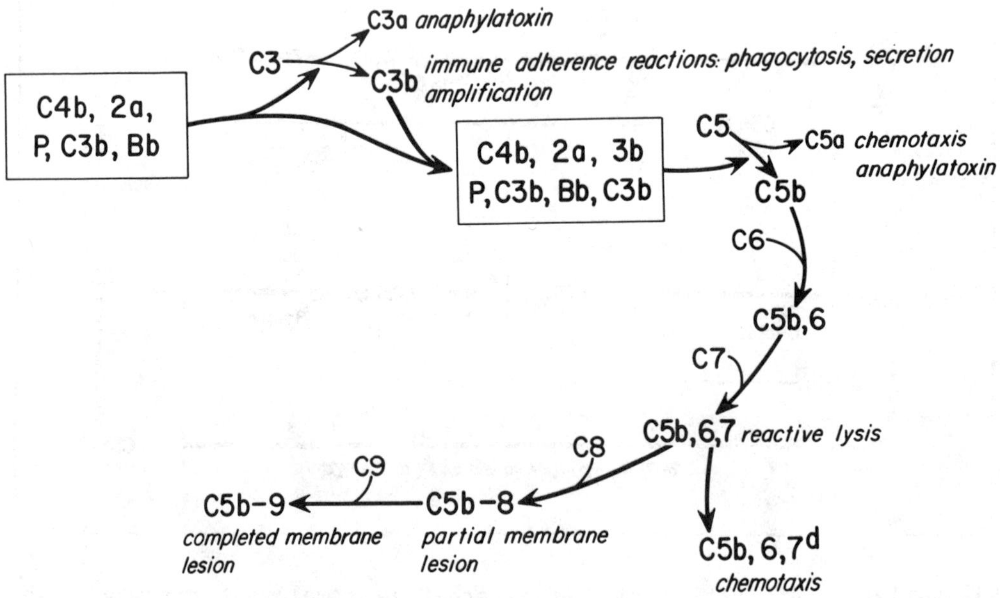

Figure 12.5. The effector sequence of the complement system. The biologically active fragments and complexes are generated as a result of cleavage of C3 and C5 by the classical and amplification C3 and C5 convertases, respectively. (Modified from Fearon, D. T., and Austen, K. F. In: Arthritis and Allied Conditions, Ninth Edition. Edited by D. J. McCarthy, and J. L. Hollander. Philadelphia, Lea and Febiger, 1979).

Third Component (C3). The structural characteristics of native C3 were noted previously. In addition to serving as a receptor for Bb and P in the stabilized amplification convertase (P,C3b,Bb), C3b is responsible for the conversion of C4b,2a and C3b,Bb to a C5 convertase state. With regard to the amplification phase, the C3b involved in converting C3b,Bb from a C3 convertase to a C5 convertase is quantitatively additional and not protected from I. C3b also has two cellular binding functions: the irreversible covalent binding to cell membranes via a metastable carbonyl available from an internal thioester and the adherence to a trypsin-sensitive receptor on many cell types.

Components 5, 6, 7, 8, and 9 (C5-9). C5 is a beta globulin consisting of an alpha chain of 115,000 molecular weight and a beta chain of 75,000 molecular weight joined by disulfide bridges. Cleavage by either classical or amplification C5 convertase releases a peptide of about 11,000 molecular weight, C5a, from the alpha chain, leaving the major fragment, C5b. C6, a beta globulin of 128,000 molecular weight, consists of a single polypeptide chain which does not undergo cleavage during participation in the effector reaction sequence. C7, a 120,000 molecular weight beta globulin, is another single chain polypeptide remaining uncleaved while expressing its role. C8, a 163,000 molecular weight gamma globulin, is composed of an 83,000 molecular weight alpha chain, a 70,000 molecular weight beta chain, and an approximately 10,000 molecular weight gamma chain. The alpha and beta chains are non-covalently linked, whereas the gamma chain is bound covalently to the alpha chain. C9 is a single chain polypeptide of alpha electrophoretic mobility and 79,000 molecular weight.

C5 may: 1) bind directly to membranes via a metastable binding site exposed with cleavage of native C5 by C5 convertases; 2) complex with C6 in the fluid phase to form C5b,6; or 3) remain in the fluid phase as C5i due to irreversible decay of the membrane binding site. Membrane-bound C5b is not stable, being subject to decay-release as C5i unless it complexes with C6. The membrane binding site on fluid-phase C5b,6, is not available until complex with C7 to form C5b,6,7, which is capable of transiently binding to unsensitized membranes, a mechanism known as reactive lysis, which extends the cytolytic effects of complement to innocent bystander cells (i.e., cells not coated with antibody). If C5b,6,7, does not encounter an apropriate membrane, the binding site of C5b decays and the complex becomes C5i,6,7, a cytolytically inactive, chemotactically active unit. Formation of membrane-bound C5b,6,7, permits binding interactions with C8 and then C9 to complete the non-covalent assembly of the C5-C9 multimolecular complex. Thus, after cleavage of C5, the reaction proceeds to completion by protein-protein interactions without further proteolysis. The C5b-8 complex inserts into the membrane to create a partial lesion, whereas the C5b-9 complex appears to form complete transmembrane channels leading to osmotic lysis of the cell.

The constituent proteins of the cytolytic complex represent a tetradecamolecular complex composed of a dimer of C5b-9 with six C9 molecules. The amphiphilic complex presents a cylindrical electron microscopic appearance compatible with channel formation in the target membrane. In addition to forming a hydrophobic channel through its interaction with phospholipids leading to impaired osmotic regulation, the dimer physically disrupts membranes. The latter mechanism accounts for a lytic action on viruses.

REGULATORY PROTEINS OF THE COMPLEMENT COMPONENT SEQUENCE

Regulation of the complement sequence occurs because of the intrinsic lability of certain essential binding steps and through the action of extrinsic control proteins. Inherent control is exemplified by the lability of certain critical protein-protein and protein-membrane interactions. The decay-dissociation of C2a and Bb from their respective C3 and C5 converstases, due to lability of their binding sites, removes the catalytic protein from the complex and eliminates function of the convertases. The lability of the membrane-binding sites appearing with generation of the C4b, C3b and C5b fragments, respectively, means that failure to achieve immediate membrane fixation results in loss of effects. The implication of this lability of binding sites involved in protein-protein interactions and protein-membrane interactions is that, to be efficient, cleavage activation must occur at or near the initiating principle.

The extrinsic control proteins of the reaction sequence include the inhibitor of the activated first component (C1INH) and C4 binding protein (C4bp), which regulate the classical activation pathway; and H, a C3b binding protein, and I, the inactivator of C3b, which together regulate activation of the alternative pathway and amplification of either pathway. An additional type of control is directed against biologically active cleavage products. The anaphylatoxin inactivator (AI) inactivates a class of low molecular weight reaction byproducts and the S-protein competes with bystander membranes for the transitory binding capacity of C5b,6,7.

C1INH. C1INH consists of a single polypeptide chain of alpha globulin electrophoretic mobility and 105,000 molecular weight with an unusually high carbohydrate content in the range of 35%. C1INH controls assembly of classical C3 convertase (C4b,2a) by binding to the light chain of C1s, thereby irreversibly inhibiting the capacity of its serine protease site to cleave C4 and C2. C1INH also blocks the esterolytic activity of C1r, thereby regulating both activation and expression of the function of the C1s subunit (Figure 12.2).

C4bp. C4bp appears to consist of non-covalent multimers of a 550,000 molecular weight monomer that, in turn, is constituted of eight disulfide-linked protomers, each of 70,000 molecular weight. This macromolecule regulates the generation and expression of classical pathway

C3 convertase, C4b,2a, by three effects: competitive inhibition of C2 binding to C4b; augmentation of the cleavage inactivation of C4b by I; and acceleration of the rate of decay of C4b,2a, by dissociation of C2a to yield C2i (Figure 12.2).

I. I, a beta globulin of 93,000 molecular weight, is composed of two polypeptide chains, an alpha chain of 55,000 molecular weight and a beta chain of 42,000 molecular weight linked by disulfide bonds. I cleaves the alpha chain of C3b without fragmentation, and the product, iC3b, cannot function to form the amplification convertase, to convert C3b,Bb and C4b,2a to C5 convertases, or to mediate immune adherence. Inactivation is followed by further cleavage with a non-complement tryptic protease such as plasmin to yield C3c and the smaller 25,000 molecular weight fragment, C3d. I cannot inactivate C3b in the bimolecular C3 convertase, C3b,Bb, although it will inactivate the additional C3b wihch converts the C3b,Bb convertase to a C5 convertase.

H. H, a beta globulin of 150,000 molecular weight, is composed of a single polypeptide chain. H regulates the generation and expression of the amplification C3 convertase, C3b,Bb, by three actions: 1) competitive inhibition of B binding to C3b; 2) augmentation of the cleavage inactivation of C3b by I; and 3) acceleration of the rate of decay of C3b,Bb by dissociation of Bb to yield Bi (Figure 12.3). Neither H alone nor I is sufficient to prevent the interaction of C3, B, D, and P from progressing to amplification. Individuals genetically lacking I are depleted of C3 and B by their amplified utilization. It is evident that three levels of control of the amplification convertase are complementary and necessary, especially in the presence of properdin stabilization. Intrinsic and H-mediated extrinsic decay release of Bb from C3b,Bb are only partially effective in preventing continuous activation of C3. Indeed, the C3b may reform new convertase with B and D unless C3b is inactivated by I. I acts only on C3b that is unassociated with Bb and this reaction is augmented by H independent of its capacity to displace Bb from C3b,Bb. Regulation by H is modulated by sialic acid on cell surfaces, since these moieties favor H binding to C3b without altering the association constant of B for C3b. Thus, in the relative absence of sialic acid, such as occurs on activating particles of the human alternative complement pathway, the random deposition of C3b from the fluid phase is followed by preferential uptake of B and cleavage activation to form C3b,Bb because of an impaired H-mediated binding to C3b.

Anaphylatoxin Inactivator (AI). AI is an alpha 2-globulin with a molecular weight of 310,000 which was recognized originally as kininase I based on its capacity to inactivate bradykinin. The enzyme consists of eight apparently identical non-covalently bound subunits of molecular weight 36,000. The inactivator, which cleaves the C-terminal arginine from C3a, C5a, C4a and bradykinin, is metal dependent. The active site is inhibited by high concentrations of epsilon-aminocaproic acid.

S Protein. S protein, an inter-alpha glycoprotein composed of a single polypeptide chain of 80,000 molecular weight, was initially recognized as a novel, non-complement protein because of its incorporation into the fluid phase pentamolecular complex of C5b-9. It now appears that S protein binds to the C5b-7 complex at its membrane binding site so that the incorporation of C8 and C9 occurs without cytotoxicity for bystander cells because the complex is unable to bind to membranes or to dimerize.

FUNCTIONS ELABORATED BY THE ACTIVATION OF COMPLEMENT

The biologic activities implicated in host defense and tissue injury and derived by complement activation stem largely from the cleavage of C3 and C5 and the assembly of the pentamolar terminal complex. These activities may be directly related to the macromolecular complex which initiated the reaction sequence or may result from alterations in the microenvironment in which the initiating complex is localized. The former would be exemplified by cytolysis of immune adherence-mediated enhanced phagocytosis and the latter by alterations in vascular permeability or by the class and number of infiltrating cells.

Functions Mediated by Cellular Receptors for Complement Fragments. The adherence of particles treated with antibody and complement to human erythrocytes, termed immune adherence, was the initial indication that specific receptors for altered complement proteins existed on human cells. This adherence reaction was mediated through C3b on the immune complex and C3b receptors on human erythrocytes; C3b receptors are also present on other human cells including those involved in the inflammatory reaction (Table 12.2). The receptor for C3b is now termed CR1. Receptors for the degradation products of C3b, iC3b (from the action of I and H) and C3d (from proteolytic cleavage of iC3b), have also been demonstrated on some cell types by particle adherence. CR2 is the name now given to a distinct receptor that preferentially binds C3d. CR3 is a third C3 receptor that strongly interacts with iC3b. C4b on immune complexes also can mediate their uptake by cells bearing C3b receptors. Likewise, iC3b can bind to CR1, but with low affinity. Thus, the term immune adherence reflects the interaction between a variety of complement fragments and specific cellular receptors and is now obsolete.

The CR1 or C3b receptor has been purified to homogeneity from human erythrocyte membranes and identified as a glycoprotein with an apparent molecular weight of approximately 205,000. Antibody to this glycoprotein inhibits C3b receptor function of neutrophils, B lymphocytes and monocytes, and immunoprecipitates a single membrane protein of the same size as that isolated from the erythrocytes. Studies of the lateral distribution and diffusion of the C3b receptor on neutrophils and monocytes have revealed that they are present predominantly in discrete clusters and do not undergo diffusive motion, suggesting

Table 12.2

Complement Receptors on Human Cells

Cell Type	Receptor CR1	CR2	CR3
Erythrocytes	+	-	-
Monocytes	+	-	+
Eosinophils	+	-	-
Neutrophils	+	-	+
Glomerular epithelial cells	+	-	-
B lymphocytes	+	+	+

C3b binds to the CR1 receptor. iC3b binds strongly to CR3 but to a lesser extent with CR1 and CR2. C3d binds to the CR2 receptor.

that they are somehow anchored to specialized areas of the plasma membrane.

Most studies of the role of the C3b receptor in the phagocytic response of neutrophils and of monocyte/macrophages have concluded that it mediates binding but not internalization of C3b-bearing targets. Sheep erythrocytes with membrane-bound C3b adhere to these effector cells but are not internalized unless they also carry IgG or have had membrane-associated sialic acid removed. The receptor on the phagocytic cells that mediates phagocytosis, in the first instance, is the Fc receptor. In the second instance, it is an uncharacterized, trypsin-sensitive membrane constituent. The monocyte recognition unit for activators of the alternative pathway is distinct from its C3b and IgG-Fc receptors and may, like the alternative complement pathway, be of particular importance to the non-immune host. Although generally benefitting the host by augmenting uptake of bacteria or immune complexes, C3b-dependent adherence of material to neutrophils and macrophages may be detrimental under certain *in vitro* circumstances that may reflect situations that occur in inflammatory diseases. Neutrophils presented with non-phagocytosable surfaces bearing IgG and C3b release lysosomal enzymes and superoxide anion extracellularly.

The CR2 receptor interacts with C3d and is found mainly in B lymphocytes. This receptor is a membrane protein of 148,000 molecular weight. A monoclonal antibody has now been found to specifically react with it. The functions of this receptors on B lymphocytes are not entirely elucidated. The production but not the maintenance of established memory is impaired in mice depleted of C3, suggesting a role for C3 fragment receptors in the development of this response. Incubation of lymphocytes with C3b causes secretion of a lymphokine chemotactic for monocytes. Addition of C3c or C3d to culture media inhibits the blastogenic response of human peripheral blood lymphocytes to antigens but not to lectin mitogens. Conversely, addition of anti-C3 antibody to primed mouse spleen cell cultures inhibits the generation of antibody-secreting cells in response to T-dependent antigens. Thus, a coherent definition of the role of C3 receptors on B lymphocytes in the regulation of the immune response is unclear at this time.

Finally, the CR3 receptor binds iC3b with high avidity. It is found in monocytes, macrophages, neutrophils, and some NK cells. A monoclonal antibody (anti-Mac-1) appears to recognize this structure which consists of a disulfide-linked integral membrane protein made up of two chains, one heavy chain of 175,000 molecular weight and a second, smaller chain of 95,000 molecular weight. The lighter chain appears to be common to another membrane structure, the LFA-1 molecule, found on lymphocytes (Chapter 7).

The Phlogistic Peptides, C3a and C5a. C4a, C3a and C5a are activation peptides generated when C4, C3 and C5 are cleaved near the amino termini of the alpha polypeptide chains by $C\bar{1}$ and the respective classical and amplification convertases. The delineation of the primary structures of the human molecules reveals sufficient sequence homology to suggest a common genetic ancestry. These peptides are classically termed anaphylatoxins because of their smooth muscle-contracting activity and their capacity to activate mast cells for mediator release. They appear to bind to specific membrane receptors. However, unlike C3a and C4a, which have well-defined functional regions localized within five to eight residues of the C-terminus, C5a function requires structural information from both the linear C-terminal and the alpha helix portion of the peptide. Thus, the receptor for C3a and the relatively inefficient C4a is distinct from that for C5a. C5a is not only more potent than C3a/C4a as an anaphylatoxin, but is the only activation peptide with chemotactic activity. Subcutaneous injection of these peptides into the human causes a wheal and flare reaction that is blocked by prior administration of H-1 blocking reagents (Chapter 14). The increased vascular permeability induced by histamine may augment local deposition of immune complexes and certainly promotes efflux of plasma proteins such as immunoglobulin and complement proteins into the extravascular site of complement activation which may augment the inflammatory reaction. A serum carboxypeptidase B, termed anaphylatoxin inactivator, decreases by one-hundred- to one-thousand-fold the histamine-releasing activities of the anaphylatoxic peptides by cleaving the C-terminal arginine from these peptides (the desARG derivatives).

A most critical phase in the generation of an injurious inflammatory reaction is the accumulation of leukocytes, which can be mediated by C5a, which induces chemotactic, secretory and adherence reactions of these cells. C5a, in nanomolar concentrations, is taken up by specific receptors on neutrophils and, when present in a gradient, as would occur when the peptide diffuses away from the site of complement activation, causes directed migration of the cells *in vitro*. Higher concentrations of C5a, particularly in the presence of the drug cytochalasin B, also stimulate non-cytotoxic release of lysosomal enzymes. The desARG derivative of C5a retains substantial *in vitro* chemotactic activity which can be augmented by the presence of an uncharacterized serum "co-factor", in contrast to its minimal histamine-releasing and spasmogenic activities. The adherence of granulocytes to capillary endothelial cells preparatory to migration to the extravascular site of inflammation may be mediated by C5a/C5a desARG. *In vitro* these peptides mediate adherence of neutrophils to various surfaces. Such an activity on C5a desARG may account for the transient neutropenia observed after rapid systemic activation of complement in animals by administration of cobra venom factor and in individuals undergoing hemodialysis with dialyzer membranes that activate complement.

Rapid *in vivo* complement activation also causes leukocytosis which follows neutropenia. C3e, a small peptide that is derived from the alpha polypeptide of C3 and is capable of releasing granulocytes from the rat femoral bone marrow, is thought to account for this biologic reaction. Consistent with this thesis is the observation that an individual who genetically lacked C3 did not develop leukocytosis with pyogenic infections.

Solubilization of Immune Complexes. An additional regulatory mechanism for the pathobiologic consequences of circulating or tissue-deposited immune complexes is their solubilization by the action of the classical and alternative pathway C3 convertases. The solubilizing effect is due to the intercalation of complement fragments into the lattice with apparent steric hindrance of the antigen-antibody interaction. As the cleavage products of the alpha chain of C3 are tightly associated with the heavy chain of immunoglobulin, possibly by covalent linkage through the metastable binding site, the critical event in solubilization appears to be the amplified deposition of C3b via the alternative pathway. The classical complement activating sequence accelerates solubilization via the alternative pathway, most likely by introducing C3b for generation of the amplification C3 convertase.

The Membrane Attack Complex, C5b-9. There are two means by which the C5b-9 complex can damage membranes. The first is the apparent formation of a transmembrane channel that allows the passage of salt, water, and even small proteins across the membrane. These changes lead to net uptake of water by a cell, resulting in swelling and gross disruption of the membrane. The lesion, as visualized by electron microscopy, is a hollow, thin-walled cylinder of approximately 10 nm internal diameter and 15 nm height with an extramembranous annulus with internal and external diameters of 10 nm and 20 nm, respectively. The second means of membrane damage is dependent on the phospholipid-binding properties of an amphiphilic complex and is prominent when large numbers of tetradecamolecular complex of C5b-9 are deposited in target membranes. Membrane damage by this means may be important for lysis of viruses whose envelope membranes do not function as osmotic barriers.

BIOSYNTHESIS AND METABOLISM OF COMPLEMENT PROTEINS

The metabolic behavior of highly purified and radiolabeled human C4, C3, C5 and B reveals a fractional catabolic rate for all four proteins in the same relatively high range. This fractional catabolic rate of about 2% of the plasma pool per hour, or 50% of the plasma pool per day indicates that these proteins are among the most rapidly metabolized human plasma proteins. Although fractional catabolic rates among normal subjects are independent of serum levels of the protein, synthetic rates for each of these complement proteins correlate well with plasma levels. Thus, in normal persons, the rate of complement component synthesis is the major determinant of the plasma concentration.

Hypercatabolism in diseases with an immunologic element, such as systemic lupus erythematosus or rheumatoid arthritis, is accompanied by compensatory hypersynthesis. In certain abnormal circumstances, such as in membranoproliferative glomerulonephritis, C3 is hyposynthesized with or without evidence of hypercatabolism. However, in most acquired diseases, reduced plasma concentrations reflect increased catabolism to a degree that overcomes compensatory hypersynthesis.

The nomenclature for genes coding for complement proteins differs in two instances from that used to describe the proteins themselves. The genes determining structural variation in B and C4, a single locus for B and two loci for C4, are known as Bf, C4A and C4B, respectively. Genetic structural polymorphisms in complement proteins have largely been defined by methods detecting differences in net surface charge (electrophoresis and isoelectric focusing). There are common genetic variants of C2, C3, C4, C6, C7, and C8, and of B of the alternative complement pathway. Available data suggest that single loci control the synthesis of C2, C3, C6, C7, C8, and B, whereas C4 is controlled by two closely linked loci, C4A and C4B. Loci for three complement proteins are very closely linked to the genes of the major histocompatibility complex (MHC) on the short arm of chromosome six (Chapter 6). Moreover, the increased association of specific histocompatibility (HLA), types with rare variants of the Bf locus in patients with juvenile onset diabetes mellitus, suggests that a gene for disease susceptibility is close to Bf on the sixth chromosome.

Elucidation of the structural polymorphisms of complement proteins has facilitated the study of complement biosynthesis *in vivo*. In patients given liver transplants, a complete change of allotype to that of the donor has occurred for C3, C6, C8 and B, indicating that more than 90% of these circulating complement proteins are synthesized in the liver. Studies of the metabolism of isotopically-labeled C3 *in vivo* and of C3 synthesis by peripheral-blood monocytes *in vitro* in patients with homozygous C3 deficiency have demonstrated that hyposynthesis is the basis of C3 deficiency. However, monocytes from unrelated C3-deficient patients produced about 25% of the C3 produced by normal monocytes, even though the serum C3 concentration in the affected persons was less than 0.1% of normal. These findings reflect the contribution of liver biosynthesis to serum C3 as compared with extrahepatic synthesis. C1, and thus its three subunits, are synthesized by gastrointestinal epithelial cell cultures, although C1q, in addition, may be macrophage-derived. The macrophage, based largely on studies with animal cells, appears to be a source of proteins involved in convertase formation. The latter may be of considerable importance in the initial events responsible for local host defenses.

In the past few years, biochemical studies of complement synthesis have revealed some of the mechanisms of translation and processing of complement proteins. C3, C4, and C5 are each synthesized as single-chain precursor proteins that undergo proteolytic cleavage to generate the multichain native complement components. These three components have other features in common, including primary structural homologies and similarities in biologic activities. Glycosylation of pro-C4 and possibly the other procomplement proteins, is required for secretion of the native molecules. Analysis of C4 protein derived from human plasma has revealed about 1% to 3% to be still in the single chain pro-C4 state, whereas the remainder exhibits the three chain structure characteristics of the post-synthetic modification apparently related to its secretion. Biochemical studies of complement deficiencies in animals have revealed at least two mechanisms. In the C4-deficient guinea pig, no pro-C4 is synthesized, although indirect evidence of the production of C4 messenger RNA has been obtained. In contrast, in the C5-deficient mouse pro-C5 is synthesized but not secreted.

COMMENTARY ON THE ROLE OF THE CLASSICAL AND ALTERNATIVE COMPLEMENT PATHWAYS IN HEALTH AND DISEASE

The insights gained concerning the role of complement in the maintenance of host integrity from the study of patients with inborn errors were in some instances predictable from *in vitro* findings and in others were without precedent. Genetically controlled deficiencies have been described for almost all the components of the complement system and for two of the natural inhibitors of this system (Chapter 15).

C3 deficiency consistently leads to marked impairment of host defenses, manifested in vivo by recurrent pyogenic and gram-negative infections and impaired leukocyte mobilization and in vitro by absent serum bactericidal, chemotactic and opsonic enhancing activity. Since such patients do mount a specific antibody response, their susceptibility is attributed to an absence of C3b-mediated alternative pathway amplification and lack of C3b-mediated enhancement of phagocytosis. Their susceptibility to recurrent infections suggests that the synergistic action of the IgG (Fc) and C3b receptors is critical to full host defense against pyogenic microorganisms controlled by phagocytosis. Homozygous I deficiency, which permits uncontrolled activation of the alternative complement pathway with secondary C3 and B deficiencies, is associated with similar susceptibility to recurrent pyogenic infection.

Deficiencies of the latter complement components, C5, C6, C7, C8, and C9 are associated with recurrent or disseminated Neisserial infections such as meningococcal meningitis and gonococcal arthritis. In these cases, the bacteremia may not be controlled in the absence of a cytolytic sequence.

Certain deficiency states, especially of C2, are associated with an increased frequency of diseases such as systemic lupus erythematosus, Henoch-Schonlein purpura, polymyositis, or glomerulonephritis. Since genes coding for three of the complement proteins (C2, C4, and B) have been linked to the MHC on the sixth autosomal chromosome, the increased susceptibility to these diseases may reflect genetically linked alterations in immune responses.

Alternatively, the advent of adaptive immunity may require an intact classical or antibody-dependent complement activating sequence in order to clear the products of the immune response. Since deficiencies in complement proteins, not linked to the MHC, namely C1r, C1s, and C1INH, are also associated with an increased apparent incidence of immune complex-mediated diseases, it seems that the problem is not limited to deficiencies of proteins coded for on the sixth chromosome. Further, as patients with C2, C4, C1r/s and C1INH deficiencies do not experience undue susceptibilities to bacterial infections of any type, it seems evident that their intact alternative complement pathway maintains normal resistance. It is thus tempting to speculate that the alternative complement pathway is the critical route for recruiting C3b and C5b-9 for microbial resistance, whereas the classical activating pathway is essential for clearing the products of adaptive immune response in the form of immune complexes.

Clinically, the most important deficiency is of C$\bar{I}$INH, which is associated with the syndrome of hereditary angioedema of the skin, gastrointestinal tract, and upper respiratory tract. In this disease, the uninhibited activation and action of C$\bar{I}$ on its substrates, C4 and C2, generates a fragment, presumably C2b, which is further processed by a plasma protease, possibly plasmin, to a vasoactive peptide. The presence of the C4bp prevents significant formation of classical C3 convertase with subsequent significant C3 cleavage. The affected patients are heterozygotes, the condition being inherited as an autosomal trait, with the half-normal amount of C$\bar{1}$INH normally synthesized being depleted secondary to its interaction with C1. Correct diagnosis may avert needless abdominal surgery or death by asphyxiation. Effective pharmacologic intervention is now available in the form of attenuated androgens that stimulate C$\bar{1}$INH production.

Although the role of complement in host integrity has been established by clinical findings in patients with inborn errors, its contribution to acquired disease processes is unproven. The acquired defects of the complement system in disease can serve as markers of tissue injury but do not distinguish secondary utilization with beneficial clearance of immune aggregates from concomitant contributions to the tissue injurious processes.

REFERENCES

Austen, K. F. Homeostasis of effector systems which can also be recruited for immunologic reactions. J. Immunol., 121:793, 1978.

Fearon, D. T., and Austen, K. F. The human complement system. Biochemistry, Biology and Pathobiology. Essays Med. Biochem., 2, 1976.

Fearon, D. T., and Wong, W. W. Complement ligand-receptor interactions that mediate biological responses. Ann. Rev. Immunol., 1:243, 1983.

Hugh, T. E., and Muller-Eberhard, H. J. Anaphylotoxins: C3a and C5a. Adv. Immunol., 26:1, 1978.

Muller-Eberhard, H. J., and Schreiber, R. D. Molecular biology and chemistry of the alternative pathway of complement. Adv. Immunol., 29:1, 1980.

Muller-Eberhard, H. J. Chemistry and reaction mechanisms of complement. Adv. Immunol., 8:1, 1968.

CHAPTER 13

Immunopathology

Immunological processes can produce inflammation and tissue injury. Immunological tissue injury can result from the immune response of the individual either to foreign antigens or to autologous components. Autoimmunity is the term used to define a reaction of the host against self. From a pathogenetic point of view, the immunological reactions that produce pathology may involve either antibodies or cellular immunity reactions such as those described in Chapter 7.

Antigen-antibody interactions may produce different kinds of tissue injury depending on the class of the antibody molecule. Antibodies of the IgG class bind to antigen, forming macromolecular complexes that fix complement (C). Under appropriate conditions, the antigen-antibody-C complexes induce severe inflammation involving neutrophils. This inflammatory reaction may lead to tissue necrosis (i.e., death of cells), disruption of the normal tissue architecture, alteration in permeability barriers, and scarring. (Antibodies of the IgM class also result in immune complexes that fix C. However, because of the small amounts of IgM in the circulation, their role is not as important relative to that of the IgG antibodies). Antibodies of the IgE type bind to antigen and induce mast cells or basophils to degranulate and to release their content of powerful vasoactive products. The vasoactive amines produce a transitory increase in vascular permeability without much of a cellular infiltrate, except for a variable number of eosinophils. These reactions, the anaphylactic reactions described in Chapter 14, are usually of brief duration, disappearing without any residual tissue damage.

Cellular immune reactions are characterized by infiltration with phagocytes brought about by mediators from T lymphocytes. These reactions, when severe, can lead to tissue damage comparable those induced by antigen-antibody-C complexes (Chapter 7).

Most immunological diseases involve mixed pathogenetic mechanisms, but frequently one mechanism of injury may predominate over another. The factors that conditions these reactions are complex and not clearly evident in all instances. These factors involve the type of antigen, the route of inoculation, the tissue where the reaction takes place, and the host response. To illustrate these points, we will describe three examples of tissue injury and inflammation produced by: 1) antigen-antibody-C complexes, 2) cellular immunity, and 3) IgE-antigen interactions.

1. The normal physiological antibody response to conventional protein or carbohydrate antigens injected into the blood may result in the formation of immune complexes in the circulation which produce tissue pathology under a special set of conditions to be described later. This process, with the resulting tissue damage, may take place in any individual capable of making a normal immune response. The immune injury in these cases is caused by circulating antigen-antibody-C complexes that produce severe acute inflammation in various vascular beds. The antibodies of the IgE class contribute to this acute inflammation in a very limited extent. Although the normal individual also develops T cell immunity to many antigens, the severe acute inflammation produced by the complexes may minimize or obscure a delayed sensitivity component.

2. Small reactive chemicals introduced into the skin form immunogenic conjugates with self proteins, many of which interact with Langerhans cells and macrophages of the dermis. T cells exhibit strong reactivity for these conjugates associated with the antigen-presenting cells and are responsible for contact sensitivity reactions (Chapter 7). This is the case, for example, for a small lipid from the poison ivy plant. This lipid complexes to self proteins and sensitizes T cells readily. The reaction of specific T cells with very small amount of antigen in the skin associated with macrophages produces the severe delayed-type inflammation. Although some antibodies can be formed against the antigen, the very small amount of antigen free in the extracellular space does not favor the formation of sufficiently large amounts of soluble antigen-antibody complexes to fix enough C to produce acute inflammation. Thus, contact with this small amount of antigen clearly favors the development of delayed sensitivity reactions and not of an Arthus reaction (see below). Again, as in the first example, contact sensitivity can be produced in any individual.

3. The last example is that of certain antigens which, upon introduction to specially sensitive individuals, usually by way of the skin or mucosal surfaces, favor a particular immune response, that of the IgE type. This is the example of an individual with the genetic predisposition to produce strong IgE antibody responses upon contact with the correct antigen. The "allergens" do not interact with tissue proteins of the mucosas but readily diffuse, thus are capable of establishing contact with IgE antibodies on mast cells to produce the allergic reaction.

Chapter 7 described cellular immunity reactions; Chapter 14 considers anaphylaxis. This chapter is concerned with: a) antigen-antibody-C reactions, and b) autoimmunity.

IMMUNE COMPLEX PATHOLOGY

Immune complexes made with IgG antibody (or IgM) can fix C and, therefore, have the potential of inducing severe inflammation and disease. Immune complexes may result from the combination of antibody with: a) soluble antigen in the circulation; b) soluble antigens in extracellular spaces; or c) antigens that form part of the structure of a tissue or a cell (i.e., tissue-fixed antigens). Soluble immune complexes usually result from the combinations of antibodies with foreign antigens, although under abnormal circumstances, the antigen may be autologous. Complexes formed against tissue-fixed antigens generally involve autoantibodies. However, there are examples of foreign antigens reacting with tissue components and forming an immunogenic complex to which antibodies can bind and produce injury. Examples of immune complex pathology involving soluble and tissue-fixed antigens are given below.

Systemic Immune Complex Disease—Acute Serum Sickness. Antigen-antibody complexes formed in the circulation disseminate and localize in various tissues and produce acute inflammation. Serum sickness is a typical example of an acute immune complex disease. It was first described by Von Pirquet in 1911 when he observed the development of symptoms in patients receiving horse anti-bacterial serum for the treatment of infectious diseases. Several days after the injection of serum, the patients developed fever, splenomegaly, skin rashes, joint pain, and proteinuria. Most of the symptoms disappeared after a few days, and the patients recovered. Von Pirquet found precipitating antibodies to the foreign serum in the patients' sera at the times when the symptoms were disappearing. However, at the peak time of symptoms, such antibodies were not found. He thought that some kind of toxic products, responsible for the symptoms, were circulating at the time that the disease developed. This prediction proved correct—indeed, the toxic products were later identified as circulating antigen-antibody complexes.

The following is a description of experimental serum sickness induced in the rabbit by injection of 200 mg of purified bovine serum albumin (BSA). This experimental model has provided a basis for the understanding of the pathogenesis of many human glomerulonephritis and vascular and connective tissue diseases (Figure 13.1).

The BSA is labeled with radioiodine, and its disappearance in the blood is measured. During the first week, the rabbit is asymptomatic; the BSA is slowly eliminated from the blood, at its normal catabolic rate. After about one week, antibody appears in the serum. This small amount of antibody immediately binds to the circulating BSA in the blood, forming small antigen-antibody complexes. No free antibody can be detected at this time since all the available antibody becomes complexed with the excess antigen. The small soluble complexes in antigen excess circulate, seed into the different tissues, localizing in their blood vessels, where they produce the pathological changes. The immune

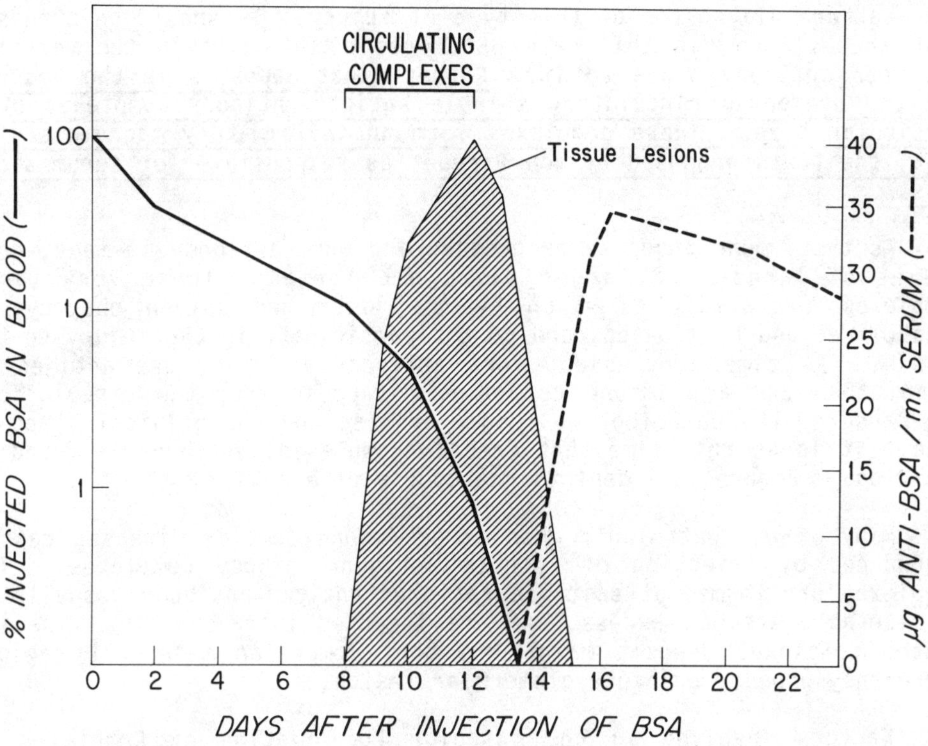

Figure 13.1. This figure is taken from the classical paper of F. J. Dixon, "Pathogenesis of Serum Sickness", published in the Archives of Pathology, 65:18, 1958. Note the rate of disappearance of the iodinated albumin, which, during the first eight days, follows a normal half-life. At about Day 8, antigen-antibody complexes are detected in the blood immunochemically, but no free antibody is detected. The shaded triangle represents the time that pathology is found in the various tissues.

---

complexes which localize in vessel walls of the various organs produce hyperplasia of the endothelium, necrosis of the vessel wall (fibrinoid necrosis), heavy infiltration by neutrophils, and increase in permeability. Lesions are very prominent in the glomerulus of the kidney, characterized by marked cellular hyperplasia, leukocyte infiltration, and leakage of protein into the uriniferous space.

In all the sites of tissue injury, the antigen-antibody complexes can be visualized by immunofluorescence. This has been an invaluable technique for the identification of immune complexes in the vessel walls and in the kidney along the glomerular capillary wall. In the renal glomerulus, Ig, C, and the antigen appear in an irregular, granular pattern diagnostic of this type of injury. It should be stressed that the antigen, in this case BSA, does not deposit in the vessels, and then antibody binds to it. Rather, what deposits in the vessels are the preformed circulating soluble antigen-antibody complexes of a particular size. These complexes form an inflammatory macromolecular unit, the toxin proposed by Von Pirquet as responsible for serum sickness.

As the immune response progresses and more antibody is made, complexes of larger and larger sizes are formed. These very large complexes are avidly taken up by the liver and spleen phagocytes, catabolized and eliminated, and do not participate in the injury to the tissue. As time progresses, more antibody is made, the antigen is eliminated, and all immune complexes disappear from the circulation. The cause of the pathology no longer exists, and the clinical symptoms wane. It is at this time that free (uncomplexed) antibody is found in the blood. Figure 13.1 depicts the course of events.

Many of the pathologic changes of immune complex diseases can be reproduced by injection of soluble antigen-antibody complexes. The complexes are formed at suitable ratio of antigen-antibody, usually in considerable antigen excess, and are injected intravenously. The injected complexes deposit mainly in the glomerular mesangial regions where they produce an acute glomerular lesion.

Factors Involved in the Vascular Localization of Complexes in Acute Immune Complex Disease. These factors are:

1. Size of the complexes: The complexes formed by one or two molecules of antigen with one or two of antibody are involved in the production of diseases. These are the size of the complexes that form whenever there is an excess of antigen. These small size complexes bind less avidly to phagocytes of liver and spleen, circulate longer, and have the opportunity to localize in blood vessels. In contrast, complexes in antibody excess are large, bind readily to liver and spleen phagocytes, and circulate poorly.

2. Vasoactive amines: There must be an increase in vascular permeability to allow the complexes to penetrate the vessel walls. This increase in permeability is thought to be produced by vasoactive amines like histamine or serotonin released by circulating platelets (Figure 13.2). An IgE antibody found in serum at this time may also be involved in the release of vasoactive amines. In tissue culture experiments, it has been found that IgE antibody can bind to circulating basophils and release factors that produce the secretion of amines from the platelets. One such factor, a small lipid named platelet-activating factor (PAF), has been identified and isolated. The formula

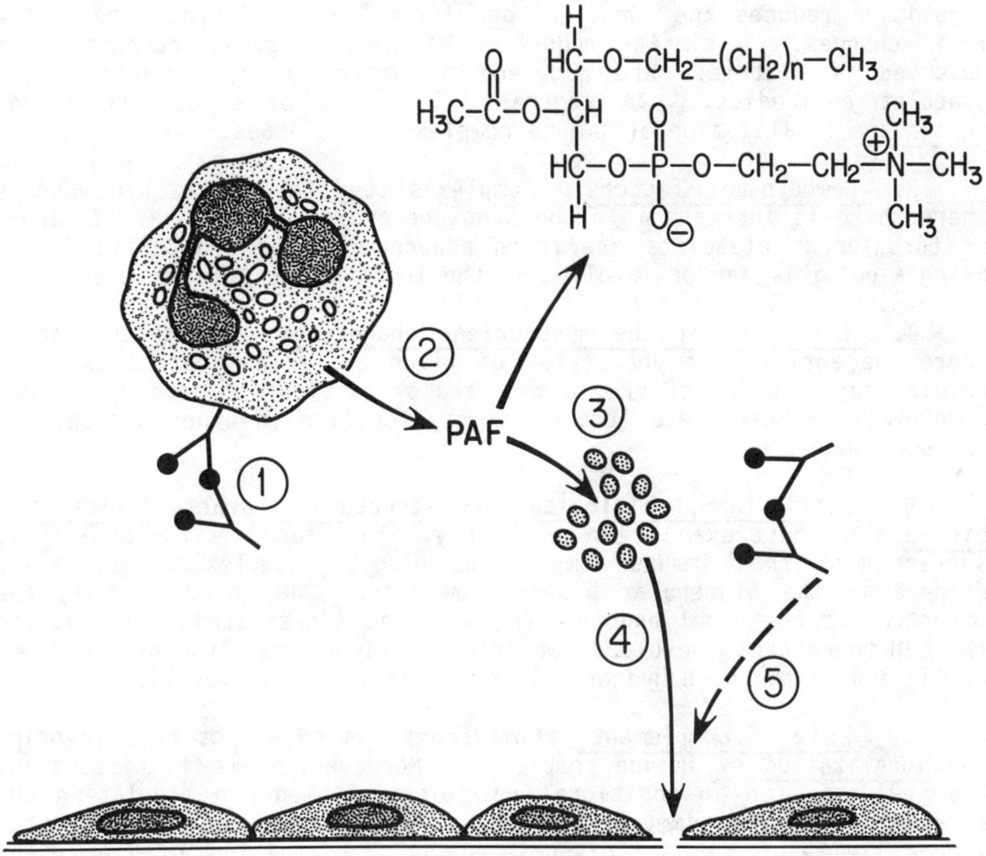

Figure 13.2. A possible mechanism for the increase in vesicular permeability in acute serum sickness. Complexes of antigen with IgE (1) bind to basophils—or other leukocytes—inducing the release of PAF (2). PAF degranulates the plateletes (3), resulting in the release of their vasoactive amines (4). The vasoactive amines contract the endothelial cells, producing gaps through which the circulating immune complexes seep and interact with the basement membranes (5).

---

for PAF (O-1-hexadecyl [or octadecyl]-2-acetyl-sn-glyceryl-3-phosphorylcholine) is given in Figure 13.2. Purified PAF causes platelets to aggregate and release their intracellular mediators, as well as prostaglandins. It also causes neutrophils to aggregate and release lysosomal enzymes and blood vessels to increase their permeability to proteins. In experimental acute serum sickness in the rabbit, administration of anti-histaminic drugs at the time of immune complex deposition reduces the localization of complexes and hence the pathologic changes. A similar reduction of immune complex deposition is observed if platelets are reduced in number by injection of anti-platelet antibodies. In contrast, injection of vasoactive amines favors the localization of immune complexes in tissues.

3. Hemodynamic factors: Complexes tend to localize in vessels where there is increase in blood pressure and/or turbulence. In areas of turbulence, platelets are found adherent to the endothelium, this being a possible factor involved in the localization of complexes.

4. The state of the mononuclear phagocytes: In circumstances where the activity of phagocytes of liver and spleen decreases (as a result, for example, of previous uptake of particulate matter), immune complexes then circulate longer and may localize in other tissues and produce damage.

5. Particular physiological and structural characteristics of a tissue: The best example is the kidney. The kidney is the organ that suffers most from immune complex pathology. Complexes are readily trapped in the glomerular basement membrane (GBM) because: a) the structure of the renal endothelium, which is fenestrated, allowing for the GBM to contact the blood directly; b) high blood flow of the glomeruli; and c) the high hydrostatic pressure in the glomeruli.

6. Role of complement: Complement has no direct role favoring the localization of immune complexes. Moreover, there is circumstantial evidence for an additional role of complement in modulating the size of circulating immune complexes. In vitro it can be shown that immune complexes can be dissociated by the addition of complement proteins that intercalate into the lattice of complexes (Chapter 12). The interesting feature is that individuals with congenital absence of C2 and C4 have a higher incidence of immune complex disease (including systemic lupus erythematosus). Perhaps the greater incidence of such diseases may be caused by the persistence of complexes that would normally disappear in individuals with an intact complement proteins.

Factors Involved in the Production of the Disease. Although the pathogenesis of all the manifestations are not clear, a great many can be explained by the activation of C with the infiltration of neutrophils. The neutrophils, as they infiltrate the vessels and engulf the complexes, release molecules that damage basement membrane, producing disease. See below, the description of the Arthus reaction.

Characterization of the Antigens. Three conditions have to be met in order for an antigen to induce acute serum sickness:

1. The antigen must be immunogenic. Poorly immunogenic antigens that induce very weak immune responses do not result in acute immune complex disease.

2. The amount of antigen administered is critical and should be relatively large.

3. Antigens should circulate for sufficient periods of time to enable the antibody to combine with it.

Strongly immunogenic antigens that immediately upon injection leave the circulation do not result in serum sickness. In this case, by the time antibodies appear in the blood, all the antigen has disappeared, and no complexes can be formed.

Chronic Immune Complex Disease. In acute immune complex disease, a large dose of soluble antigen is introduced, and disease develops as a result of the rapid formation of many small immune complexes seeding to various tissues. Tissue pathology can also develop by repeated administration of very small amounts of antigen. After a certain time, the continuous formation of immune complexes produces tissue injury. The most important factor for the development of chronic immune complex disease is continuous antigenemia. The ratio of antigen to antibody is also an important factor since complexes in antigen excess are the ones most likely to deposit in vascular beds.

The model of chronic serum sickness was carefully studied by Frank J. Dixon and associates who established the conditions for developing immune complexes and tissue injury. Rabbits were injected daily with BSA and the titer of antibodies measured periodically. Three patterns of response were observed:

1. No antibody response and no chronic serum sickness: These were rabbits that, upon repeated injection with BSA, became tolerant, did not form antibodies, and, hence, could not form immune complexes.

2. High antibody responders, limited disease: These rabbits made very high antibody titers; the dose of injected antigen was not sufficiently large to produce complexes in antigen excess. The large complexes in antibody excess were rapidly trapped by the liver phagocytes. High dose of antigen, however, did result in the production of a large number of complexes sufficient to be trapped in some tissues and produce some weak inflammation.

3. Low or average antibody responders, moderate renal disease: These were rabbits that made an average or minimal response. Depending on the dose of antigen, immune complexes in antigen excess were formed, and these localized mainly in the kidney.

The primary tissue that develops chronic immune complex disease is the kidney. The complexes become deposited along the GBM and accumulate in the epithelial side where they can be identified as electron-dense deposits. By immunofluorescence, the complexes are visualized as irregular, granular deposits along the glomerular capillary walls. The end result of chronic immune complex deposition is chronic renal insufficiency with marked proteinuria, azotemia, and, eventually, renal failure.

Local Immune Complex Pathology: the Arthus Reaction: The Arthus reaction is an acute immune complex vasculitis, usually induced in the skin, characterized by severe damage to blood vessel walls and an increase in vascular permeability. The reaction is produced by the injection of antigen into the skin of an immune individual with circulating antibodies to the antigen. The reaction peaks four to ten hours after injection and consists of an area of edema with severe hemorrhage and, in severe cases, ulceration. Histologically, the hallmark of the reaction is a severe infiltration of neutrophils along vessel walls, with extravasation of proteins and red cells into the extravascular space. Occasional vessels thrombose. The reaction results from the formation of immune complexes—the antigen injected into the skin plus the serum antibody—along vessel walls. The complexes can be easily identified by immunofluorescence. To elicit an Arthus reaction, the amounts of antigen have to be sufficiently large to produce an inflammatory reaction of a magnitude such that the vessel walls are injured. (A very small amount of antigen injected into the skin will not elicit a significant Arthus reaction yet may trigger a delayed sensitivity reaction.) (See Chapter 7 for a comparison.)

Pathogenesis of Arthus Reaction. The following steps take place:

1. Antibody binds to antigen along vessel walls.

2. Immune complexes fix C (by classical or alternative pathway).

3. Chemotactic factors are formed.

4. Neutrophils are attracted and bind to the immune complexes via their surface C3 receptor.

5. Neutrophils phagocytose the complexes.

6. During phagocytosis, enzymes and inflammatory chemicals from neutrophils are secreted, causing vessel wall damage.

Neutrophils contain cathepsin D and E, which are acid hydrolases that degrade proteins; elastase and collagenase, active at neutral pH; and a variety of cationic peptides of 2,000 to 5,000 daltons which: a) have bactericidal activity; b) can dilate vessel walls and contract smooth muscle; and c) release histamine from mast cells. Neutrophils can also release oxygen radicals like hydrogen peroxide, the superoxide anion, and the hydroxyl radical which can produce damage to endothelial cells.

Hence, the injury in immune complex vasculitis is mediated by C via the presence of activated C3 and the release of chemoattractants. Experimental manipulations that eliminate serum C abrogate Arthus reactions. In the absence of neutrophils, antigen-antibody-C will still form, some slight increase in permeability to proteins may take place, but severe injury will not develop.

Immune Complex Pathology Involving a Tissue-Fixed Antigen: Anti-GBM Nephritis: In the early 1930's the experimental model of nephrotoxic serum nephritis was developed by the Japanese investigator Masugi (Figure 13.3). The model consists of producing glomerulonephritis by injecting an experimental animal with antibodies to its own GBM. For example, antibodies to GBM are produced by immunizing rabbits with GBM isolated from rat kidney; the rabbit antibodies to GBM are then injected into rats. These antibodies circulate briefly because they are immediately removed as they are fixed to the GBM of the rat. Bound to the GBM, the antibodies then fix C. The antibodies can be identified, by immunofluorescence, bound in a continuous homogeneous pattern, all along the glomerular capillary wall. A few hours after binding of anti-GBM, neutrophils infiltrate the glomerular capillaries and produce

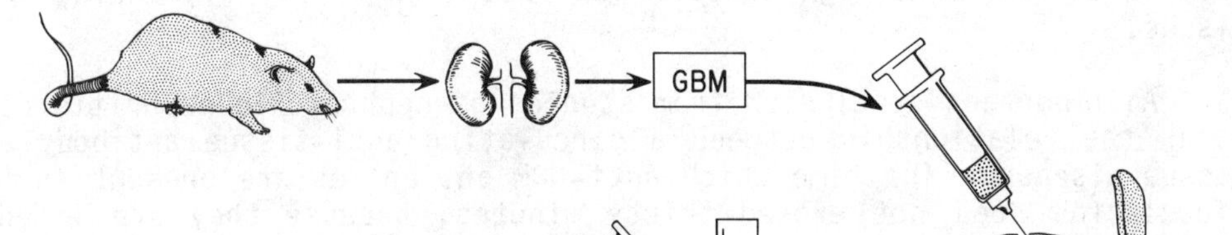

Figure 13.3: Antibodies against the GBM of rats can be made in rabbits. These antibodies when injected into rats produce nephritis. The nephrotoxic serum nephritis develops in two stages.

damage to the GBM, which then leaks plasma proteins. A great part of this early glomerular injury is caused by these infiltrating neutrophils that injure the capillary wall in a process analogous to the Arthus reaction. In the absence of neutrophils, glomerular injury is decreased, despite the fact that the antibodies are bound to the kidney, together with C. It is also apparent that not all the glomerular injury in nephrotoxic nephritis is associated with neutrophils and C fixation. High levels of antibodies can produce proteinuria in the absence of circulating neutrophils or serum complement.

The injury in nephrotoxic nephritis takes place in two stages. The first stage is the anti-GBM binding to the glomerulus as described above. A few days after injection, however, proteinuria, an indicator of glomerular injury, decreases but later reverts to a high level. This second phase of glomerular damage is produced as a result of the host antibody response to rabbit IgG bound to the GBM. The host antibodies react with the nephrotoxic IgG which persists bound to the GBM and is now acting as an antigen bound to the glomerulus. The second phase develops slowly and is independent of neutrophils. This is an example of how a foreign protein can result in injury by binding to a tissue.

An important conclusion from studies of nephrotoxic nephritis concerns the relationship between a circulating anti-tissue antibody and tissue disease. The time which anti-GBM antibodies are present in the circulation does not exceed thirty minutes, because they are immediately removed by the kidney antigens readily accessible to the blood. This short time contrasts with the five-day half-life of normal rabbit IgG, or of antibodies to antigens not readily available in the circulation, such as mitochondrial antigens. The anti-mitochondrial antibodies, for example, also have a normal catabolic half-life of five days. An important conclusion is that <u>the level of circulating antibody to a tissue antigen does not correlate with and cannot allow a prediction of the degree of tissue injury</u>. In the example given, the anti-GBM antibodies are immediately removed, while the anti-mitochondrial antibodies, which do not produce injury, remain in blood.

EXAMPLES OF IMMUNE COMPLEX DISEASES

Acute and chronic serum sickness, the Arthus reaction, and nephrotoxic serum sickness, are the four classical examples of immune complex pathology. To summarize, these models show that: 1) soluble immune complexes formed in the circulation following injection of <u>large</u> amounts of antigen produce an acute systemic vasculitis; 2) <u>small</u> amounts of antigen <u>persisting</u> in the circulation for long periods of time result in severe and chronic disease; 3) a large <u>local</u> accumulation of soluble immune complexes is highly inflammatory; and 4) immune complexes involving antibodies specific for antigens that are not circulating but are exposed as parts of tissue structures, can induce severe cell or tissue injury. Many diseases of man and animals result from immune complexes. A few selected examples are listed below.

Examples of Pathology Involving Circulating Immune Complexes. The following antigens have been found involved in immune complex disease:

1. Foreign serum or protein (serum sickness): In clinical medicine, serum sickness occurred frequently in the pre-antibiotic era when antisera from horses immunized with bacteria or their products were used to treat infectious diseases.

2. Bacterial antigens: Immune complex pathology can be found associated with a number of infectious processes when there is: a) acute release of bacterial products and/or b) the persistence of an infectious process for long periods of time, leading to continuous exposure to soluble microbial antigens. Post-streptococcal glomerulonephritis is an immune complex glomerulonephritis seen in some children a few days following infection usually with Type 12 hemolytic streptococcus. The exact nature of the antigen localized in glomeruli is not clear. The nephritis is an acute proliferative process with heavy deposits of immune complexes. About 95% of the children recover after four to six weeks. Immune complexes have also been found in glomeruli of patients with chronic infections such as post-streptococcal endocarditis, pneumococcal otitis, secondary syphilis, and ventriculoatrial shunts infected with staphylococci.

Lepromatous leprosy is an example of a chronic infectious process with a large bacillary load and chronic antigenemia in which symptoms of immune complex disease occur frequently. In this disease, tissue macrophages are highly infected with bacilli. The macrophages cannot eliminate them, most likely because of a deficient cellular immune reaction. Frequently, patients have the acute leprosy reaction which develops spontaneously or following treatment with microbicidal drugs. This reaction is characterized by red nodules in skin, arthritis, and proteinuria resulting from the sudden release of leprosy antigens and their combination with antibodies to form immune complexes.

3. Parasitic antigens: The best-known example is Plasmodium malarie infection seen in children of West Africa where severe nephritis develops. The nephritis is an immune complex disease formed by complexes of antibody with soluble malaria antigens.

4. Viruses: A number of animal viruses can produce severe immune complex disease. In many of these, the virus persists in the circulation without producing much effect until such a time as immune complex pathology develops. One of the best examples is experimental lymphocytic choriomeningitis (LCM) infection. The association between LCM virus infection and the host immune response is complex and involves both immune complex formation as well as cellular immune reactions. The LCM virus is a non-cytopathic RNA virus that infects cells of the meninges and the nervous system. Intracerebral infection of adult mice

produces a severe choriomeningitis with involvement of the central nervous system and eventual death. The disease is produced by T cells that react with the virus associated with the membrane of the cells. Thus, intracerebral infection of adult mice with LCM virus followed by X-irradiation or by immunosuppressive drug treatment results in systemic viremia but no disease: the virus replicates in the brain and eventually spreads throughout all tissues; the mice will not suffer clinical disease. However, reconstitution of these immunosuppressed mice by transplanting T lymphocytes from LCM-immune mice results in the development of acute disease.

A second very interesting situation with regards to immune complex formation occurs in mice made partially tolerant to LCM virus. No acute disease develops in infected newborn which become partially tolerant to the virus and develop viremia (Chapter 9). However, tolerance to the virus is not absolute, and a small antibody response slowly develops with time. This small response, together with the excess circulating virus, forms the basis for immune complex formation, which results in chronic severe immune complex glomerulonephritis. Thus, it is the host, either by a rapid T cell response or by immune complex formation, that is responsible for all the pathology of the LCM disease!!

Other examples of immune complex diseases associated with viral antigens have been identified. These include Aleutian disease in mink, a viral disease similar to LCM, and equine infectious anemia of horses. What about humans? Particular attention has been given now to infection with hepatitis B virus, responsible for about half the cases of viral hepatitis. The process starts with infection of liver cells, followed by a brief period of viremia with virus and free viral antigens in blood. A surface antigen from the virus has been readily identified in blood during this period of time. This brief period is then followed by the presence of antibodies to viral components such as the surface antigen and core antigens of the virus. Thus, in this infection, there is a time period when viral antigens may be present in the circulation at the time when antibody is formed. The clinical symptoms in hepatitis involve not only the liver but may include other organs such as the joints and the kidneys. The extra-hepatic symptoms, found in about one-quarter of the patients, resemble serum sickness and appear to be caused by immune complexes. Some patients also have been found with severe vasculitis and glomerulonephritis. Lastly, there is speculation that the damage to the liver cells may also involve the immune response, in particular, the cytolytic T cell response, in a process akin to the LCM infection described above. This has not been proven.

5. Autologous antigens: Systemic lupus erythematosus (SLE) is a frequent autoimmune disease in which the patients make antibodies to a number of autologous constituents. Patients with SLE have a generalized increase in the production of autoantibodies. Prominent among

these are antibodies to native DNA, single-stranded DNA, a variety of nucleoproteins, cytoplasmic components, and to antigens in platelets, red cells, and neutrophils. Many of these antibodies do not cause direct injury to cells because they cannot cross the cell membrane to bind to their target antigen. However, the autoantibodies may combine with antigens in the blood or extracellular tissue fluids and form immune complexes that result in tissue injury. The antigens are released from normal cells during the course of their normal turnover. Indeed, in SLE antibodies bind to trace amounts of nucleic acids in serum to form immune complexes that deposit in GBM, in blood vessels of various tissues, and in the skin. The complexes of DNA-anti-DNA found in the GBM of lupus patients are the major component responsible for renal injury. Antibodies to platelets, red cells, or neutrophils produce a depletion of these cells with important functional consequences.

A disease very similar to SLE develops spontaneously in several strains of inbred mice. Particularly notable is a strain developed in New Zealand and named New Zealand Black (NZB). The NZB mice develop a number of autoimmune traits: severe hemolytic anemia, antibodies to single- and double-stranded DNA, and immune complex disease. The immune complex disease develops best in F1 crosses between NZB and a second New Zealand strain, the New Zealand White. Several genetic factors play a key role in this autoimmune disease. NZB mice are infected with murine leukemia virus, which are thought to influence autoimmune responses, by means not yet clear, and also to contribute antigens for formation of immune complexes.

The reasons for the immunological abnormalities in human and murine SLE is not known. The disease predominates in females—about 80% of cases. In the NZB mouse, castration results in increased incidence of disease in the male, while giving androgens retards the disease in the female. Concerning the cellular abnormalities, the thinking at present is that there is a generalized polyclonal stimulation of autoreactive clones of B cells resulting in multiple autoantibodies. Some argument has been raised about the possibility that the B cells' abnormality is caused by a dysfunction in regulatory T cells with an imbalance towards more helper T cells and less suppressor T cells. There is no consensus on this point among those investigating SLE. There is a recent finding that T cells secrete factors that result in maturation of B cells, implying that the primary defect is at the level of the T cell.

Another example of immune complex formation involving autologous antigens is the Heymann nephritis of rats. This immune complex disease is produced by immunization of rats with an autologous preparation of membranes from renal tubular cells. A few weeks after immunization, the rats make autoantibodies to the tubular cells, the antigen being localized to the apical portion facing the lumen of the tubules. These antibodies do not bind to the cells but will bind to trace amounts of the antigen found in the circulation, forming immune complexes that produce glomerular disease. A few cases of immune complex nephritis of man have been found involving an antigen of renal tubular cells.

6. Unknown antigens: A great many forms of glomerular diseases in man are caused by deposition of immune complexes along the GBM. In the majority of cases, the immune complex pathogenesis is based on immunofluorescent studies which disclose a typical "granular" deposition of Ig, with or without C, along GBM, in a picture identical to that described for the experimental models of acute and chronic immune complex diseases. In most cases, the antigens responsible for the formation of the complexes are not known. It is most likely that these glomerular immune complexes diseases involve a myriad of different antigens; some perhaps resulting from viral or bacterial infections, some derived from autologous constituents. The glomerular diseases involving immune complexes have various types of pathologic pictures varying in their degree of severity, in the extent of associated inflammatory reaction, and in the extent of deposition of immune complexes.

Certain forms of vasculitis are associated with deposits of immune reactants in vessel walls and are thought to be caused by immune complexes. Vasculitis can be associated with known immune complex diseases involving the kidney like in SLE. Polyarteritis nodosa is a subacute or chronic disseminated vascular disease characterized by necrotizing inflammation of medium and small arteries. The etiology and pathogenesis are unknown; but because Ig, C, and fibrin have been found in the lesions by immunofluorescence, the speculation has arisen that it has an immune complex pathogenesis.

Examples of Local Immune Complex Pathology. Rheumatoid arthritis is a chronic inflammatory disease of the joints believed to have an important immune complex component. The evidence for immune complexes involves the finding in joint fluids of antibodies to autologous IgG, together with neutrophils. The joint fluids have a low level of C proteins, presumably because these are fixed to the antigen-antibody complexes. The antibodies to IgG are of the IgM or IgG class and react with IgG that is complexed to antigen or chemically polymerized. These antibodies are called rheumatoid factor. Rheumatoid factor can be considered as an autoantibody. The thinking is that these autoantibodies develop to antibodies forming immune complexes with a microbial agent. The reasons for the localization of complexes in the joint remains unexplained. However, it is well established in experimental animals that immune complexes injected into the joint fluid result in severe acute inflammation that affects the synovial lining.

Other examples of immune complex formation at a local site are the hypersensitivity pneumonitis. These result from inhaling ambient air containing a high amount of antigen to which the individual is immune. The antigen-antibody complex that forms in the alveoli of the lung produces a severe inflammation with acute respiratory distress. Many clinical cases have now been reported in individuals exposed to antigens bound to dusts or particles such as fungi or proteins. Farmers' lung disease is one such example that develops upon inhalation of dust from hay contaminated with saprophitic fungi. Sugar cane workers develop a similar disease upon immunity to thermophilic actinomycetes contained in the sugar cane. Pigeon breeders frequently develop lung disease as they become immunized to the pigeon IgA abundant in the birds' droppings. Recently, several cases have been reported of hypersensitivity pneumonitis resulting from inhalation of fungi from contaminated humidifiers and air conditioners.

Examples of Tissue-Fixed Immune Complex Disease. Many autoimmune responses develop against tissue antigens and can cause diseases (see below). A most important consideration is whether the antigen is accessible to the antibodies. Autoantibodies to red cells, neutrophils, and platelets bind to these circulating blood cells, readily depleting them from the circulation. These autoantibodies are responsible for many cases of autoimmune hematological disorders. An interesting point to bring out is the cases of some drugs which combine with blood elements to form cell-bound antigens. Drug-induced hemolytic anemia or thrombocytopenia have been reported upon administration of phenacetin, quinidine, aspirin, and sulfonamides. In these cases, it can be documented, in the laboratory, that the red cell or the platelet are lysed by the patient's antibodies only in the presence of the drug, which somehow associates with the membrane of the cell.

AUTOIMMUNITY

Autoimmunity is an immune reaction to self components. It can be viewed as a breakdown of the tolerant state to autologous constituents. Some aspects of tolerance to self were mentioned in Chapter 9. Autoimmune reactions can develop spontaneously in man, and can also be induced to a number of tissue antigens using experimental animals appropriately immunized. Autoimmune reactions can be manifested by autoantibody production and/or by cellular immune mechanisms (i.e., T cell immunity). The immune complexes and/or cellular immune processes can produce tissue damage and disease. Autoimmune reactions, however, can also be harmless. There are many instances of autoimmune reactions to intracellular antigens inaccessible to antibodies or to T cells, and which, therefore, do not relate to disease.

The capacity to induce an autoimmune reaction varies from antigen to antigen. An important point is that self tolerance is maintained best in conditions where the self-antigen, even in trace amounts, is accessible to the circulation, hence, to the immune cells. The following statements can be made:

1. Autoimmunity to serum proteins is never found. Apparently, the high levels of serum proteins maintain a very effective tolerant state. In the cases of congenital absence of a serum protein, the deficient individual is capable of making antibodies if immunized with the absent protein. In Chapter 9 we gave the example of guinea pigs

with a genetic deficiency of C4 which, upon immunization, easily made anti-C4 antibodies. Hence, the capacity to respond appears to be present, but it is blocked in some way in the normal individual. In analogy to tolerance to foreign proteins, the high level of serum proteins may produce tolerance at the B and T cell level. A recent study has shown the presence in lymphoid organs of B cells reactive to C5, a protein of the complement system found in serum in small amounts. The normal individual, however, is tolerant and will not activate its B cells because of a lack of help from T cells. The experiments of Triplett described in Chapter 9 are also relevant to this point.

2. It is easy to make autoantibodies to many intracellular components. Apparently, the state of tolerance to these antigens is poor, and one makes easily an immune response to them. Perhaps the fact that the intracellular antigens remain "hidden" from immune cells explains this lack of tolerance. For example, autoantibodies to intracellular components of heart of liver cells are made following cell death as a result of poor blood flow or toxins. In ischemic heart injury, autoantibodies to heat proteins are found in serum. Necrosis of liver cells by carbon tetrachloride results in production of autoantibodies to mitochondrial proteins. In these cases, autoantibodies do not cause injury because they are directed to cytoplasmic components.

3. Immune reactions to many tissues can be induced only following strong immunization measures, such as:

a. incorporation of autologous tissue with "adjuvants" like Freund's adjuvant (the water-in-oil emulsion containing dead virulent tubercle bacilli). Incorporation of myelin basic protein, sperm proteins, and thyroid proteins, for example, results in the production of antibody and T cell immunity. The basis for induction by the antigen in adjuvant is not known. It does imply that B and T helper cells are found reactive to the autologous proteins. Whether they are found in limited number and controlled in some way by a level of Ts can be argued, inasmuch as they remain inoperant under physiological conditions. The adjuvant could conceivably boost helper T cell function. In some mouse strains, repeated injection of mouse thyroglobulin without adjuvant can eventually result also in autoimmunity and thyroiditis.

b. introducing an element of foreignness into the autologous proteins, for instance by conjugating a new foreign molecule to them (such as a hapten) or by denaturing the autologous proteins. Another way to bypass unresponsiveness to autologous components is by immunizing with a similar tissue protein from a different species which shares cross-reactive antigens. For example, rabbit thyroglobulin and human thyroglobulin share antigenic determinants, but each has specific determinants of its own. Immunization of rabbits with human thyroglobulin is possible since a human protein is immunogenic in the rabbit. Upon such immunization, however, the rabbit will make autoantibodies to the antigens shared between rabbit and human thyroglobulin. One way to interpret this phenomenon is in the light of the information available on T-B collaboration and tolerance (see Table 9.2 in Chapter 9). In these instances, the normal individual has B cells reactive to autologous thyroglobulin, a point which has been proven, but may have limited helper T cells. Introduction of a foreign determinant in the molecule, such as the cross-reactive determinants, allows clones of T cells reactive to this new determinant to be activated.

Examples of Autoimmune Diseases in Experimental Animals

1. Anti-GBM antibody-induced glomerulonephritis: Immunization of an animal with foreign GBM, in order to produce antibodies for nephrotoxic serum nephritis, also leads to the production of autoantibody that fixes to autologous GBM and induces severe nephritis in the immunized animal. In our example shown in Figure 13.3, the rabbits immunized to rat GBM had some antibodies which caused nephritis.

2. Experimental allergic encephalomyelitis: Immunization with a basic protein from myelin induces an acute disseminated disease of the nervous system with mononuclear cell infiltrates and demyelination. It is caused by T cells via a cell-mediated mechanism.

3. Thyroiditis: Immunization with heterologous thyroglobulin induces inflammation in the thyroid gland. Autoantibodies to thyroglobulin and T cell immunity are involved in the pathogenesis of this disease. Thyroiditis can also be produced by immunization with chemically modified autologous thyroglobulin or, in some species, with autologous thyroglobulin in Freund's adjuvant.

4. Aspermatogenesis: The testes offers an example of how anatomical features condition the kind of pathological lesion. The testes is formed by seminiferous tubules, where the sperms develop, and a collecting system of ducts. The seminiferous tubules end up in short, straight tubules which connect with the rete testes, a sac-like structure that collects the sperm. The seminiferous tubules are impermeable to plasma proteins but not the rete testes, which contains them. Immunization with sperm in adjuvants induces both the formation of autoantibodies to sperm and T cell immunity. The autoantibodies bind to the sperm in the rete testes, producing acute inflammation. However, they cannot gain access to the tubules. On the other hand, the immune T cells actively penetrate into the tubules where they produce a cellular immunity reaction that results in the death of the germinal epithelium.

5. Other autoimmune reactions include those to adrenals, pancreas, peripheral nerve, and lens tissue.

Human Diseases with an Autoimmune Component

1. Anti-GBM nephritis: A rare, severe, sometimes fatal disease in which the individual makes autoantibody to its GBM. It can be accompanied by pulmonary damage (Goodpasture syndrome). The anti-GBM cross-react with lung basement membrane and can produce a severe inflammation in the lung. The antibodies are found deposited in a smooth, linear pattern all along the GBM and along lung alveoli. The anti-GBM antibodies fix complement and attract neutrophils. These autoantibodies isolated from blood can transfer the disease to monkeys. (The autoantibodies crossreact with monkey GBM.)

2. Post-rabies vaccine encephalitis: Following immunization with attenuated rabies virus in spinal cord, some individuals develop an encephalitis identical to that induced in experimental animals by immunization with brain.

3. Chronic thyroiditis: Hashimoto's disease is characterized by enlargment of the thyroid, heavy infiltration of the gland by mononuclear cells, and a variety of autoantibodies to thyroid proteins.

4. Autoimmune hemolytic anemia: Patients develop autoantibodies spontaneously; the autoantibodies can be found in the red cells by an anti-Ig reagents (Coombs test).

5. SLE: Explained earlier.

6. Idiopathic thrombocytopenic purpura: This disease is characterized by a drastic reduction in the number of platelets as a result of autoantibody. The platelets coated with antibody are removed by splenic macrophages.

7. Autoimmune anti-receptor diseases: These are autoimmune diseases in which autoantibodies are directed to cell surface receptor molecules involved in cell-to-cell communication and/or hormone-receptor interactions. The best studied is myasthenia gravis, a condition characterized by weakness and fatigue of voluntary muscles, sometimes severe enough to result in paralysis. The disease can affect all skeletal muscles. The basic problem in myasthenia is an interruption of the normal neuromuscular transmission as a result of autoantibodies directed to the aceytylcholine receptor. The number of receptors in the neuromuscular function is reduced, most likely from the repeated modulation by the antibody (in a way similar to the capping described in Chapter 5 for the B cell). Myasthenia gravis can be induced in rabbits by immunizing with the membranes of the electric eel, which are very rich in the aceytylcholine receptor. Antibodies to the receptor can transfer the symptoms to normal individuals.

A second disease caused by an anti-receptor antibody is Graves disease. This is a disease caused by an increased production of thyroid hormones resulting in symptoms of hyperthyroidism (increased metabolic rate, loss of weight, restlessness, palpitations, etc.). The autoantibodies bind to the thyroid acinar cell, to or very close by, the receptor for the thyroid-stimulating hormone, a polypeptide made in the pituitary and responsible for stimulating the cell to produce thyroid hormones. The anti-receptor antibody, in fact, takes the place of the hormone and stimulates the cell to increase cyclic AMP, an event that results in increased production of the hormone. Why some antibodies stimulate the cell as in Graves disease, while others do not and, moreover, block the action of the hormone, is not known.

Other anti-receptor diseases include the rare cases of insulin-resistant diabetes, in which antibodies to the insulin receptor result in the severe diabetes. Insulin-resistant diabetes is accompanied by a skin disease, acanthosis nigrican. A few cases of autoantibodies to the beta adrenergic receptors have been reported which may be important in those cases of bronchial asthma. The autoantibodies, by blocking the site of binding of catecholamines, prevent a normal bronchodilatory response, therefore, favoring the effects of alpha adrenergic agonists.

8. <u>Pemphigus:</u> <u>Pemphigus vulgaris</u> is a chronic disease of the skin and mucous membranes characterized by the presence of soft blisters on an otherwise normal skin. The blisters are vesicles that form within the epithelium as a result of detachment (called acantholysis) of the cells in the middle layers, leaving intact a row of basal cells adherent to the connective tissue. These bullae readily break upon mechanical pressure, leaving a denuded area that heals poorly and is prone to infection. Pemphigus is caused by an autoantibody that binds to the surface of the epidermal cells, apparently to the surface "cement". It is thought that the antibody may stimulate a protease that may then be responsible for the acantholysis. In pemphigus the autoantibodies can be found bound to the skin of the patient or in the circulation. The antibodies injected into neonatal mice reproduce the skin pathology. A different type of bullous skin disease is <u>bullous pemphigoid</u>. In these cases, the bullae are found between the basal layer of the skin and the collagenous basement membrane. The autoantibodies are found bound to the basement membrane.

REFERENCES

Cochrane, C. G., and Koffler, D. Immune complex disease in experimental animals and man. Adv. Immunol., 16:185, 1973.

Larsen, G. L., and Henson, P. M. Mediators of inflammation. Ann. Rev. Immunol., <u>1</u>:335, 1983.

Miescher, P. A., and Muller-Eberhard, J. H. <u>Textbook of Immunopathology</u>, second edition, Grune and Stratton, New York, 1976.

Moller, G., ed. Models of Autoimmune Disease. Edited by G. Moller, Immunol. Rev., Volume 55, 1981 (ten excellent chapters that include analyses of lupus, autoimmune diseases of red cells, nervous system, kindey, thyroid, and testes).

Oldstone, M. B. A., and Dixon, F. J. Immune complex disease in chronic viral infections. J. Exp. Med., 134:32s, 1971.

Unanue, E. R., and Dixon, F. J. Experimental glomerulonephritis. Immunologic events and pathogenetic mechanisms. Adv. Immunol., 6:1, 1967.

Weigle, W. O. The induction of autoimmunity in rabbits following injection of heterologous or altered homologous thyroglobulin. J. Exp. Med., 121:289, 1965.

Weigle, W. O. Analysis of autoimmunity through experimental models of thyroiditis and allergic encephalomyelitis. Adv. Immunol., 30: 159, 1980.

CHAPTER 14

Immediate Hypersensitivity Reactions and Anaphylaxis

A normal component of the immune response to thymic-dependent antigens is the production of small amounts of IgE antibodies. Although the physiological significance of these IgE antibody production is not well known, the role of these antibodies in producing anaphylaxis and allergies is well established.

The phenomenon of anaphylaxis was described initially by Richet and Portier in 1902 when they studied the antitoxic immunity of dogs to a poison obtained from sea anemones. They carried out their experiments while on a cruise in the Mediterranean on the boat of the Prince of Monaco. There was, indeed, a serious advantage in those days in carrying out research in immunology as compared to modern times. Richet and Portier found that dogs previously immunized with the poison exhibited severe vascular shock and collapsed and died within a few minutes after reinjection of an amount of the poison far below the lethal dose. Because this response was the reverse of immunity in which the animals are in a prophylactic state, the phenomenon was called anaphylaxis, the opposite of immunity. Since that time, the mechanisms involved in anaphylaxis have been intensively studied. Anaphylactic reactions occur in practically every mammalian experimental species as well as in humans, and can be divided into: 1) systemic reactions that result from the rapid intravenous introduction of the antigen to sensitized individuals; and 2) local reactions elicited by introducing the antigen locally, as in the skin.

From the early times, it was clear that anaphylactic reactions are the result of an immune response to an antigen or sensitization to this antigen. This conclusion derived from the observation that an interval is required between the first and second injections of antigen in order for anaphylactic sensitivity to develop. The time interval between the injections is in accord with the time required for the formation of antibodies. Furthermore, anaphylactic sensitivity can be transferred passively by administration of antiserum from sensitized animals. Thus, normal guinea pigs that receive antibody from sensitized guinea pigs, followed twenty-four hours later by the specific antigen, will develop anaphylactic shock, which cannot be distinguished from that observed in actively sensitized animals.

Table 14.1

Model of Anaphylactic Phenomena: Stages of the Reaction

1. Immunization with production of anaphylactic antibody.
2. Sensitization of cellular elements: mast cells and basophils.
3. Triggering of cellular elements by antigen-antibody reaction at the cell surface.
4. Release of chemical mediators.
5. Stimulation of smooth muscle contraction by vasoactive amines and effects on endothelial cells and small vessels.
6. Symptoms in shock organs.

All anaphylactic phenomena can be analyzed according to a model involving six defined steps, as shown in Table 14.1. The first step is the production of a special sensitizing antibody following immunization. This antibody is usually of the IgE class of antibodies. The second step is the sensitization by the anaphylactic antibody of specialized cellular elements involved in inflammation: mast cells and blood basophils. The third step concerns the triggering of these elements by specific antigen reacting with the cell-bound anaphylactic antibody at the cell surface, followed, in the fourth step, by the release of the mediators. The fifth step is the stimulation of smooth muscle contraction at the local site or throughout the organism by the vasoactive amines, and the effect of vasoactive amines on endothelial cells of small vessels, resulting in the symptoms of anaphylactic shock. These symptoms vary from species to species according to the sensitivity of the smooth muscles of different organs. The organs that are particularly sensitive to anaphylactic shock are called the shock organs.

SYSTEMIC ANAPHYLACTIC REACTION

We shall first begin by describing the systemic anaphylactic reactions that develop in different experimental animals and in humans. These follow the systemic administration of antigen to an individual with anaphylactic antibodies to the antigen in question. In spite of the fact that all anaphylactic phenomena follow precisely the pattern of events we have just described, the phenomenology of anaphylactic reactions vary from species to species according to the type of organ primarily involved in the reaction. The guinea pig, within minutes after injection of antigen, becomes restless, its hair bristles, and it has difficulty in breathing. Finally, the guinea pig urinates and defecates, undergoes systemic convulsions, and dies in a cyanotic state. The whole process takes no longer than two to three minutes. The phenomena of anaphylaxis in the guinea pig are largely the result of the spastic contraction of the smooth muscles in their bronchial tree, leading to an incapacity of the animal to exhale the inhaled air. At autopsy, the lungs are found to be markedly distended and do not collapse. The other symptoms, such as the bristling of the hair, are caused by the contraction of smooth muscle in the hair follicles; urination and defecation are caused by smooth muscle contraction in the gut and bladder. The major shock organs in the guinea pig, however, are the bronchi of the lungs which are the cause of asphyxia and death.

In other animal species such as humans, rats, and mice, the symptoms of anaphylactic reactions include, besides those attributed to bronchospasm, those of vascular collapse. There is a precipitous drop in blood pressure, the subject becomes cold and clammy, and undergoes vascular shock. This is caused by vasodilation of venules and generally of the whole vascular tree and increase in vascular permeability with loss of fluids and proteins from the circulation. In species like the dog or the rabbit, there is a severe contraction of smooth muscles in critical areas of the circulation. For instance, in the dog, the smooth muscles of the hepatic veins constrict causing a marked deficit in venous return to the heart and vascular collapse. In the rabbit, the smooth muscles of the pulmonary arteries are the main targets for the vasoconstriction resulting again in diminished return of blood to the heart and vascular collapse. In humans, symptoms develop within minutes of receiving the antigen. The symptoms may include respiratory distress resulting from intense bronchoconstriction, edema of the larynx, presence of urticaria (hives) in the skin, gastrointestinal symptoms (vomiting, cramps, diarrhea), and vascular collapse. Table 14.2 is a summary of acute anaphylaxis in different species.

PASSIVE CUTANEOUS ANAPHYLAXIS

Local anaphylactic reactions, particularly in the skin, have been very useful to study anaphylactic phemonena. It was discovered very early by allergists that the injection of serum from sensitized individuals into the skin of a normal volunteer would result in passive sensitization, locally, at the site of injection. Antigen challenge twenty-four to forty-eight hours later resulted in an acute inflammation, characterized by increased vascular permeability, redness, and leakage of proteins from the blood. Skin testing is still a common procedure used in medical practice for diagnosing allergies. Usually, the individual presumed to have an allergic reactivity to an antigen, and therefore to have IgE bound to cells in its skin, is injected

Table 14.2

Systemic Anaphylactic Reactions

Species	Shock Tissue-Organ	Mediators	Symptoms
Guinea pig	Lung (Bronchioles)	Histamine SRS-A	Asphyxia Convulsions Cyanosis Urination Defecation
Rat	Intestine Vascular System	Histamine Serotonin	Vascular collapse Cyanosis Defecation
Mouse	Intestine Vascular System	Histamine Serotonin	Vascular collapse Cyanosis Defecation
Rabbit	Pulmonary arteries	Histamine Serotonin	Vascular collapse Convulsions
Dog	Hepatic veins	Histamine Serotonin	Vascular collapse Urination Defecation
Human	Lung (Bronchioles) Larynx Vascular system	Histamine SRS-A	Vascular collapse Asphyxia Cyanosis

intradermally with very minute amounts of the antigen. A positive reaction is characterized by an area of swelling and slight redness at the site of injection, developing within minutes of the injection.

The same type of passive cutaneous anaphylaxis has been demonstrated in experimental animals such as guinea pigs, rats, and mice. Local, passive cutaneous anaphylaxis (PCA), is caused by the same classes of antibodies as systemic anaphylaxis. A latent period is necessary before passive sensitization becomes effective. That is, following the passive transfer, either systemically or locally, of antibodies from sensitized individuals, a period of time is required for effective sensitization. This period varies from several hours to one or two days, depending upon species and the class of antibodies. This latent period is explained by the time required for the antibodies to bind to tissue mast cells.

THE ANAPHYLACTIC ANTIBODIES

There are generally two classes of antibodies responsible for anaphylactic reactions. The major class of antibody responsible for hypersensitivity reactions in all mammalian species is the IgE class of antibodies (also called reagins). IgE antibodies have been identified in dogs, rabbits, rats, mice, monkeys, and man. These antibodies are present in the serum in very low concentration, in the microgram/ml range, and are also found bound to mast cells and basophils. Their presence in low concentration in the serum is because of their very low level of synthesis and not because of their strong binding to mast cells and basophils.

The production of IgE antibodies is dependent on the helper function of immune T cells. Thymus-independent antigens are not able to stimulate the synthesis of antibodies of the IgE class. It is probable, though not firmly established, that a special population of helper T cells regulate the synthesis of IgE antibodies. These IgE helper T cells may be distinct from the helper T cells that regulate synthesis of IgG antibodies. The IgE antibodies are also under very strict regulation by suppressor T cells. These suppressor T cells selectively control the amount and time of production of IgE antibodies without influencing IgG antibody production. Factors from T helper and suppressor cells have been produced that enhance or inhibit IgE. Whether an imbalance of these is responsible for the states of allergy has been speculated and is under current investigation.

In addition to IgE antibodies, there is another class of antibodies that mediates anaphylactic reactions in certain species of mammals. Fast-migrating IgG (or 7S gamma-1) immunoglobulins which do not bind complement through the normal classical pathway, are able to mediate anaphylactic reactions in guinea pigs and mice. The gamma-1 subclass of antibodies, in contrast to IgE antibodies, is synthesized in large amounts by their respective species and is found in the serum in milligram amounts per ml. However, their binding to mast cells is weak compared to the IgE class of antibodies. Other differences between the gamma-1 and IgE anaphylactic antibodies are their sensitivity to heat. The ability of IgE antibodies to sensitize is destroyed by heating at 56 degrees C, but not that of gamma-1 antibodies. The latent period is considerably longer for sensitization for passive cutaneous anaphylaxis by antibodies of the IgE class than for antibodies of the gamma-1 class. However, once sensitized by IgE antibodies, the tissues remain reactive for extended periods of time (for days and sometimes weeks), because the binding of IgE antibodies to mast cells is very strong. IgE antibodies also have a somewhat larger molecular weight than antibodies of the gamma-1 class, because of their larger H-chain.

Both IgE and gamma-1 antibodies sensitize only the species of origin. For instance, human IgE antibodies bind to and sensitize human mast cells but not guinea pig, rat, or mouse mast cells. Similarly, guinea pig, rabbit, or mouse IgE antibodies will not sensitize human mast cells and will not sensitize each other's mast cells, with the exception of mouse antibodies being able to sensitize the rat. On the whole, it appears, therefore, that the IgE and the gamma-1 antibodies are species restricted. They have been called homocytotropic. However, it has been known for a long time that antibodies from some species sensitize a different species for anaphylaxis. For instance, human and rabbit antibodies sensitize guinea pig for anaphylaxis very effectively. In all these instances, however, the class of immunoglobulin that sensitizes the foreign species is the conventional IgG class of antibodies which is not a sensitizer in its own species. These types of reactions are referred to as mediated by heterocytotropic antibodies.

SENSITIZATION OF MAST CELLS AND BASOPHILS

The anaphylactic reactions, whether systemic or local, are the result of the sensitization of mast cells and basophils by anaphylactic antibodies of the IgE or gamma-1 class. Such antibodies have been demonstrated on the surface of these cells which have been shown to have binding sites for the Fc fragment of the antibodies. The IgE antibodies bind to a specific receptor protein that has now been isolated from the mast cell. The receptor is an integral membrane protein made up of two chains. The alpha chain, of about 45,000 daltons, is non-covalently associated with a beta chain of about 30,000 daltons. IgE binds to the alpha chain.

The release of amines from mast cells is brought about not only by the interaction with specific antigen to which the antibodies are directed but also can occur following the administration of an antibody directed against the anaphylactic antibodies bound to mast cells. Thus, local and systemic anaphylactic reactions can be elicited with anti-IgE antibodies or anti-gamma-1 antibodies reacting with the anaphylactic antibodies bound to mast cells.

Triggering of Mast Cells by Antigen-Antibody Reactions. The interaction of anaphylactic antibodies on the surface of mast cells with antigen or with specific antibodies directed to the anaphylactic antibodies causes a signal to be registered on the membrane of the cell that results in the release of the mediators. The triggering of mast cells by the interaction between the anaphylactic antibodies with antigen requires the binding of several adjacent antibody molecules on the cell. For instance, only antigens that are polyvalent are able to cause mast cell degranulation. Since many antigens have multiple antigenic determinants, and since mast cells bind anaphylactic antibodies of all specificities by their Fc fragments, most antigens function as polyvalent antigens.

The requirement for cross-linking in the degranulation of mast cells has been well documented using antibodies to IgE. For example, human mast cells with IgE bound to the IgE receptor degranulates upon addition of a bivalent rabbit anti-human IgE antibodies. The anti-IgE will cross-link two adjacent IgE molecules, form a microaggregate on the membrane, and trigger the signal that produces the release of granules. No degranulation occurs if an Fab fragment of the anti-IgE antibody is used. The Fab fragment will bind to the IgE antibody without producing major changes in the cell. Cross-linking produces either a steric effect on the receptors or induces a local change in the membrane that initiates the reaction.

The release of vasoactive amine mediators by mast cells is an active process requiring energy. The reaction requires calcium, has a pH optimum from 7.5 to 7.9, and proceeds best at 37 degrees C to 38 degrees C. The mast cells are inactivated at 45 degrees C. A number of biochemical reactions are triggered by antigen or anti-IgE antibodies. Within fifteen seconds, there is a rapid and very transitory rise in the intracellular levels of cyclic AMP. At about the same time, methylation of membrane phospholipids takes place as a result of activation of methyltransferases. Methyl groups donated by S-adenosyl-methionine are incorporated into phosphatidylethanolamine, converting it to phosphatidylcholine. This change decreases membrane fluidity which may be a factor in promoting some of the biochemical changes. The rise in cyclic AMP as a result of activation of adenylate cyclase will phosphorylate cytosolic and membrane proteins by way of a cyclic AMP-activated protein kinase. The contraction of microfilaments may be stimulated in this way, resulting in the movement of the mast cell granule from the cytosol to the plasma membrane. The activation of adenylate cyclase and methyltransferases may be related. Pharmacological inhibition of methylation will inhibit the fifteen-second rise in cyclic AMP.

Two other early biochemical events include a rapid rise in cell calcium derived from the extracellular medium and an activation of a serine-protease. Inhibition of the enzyme results in decrease in granule release. Following these very rapid changes, there is a release of products derived from arachidonic acid—prostaglandins and leukotrienes.

The release of vasoactive amines results from the extrusion of the granules into the environment. Mast cells and basophils have large granules easily observed under the microscope. These granules contain vasoactive amines such as histamine as well as heparin bound to a protein complex (Figure 14.1). When the granules are extruded outside the cells by an active process, the histamine and the heparin are released from the granules by an ion exchange process at the neutral pH of body tissues. In humans, the mast cells have a distinct crystalline structure. Interestingly, this structure becomes amorphous, solubilizing in stimulated cells even before the granule is extruded.

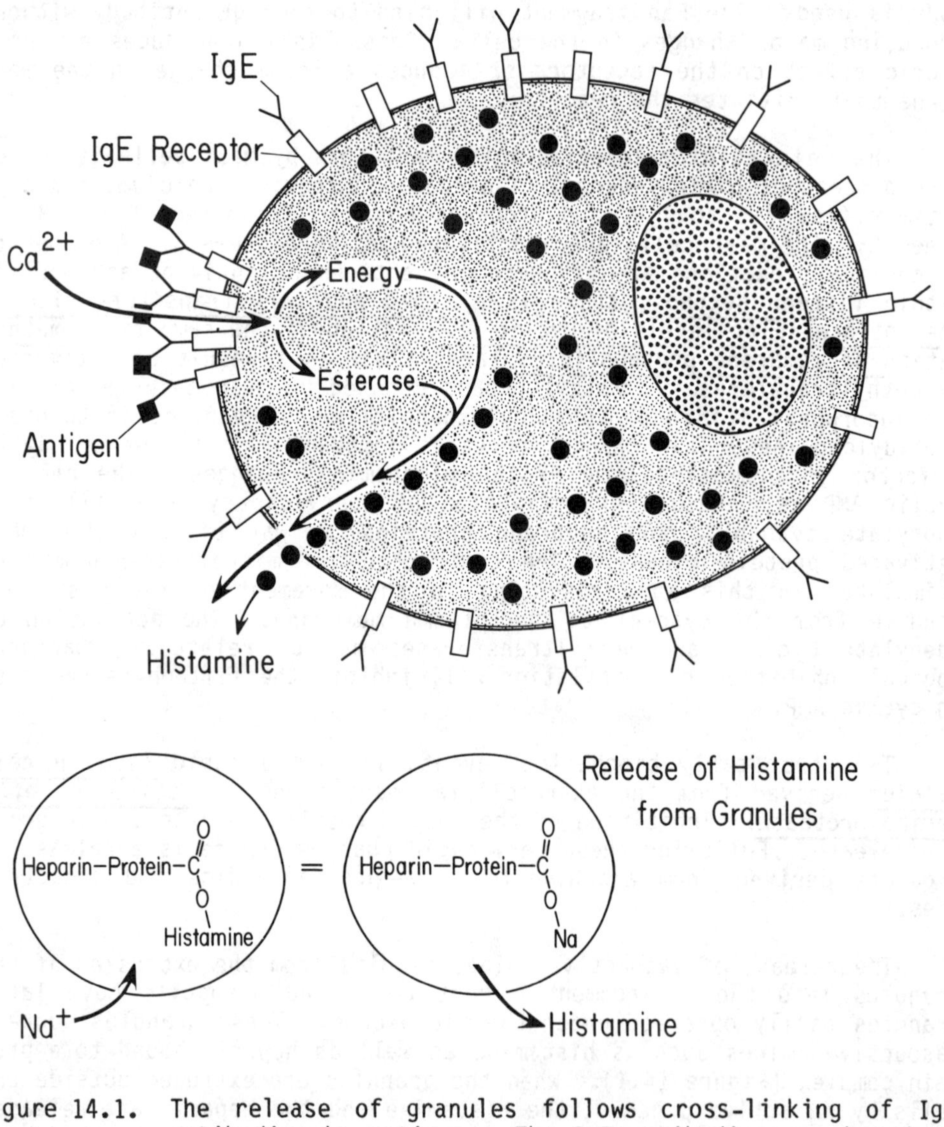

Figure 14.1. The release of granules follows cross-linking of IgE antibodies by antigen. The IgE antibodies are bound to the mast cell by a specific receptor.

The release of vasoactive amines by mast cells can be affected by a variety of hormonal agents. For instance, beta adrenergic agonists such as epinephrine and isoproterenol, and prostaglandins of the E class inhibit histamine release. These drugs may act by activating membrane-bound adenylcyclase and increasing the level of cyclic AMP in the cells for sustained periods of time. Also, drugs such as methylxanthines which affect the level of cytoplasmic phosphodiesterase inhibit the release of vasoactive amines.

MEDIATORS OF ANAPHYLACTIC REACTIONS

The chemical mediators have been studied mainly in cultures of cells (mast cells or basophils) or organs (like fragments of guinea pig or human lung) challenged with antigen or with anti-IgE antibodies. The number of mediators is extensive, and many have been isolated and studied in pure form. Although some molecules stand out by their very powerful action, the overall symptoms of anaphylaxis and allergy probably result from their composite effects. These various mediators are modulators of the basic inflammatory response. In the allergic and anaphylactic reactions, their effects predominate. In non-allergic inflammation, their effects may be more limited and mixed with the combined effects of other cellular and humoral mediators.

There are two major classes of chemical mediators responsible for anaphylactic and allergic reactions. The preformed or primary mediators are the molecules stored in the mast cell or basophil granules and released seconds after contact with the antigen. The preformed mediators include four major kinds of molecules: 1) a major vasoactive amine— either histamine or serotonin, or both; 2) chemotactic factors for granulocytes; 3) enzymes; and 4) a proteoglycan represented by heparin in the mast cell and chondroitin sulphate in the basophil. The secondary mediators are molecules synthesized by mast cells or basophils or other inflammatory cells following the interactions with antigens. The principal secondary mediators are lipid derivatives and include the leukotrienes and the platelet-activating factor.

Preformed Mediators: Histamine is a basic amine derived from the decarboxylation of histidine; it is found in mast cell and basophil granules and also in platelets. Injection of histamine into guinea pigs reproduces the symptoms of acute anaphylaxis. Furthermore, many of the symptoms of acute anaphylaxis can be blocked by injection of anti-histaminic drugs, a family of molecules that compete with histamine for its binding site in tissues. Histamine acts on smooth muscles and on the blood vessels and also on some exocrine glands and leukocytes. With some exceptions, it generally stimulates intense contraction of smooth muscle. This contraction of smooth muscle is responsible for the bronchoconstriction observed in acute anaphylactic reactions.

The effect of histamine on smooth muscle can be reproduced *in vitro*. For example, the guinea pig uterus or a strip of small intestine from sensitized guinea pig when suspended in a warm saline solution readily contracts upon addition of antigen (Schultz-Dale reaction). This contraction is produced because antigen releases histamine from the tissue mast cells by the mechanisms described previously. Similar contraction is observed following the direct addition of histamine to the salt solution.

The effect of histamine on blood vessels is primarily on the endothelial cells and on the vessel wall. The endothelial cells contract, exposing bare areas of vessel wall to the blood, causing an increase in vascular permeability to larger molecules. Also depending upon the type and species, blood vessels dilate or constrict upon addition of histamine. Usually, large vessels constrict, while arteriole, venules, and capillaries dilate, causing a drop in blood pressure.

The many effects of histamine are mediated by two different kinds of receptors on tissues, the H1 and H2 receptors, distinguished through the antagonistic effects of various kinds of anti-histamine drugs. H1 receptors mediate most of the common effects of histamine on smooth muscle and blood vessels, whereas H2 receptors mediate the effects of histamine in increasing gastric secretion or heart rate (Figure 14.2).

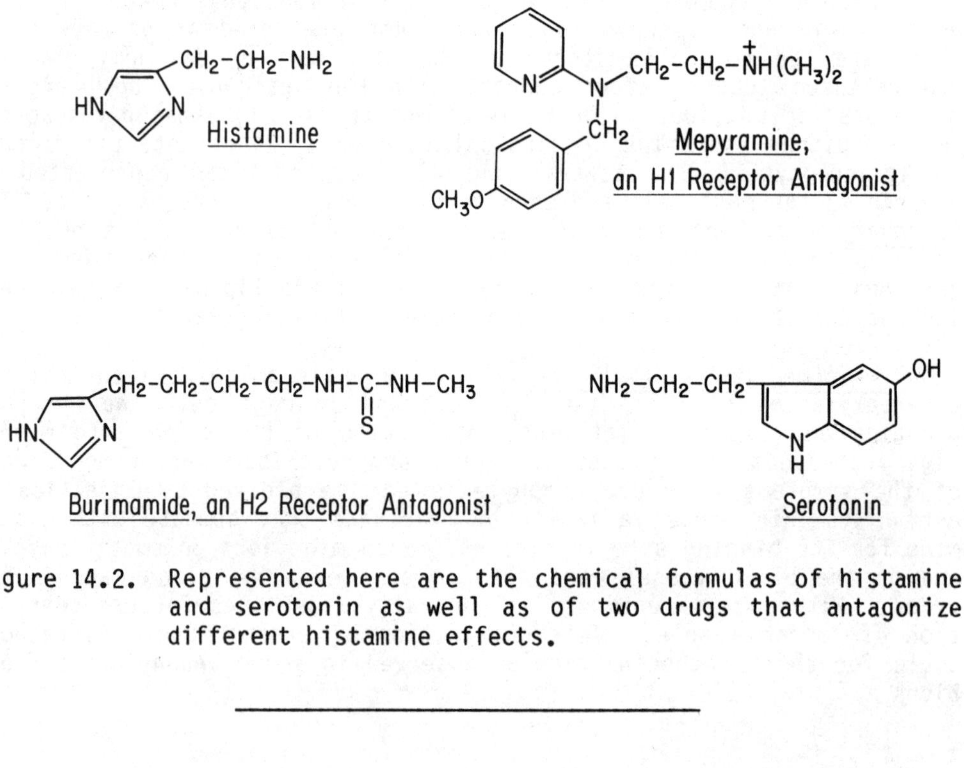

Figure 14.2. Represented here are the chemical formulas of histamine and serotonin as well as of two drugs that antagonize different histamine effects.

Histamine has also been shown to have effects on leukocytes and lymphocytes. In eosinophils, it selectively increases the number of surface receptors for C3b, in a process inhibited by H1 antihistamines, and also induces chemotaxis. Some suppressor T cells appear to be activated by relatively high doses of histamine. The biological significance of these effects is not known.

Serotonin (5-hydroxytriptamine) is found in mast cells of the rat and the mouse where it has a major role, similar to histamine in humans and guinea pigs. Serotonin causes an increase in vascular permeability and usually vasoconstriction. (Histamine is also found in mast cells of rodents, but it has little biological effect on target tissues, which contrasts with the profound effects of serotonin.) In man, serotonin is not involved in anaphylaxis although is it found in platelets and in the enterochromafin cells of the small intestine where most likely it has a physiological effect.

The chemotactic factors derived from mast cells and basophils are active towards granulocytes. The eosinophil chemotactic factors are two tetrapeptides (val-gly-ser-glu and ala-gly-ser-glu) active on eosinophils and, to lesser extent, on neutrophils. They also increase the expression of C3 receptors in eosinophils, as well as potentiate the synthesis of oxygen-derived products. Other less well-characterized molecules have been found with chemotactic activities for eosinophils and neutrophils.

Several enzymes are released with the granules. Their composition varies with the cells and the species. Included are a chymotrypsin-like and tryptic-like enzyme, beta-hexosaminidase, alpha-glucuronidase, an aryl-sulfatase and an enzyme that generates vasoactive peptides from plasma. Although the role of these different enzymatic activities is not known, it is very apparent that the granule contains a large array of potentially inflammatory molecules aside from the powerful histamine and serotonin.

All mast cell and basophil granules contain a proteoglycan. Heparin, found in the mast cell, has anti-coagulant activity and anti-complementary activity. Its polyanionic nature is responsible for the metachromasia of the granules.

Secondary mediators: The leukotrienes (LT) are a major set of mediators produced in the anaphylactic and allergic reactions. The LT were first identified in lungs from guinea pigs undergoing anaphylactic reactions and characterized as low molecular weight molecules that produced a slow contraction of smooth muscle in the Schultz-Dale assays. This contraction was not inhibited by anti-histaminics. The material was named as slow reactive substance of anaphylaxis or SRS-A. SRS-A is now known to be comprised of three distinct molecules, each derived from the other: LTC-4, LTD-4, and LTE-4. LT are derived, like prostaglandins (PG), from arachidonic acid. Arachidonic acid is esterified to the second carbon of glycerol in membrane phospholipids and released by the action of a Ca-dependent enzyme, phospholipase A-2. The released arachidonic acid can be metabolized via cyclooxygenase to produce various biologically active compounds such as the prostaglandins E-2, I-2, D-2, F-2-alpha, and thromboxane A-2. Arachidonic acid is also metabolized by lipoxygenases. The action of lipoxygenase on carbon 5 results in the production of 5-hydroxy-eicosatetraenoic acid (5-HETE) which can be converted to leukotriene A-4 (LTA-4) or B-4 (LTB-4). LTA-4 can react with glutathione to form LTC-4 and eventually LTD-4 and LTE-4 (Figures 14.3 and 14.4).

The molecules derived from the lipoxygenase pathway of metabolism of arachidonate have a number of biological activities. Five-HETE and 12-HETE (another HETE compound where lipoxygenase has acted on carbon 12) have chemotactic activity for neutrophils and also produce release of lysosomal enzymes. LTB-4 is one of the most potent chemoattractants for neutrophils and mononuclear cells known so far, being about one-hundredfold more potent than the HETE compound and tenfold more active than C5a. LTB-4 induces an increase in cyclic AMP. It also induces release of prostaglandins.

LTC-4, D-4, and E-4 (the SRS-A compounds) have a very potent effect in contracting smooth muscles particularly from lung tissue. This bronchoconstrictive effect of the SRS-A compound is more potent than that of histamine. Because of this powerful effect, the LTC-4, D-4, and E-4 compounds are thought to be a major cause of the lung changes in anaphylactic reactions and in allergic reactions such as allergic bronchial asthma. These compounds also increase the production of mucus in the lung and have effects on blood vessels such as increases in vascular permeability, particularly of post-capillary venules, and vasoconstrictive effect on arterioles.

LT are produced by a number of cells, including mast cells, basophils, and macrophages. In the lung, the LT are produced by mast cells and also be alveolar macrophages, but the extent to which each participates in IgE-mediated reactions is not known.

In IgG-mediated reactions, various PG and thromboxanes are also produced. The mast cell is a unique cell in producing large amounts of PGD-2. PGD-2 and thromboxane A-2 also have bronchoconstrictive effects. PGE-2, on the other hand, can inhibit mast cell degranulation. It is thought that PG production is a secondary event that follows the release of granules and the production of the LT. For example, addition of inhibitors of histamine and LT to lung fragments challenged with antigen results in inhibition of PG production.

The last mediator to be considered is the platelet-activating factor (PAF) which is thought to derive from membrane phospholipid. Its chemical formula was shown in Chapter 13. PAF is a major component in systemic anaphylaxis in rabbits, causing release of mediators from platelets. Its function in other species is now being studied. In its purified form, PAF agglutinates platelets and neutrophils and can

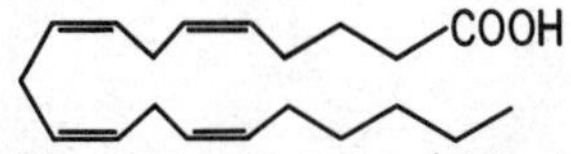

Arachidonic Acid (20:4)

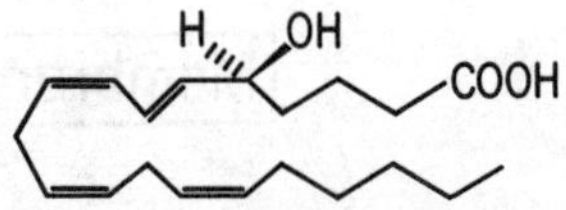

5-Hydroperoxyeicosatetraenoic Acid

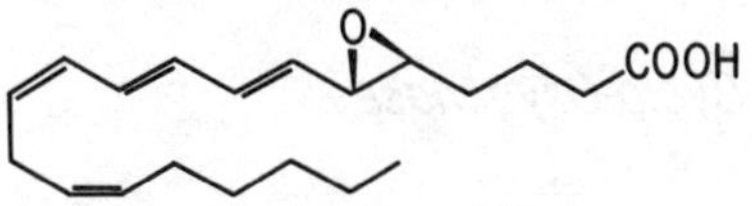

Leukotriene A_4

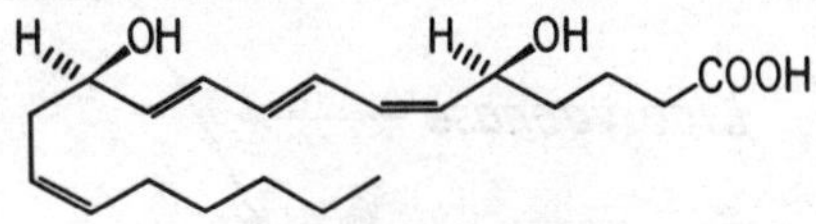

Leukotriene B_4

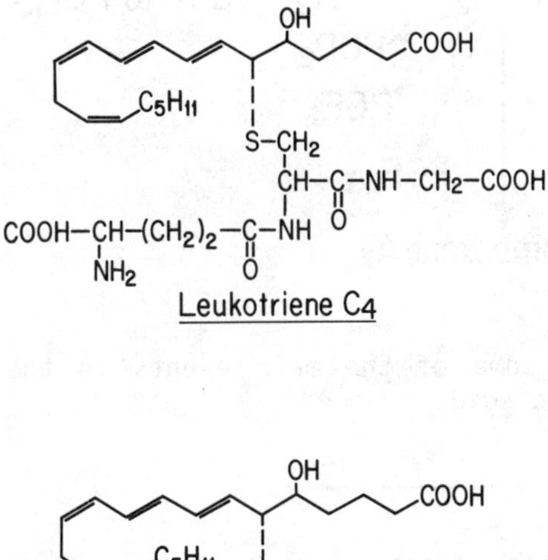

Leukotriene C_4

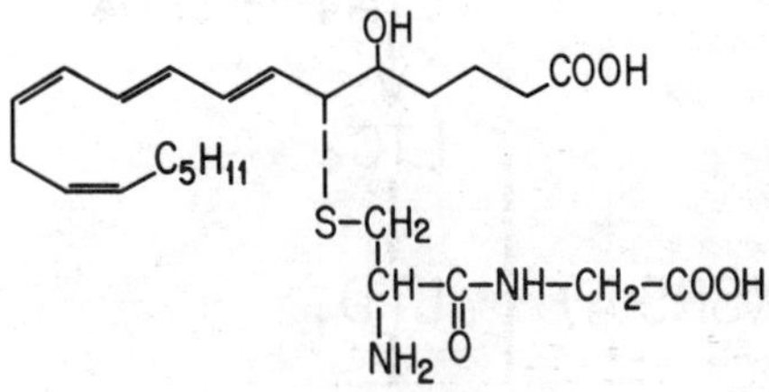

Leukotriene D_4

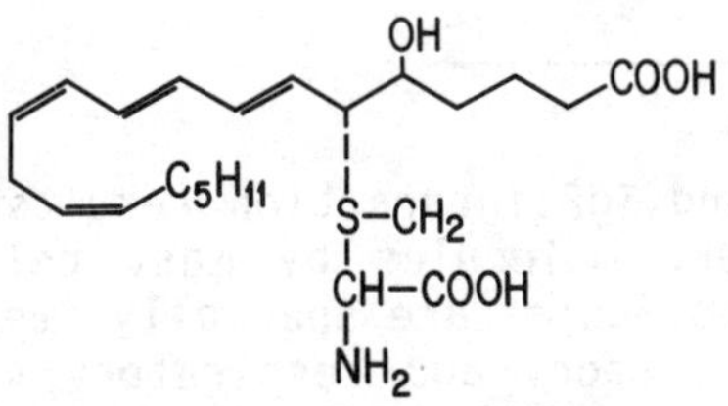

Leukotriene E_4

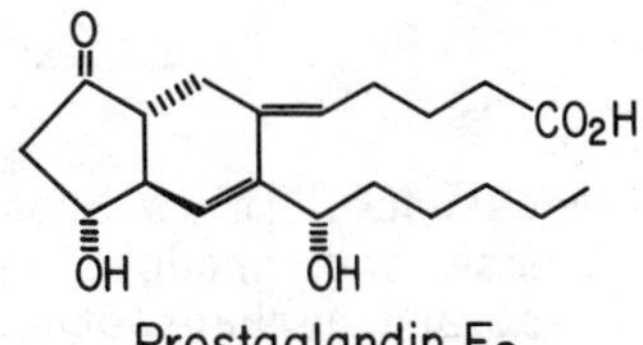

Prostaglandin E_2

Figure 14.3. Chemical formulas of leukotrienes, HETES, and prostaglandin E.

---

produce smooth muscle contraction. Injected into rabbits, PAF can produce the respiratory and vascular symptoms of acute anaphylaxis. PAF is believed to be produced by neutrophils, basophils, and macrophages following interaction with antigen-antibody or with C5a.

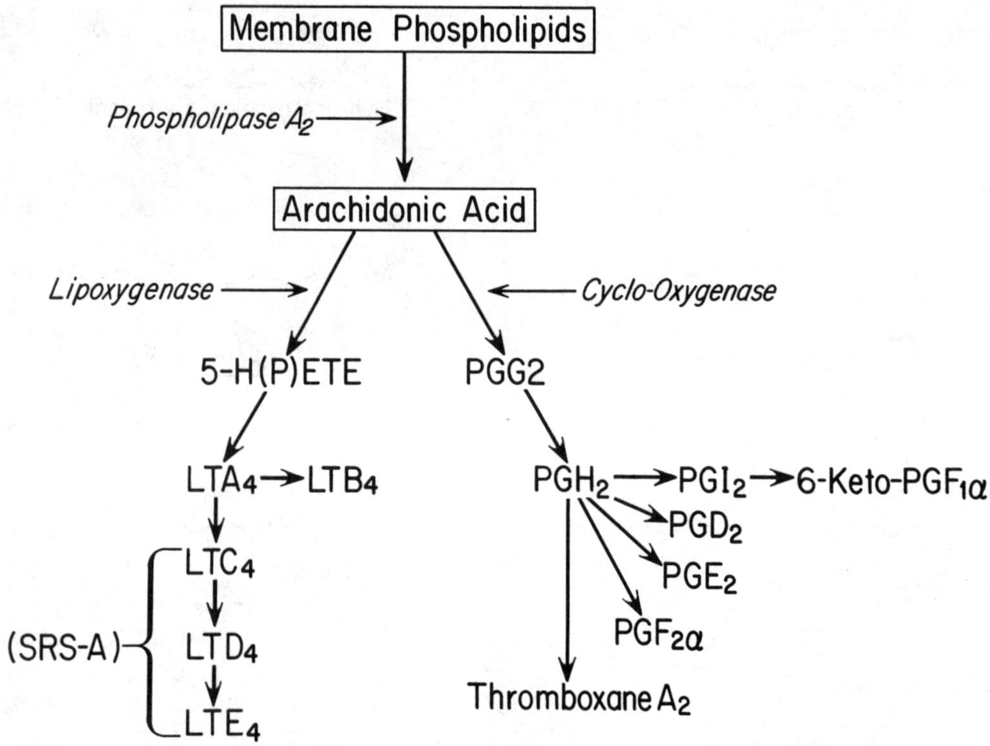

Figure 14.4. This figure represents some of the main events in the metabolism of arachidonic acid.

In essence, it is apparent that ligand-IgE interaction results in the release and production of very potent molecules by mast cells, basophils, and perhaps other cells. The molecules are specially important because of their effect in the circulatory and respiratory systems. Exactly how the molecules interact among each other in the production of all the manifestations is not clear, but their activity is not in question. Fortunately, the time that these molecules are active in tissues is short, being rapidly inactivated by tissue enzymes and other proteins. For example, histamine is rapidly eliminated, losing all its biological effect.

The Role of Complement: A relationship between anaphylactic reactions and the complement system was long suspected. This relationship is now well understood to be quite limited. None of the anaphylactic antibodies that bind mast cells activate the complement pathway directly. Niether IgE nor gamma-1 antibodies do so, and complement is not required for the release of vasoactive amines from cells upon their interaction with antigen. There is, however, a pathway for the release of vasoactive amines which involves complement components, but it is far less effective. For instance, the split products of C3 and C5, C3a and C5a, respectively, degranulate mast cells. Therefore, as a product of the classical antigen and antibody reactions with complement, these active fragments from C3 and C5 are released and trigger inflammatory reactions. However, it must be emphasized that this is a secondary mechanism as far as immediate hypersensitivity and anaphylaxis are concerned. This pathway requires a much larger concentration of antibodies than are needed for the release of active amines through the action of the anaphylactic antibodies.

SIGNIFICANCE OF ANAPHYLACTIC REACTIONS: ALLERGY IN MAN

As was mentioned before, the IgE antibodies represent the main class of anaphylactic antibodies of most species, including the human. The IgE response is a usual component of conventional immune responses to thymic-dependent antigens. Indeed, an individual challenged with a protein, for example, will make IgM and IgG antibodies but also will produce IgE antibodies, albeit briefly and in low amounts. Upon secondary boost by parental or intravenous immunization, a secondary response is produced. This response is predominantly IgG but also has a minor component of IgE antibodies.

What is the physiological significance of IgE antibodies? In Chapter 3 we speculated that perhaps the IgE antibodies are particularly important in maintaining immunity in the mucosas, for example, in the gastrointestinal tract. The anaphylactic component may be perceived as a fundamental mechanism of defense which initiates inflammatory reactions locally and helps bring, at the site of invasion of foreign organisms, the humoral and cellular elements of an immune defense reaction.

The IgE antibodies can be operating in two ways in resistance to parasitic infection. They can, by mediating the degranulation of mast cells, induce the release of eosinophilic chemotactic factors. The ECFA will attract eosinophil and also increase their representation of Fc receptors. The IgE antibodies may also mediate the attachment of the eosinophil to the parasite. (The eosinophils contain Fc receptors for IgG as well as for IgE.) This attachment results in the release of basic proteins that are lethal to some parasites. This mechanism of killing operates against several parasites like the larvae of *Schistosoma mansoni* and *Trichinella spiralis*. Limited experiments have shown that depression of the IgE antibody response or lowering the level of eosinophils reduces the resistance to these two parasitic infections.

There are two situations in which the symptoms associated with an anaphylactic antibody response predominate to the point of being detrimental to the individual. One situation is the response to conventional thymic-dependent antigens in species of animals like the guinea pig where the gamma-1 type of antibody is the major anaphylactic antibody. The second situation is the allergic state in man, or in other species, associated with IgE antibody production.

Immunization of guinea pigs with regular protein antigens consistently results in the strong production of antibodies of the gamma-1 class as well as the IgG antibodies that are slow migrating (termed gamma-2 in the guinea pigs). Invariably, the intravenous challenge of all immune guinea pigs with antigen results in acute anaphylaxis. Thus, because of the strong production of gamma-1 antibodies, the guinea pig is highly susceptible to anaphylaxis to the point where even parental immunization with small amounts of antigens may elicit the response.

The second situation is the allergic state in man. Allergy is the term first used by Von Pirquet in 1906 to denote a state of abnormal reactivity to a foreign antigen. The term allergy should be restricted to systemic or local anaphylactic reactions produced by IgE antibodies. Allergic reactions are common. They follow the sensitization or exposure to certain antigens (allergens) to which the individual mounts a selective or predominant IgE antibody response. Allergens immunize in very small amounts; in fact, many are airborne particles, a few of which establish contact with the mucosa of the nose, of the lower respiratory tract, or with the skin. The allergic individual shows a marked propensity to mount a vigorous IgE response, particularly to the small amounts of allergens introduced by way of the mucosas. Allergic or "atopic" individuals, a term coined by Coca many years ago and still used by allergists, may be numerous in some families, indicating a genetic influence. Genetic control of IgE responses has been found in experimental animals and in man.

Systemic anaphylactic reactions in man are dramatic because of their suddenness and severity. Nowadays, the most frequent cases follow exposure to drugs to which the individual has been sensitized, penicillin, for instance. Allergic reactions to insect stings can also result in severe systemic reactions.

The local allergic reactions include allergic rhinitis (hay fever), some forms of asthma, urticaria and eczematous dermatitis, and intestinal allergies. Allergic rhinitis is characterized by marked congestion of the nasal mucosa following exposure to airborn allergens. The mucosa is edematous and infiltrated with eosinophils, the typical leukocyte of allergic reactions. The most frequent allergens producing allergic rhinitis are plant pollens, dander, or fungal material. A frequent culprit in the U.S.A. is the pollen from ragweed. Several proteins have been isolated from ragweed extracts, one of which (called antigen E) is responsible for stimulating the IgE antibody response.

Asthma results from an impairment of normal air flow caused by bronchoconstriction. Many cases of asthma, principally those developing in young patients, result from a state of allergy to airborne antigens. However, allergic asthma has a complex pathogenesis not entirely explained by just the allergic state and perhaps involving other factors, including defects in beta adrenergic receptors.

A few comments on the treatment of allergic reactions are indicated. The treatment of acute anaphylactic reactions can be a life-saving procedure because a person with acute anaphylaxis can die from such an experience. This is particularly the case for individuals hypersensitive to the antigens of the bee sting or other insects, or for individuals injected indiscriminately with drugs to which they are very highly hypersensitive such as penicillin. It is essential to know what to do in these conditions and what drugs to use to counteract the very serious and dramatic anaphylactic reactions which are life-threatening. Fortunately, nature has provided us with a physiologic antagonist of the vasoactive amines responsible for the symptoms of anaphylactic reactions. Such antagonists are the catecholamines, such as epinephrine and isoproterenol, which must be administered immediately to a patient in anaphylactic shock. Epinephrine acts as an antagonist of histamine in various ways. It inhibits the effect of histamine on smooth muscles and causes the relaxation of precisely those muscles which histamine contracts. (In experimental work, it is a dramatic experience to save a guinea pig from anaphylaxis after the onset of the shock by the administration of a sufficient dose of epinephrine that will cause the relaxation of the bronchial muscles.) In addition, as stated earlier, catecholamines decrease the release of vasoactive amines from mast cells and inhibit the effect of histamine on vascular permeability and vascular tone and, therefore, prevents vascular collapse. In addition, we have at our disposal the anti-histaminics which inhibit the effects of histamine at its site of action. Anti-histaminics must be administered parenterally, immediately, to an individual suffering from an acute anaphylactic reaction.

We must also discuss another form of therapy, that of the common allergic reactions. Immunization for extended periods with the sensitizing antigen administered in increasing dosage (inappropriately termed desensitzation) is very effective in preventing the symptomatology of hay fever and other types of seasonal hypersensitivity. The therapy depends upon the synthesis of specific antibodies of the IgG class of sufficiently high affinity to bind the antigen and prevent it from reaching the IgE on the sensitized mast cells. The success of the treatment has been directly correlated with the presence in the serum of patients of a sufficient level of high affinity, blocking, IgG antibodies of the type just mentioned. Such treatments carried out over a period of years are very effective and very safe.

REFERENCES

Austen, K. A. Biologic implications of the structural and functional characteristics of the chemical mediators of immediate-type hypersensitivity. Harvey Lect., 73:93, 1979.

Bach, M. K. Mediators of anaphylaxis and inflammation. Ann. Rev. Microbiol., 36:371, 1982.

Becker, E. L. Nature and classification of immediate-type allergic reactions. Adv. Immunol., 13:267, 1971.

Bloch, K. J. The anaphylactic antibodies of mammals including man. Progr. Allergy, 10:84, 1967.

Ishizaka, K. Identification of gamma-E antibodies as a carrier of reaginic activity. J. Immunol., 99:1187, 1967.

Ishizaka, K. Cellular events in the IgE antibody response. Adv. Immunol., 23:1, 1976.

Ishizaka, T. Biochemical analysis of triggering signals induced by bridging of IgE receptors. Fed. Proc., 14:17, 1982.

Samuelsson, B. Prostaglandins, thromboxanes, and leukotrienes: formation and biological roles. Harvey Lec., 75:1, 1979.

CHAPTER 15

Immunodeficiency Diseases

We consider in this chapter examples of primary and secondary immune deficiency diseases. We will also discuss defects of complement proteins and of phagocytic cells.

PRIMARY IMMUNODEFICIENCY DISEASES

The primary specific immunodeficiency diseases are a group of hereditary or acquired defects. Patients affected with these diseases cannot mount specific immune responses and are very susceptible to infection. The primary specific immunodeficiencies all result from an absence, or maturation failure, of B cells and/or T cells. Although seventeen distinctive immunodeficiencies are recognized, only the most important ones are described below.

X-Linked Agammaglobulinemia (congenital agammaglobulinemia; Bruton's disease). Congenital agammaglobulinemia is transmitted as an X-linked phenomenon. Only males are affected. Affected boys have no B lymphocytes in their blood, bone marrow, spleen, or lymph nodes. The lymphoid tissues lack germinal centers. There is a complete absence of plasma cells in lymph nodes, gut, spleen, and other tissues where plasma cells are ordinarily found. The largest collection of B cells in the normal child is found in the tonsils. Consequently, the tonsils of children with X-linked agammaglobulinemia are very tiny, and this is one of the major diagnostic features of the disease. The serum contains no detectable IgM, IgA, IgD, or IgE. The IgG level is less than 10% of normal (less than 50 mg per dl). No specific antibody responses occur following injection of antigen.

The thymus gland is normal. T cells are normal in number and function. Affected males have normal delayed-type hypersensitivity, skin contact-type hypersensitivity, and normal allograft rejection.

The primary culture defect lies in the B cell lineage which shows a maturation block in the differentiation of early-pre-B cells to B cells. The pre-B cells are cells that have no surface immunoglobulin but yet express the heavy chain in their cytoplasm. Subsequently, the genes for the light chain are expressed, and the immunoglobulin molecule is assembled, as the cell matures to a B cell. The X-linked agammaglobulinemic boys have a normal number of pre-B cells, but these pre-B cells do not develop into mature B cells. Defects in translocation of VH genes have now been reported, implying that the genetic defect may reside in the correct assembly of H chain genes.

Because the transplacental acquisitions of IgG but not other Ig's is so effective, boys with have X-linked agammaglobulinemia are passively protected by maternal gamma globulin for the first six to nine months of life. After this, they have frequent infections of the middle ear (otitis media), the lungs (pneumonia), the skin (pyoderma), and sometimes the meninges (meningitis). The causative organisms in descending order of frequency are Hemophilus influenza, Diplococcus pneumoniae, Staphylococcus aureus, and Streptococcus pneumoniae. On the other hand, affected boys have no unusual susceptibility to infection with most fungi, parasites, enteric bacilli, and viruses. They do have frequent manifestations of collagen disease such as swollen joints resembling rheumatoid arthritis. Several patients have developed a fatal myositis and meningoencephalitis due to rare types of Echo virus. The patients also develop problems in clearing the attenuated poliomyelitis virus, a clear implication of the role of antibodies in this viral infection (Chapter 7). Among parasites, several cases have been reported with severe infection with Giardia lambdia, a small intestinal protozoa that usually does not cause serious disease.

Treatment with gamma globulin injections completely prevents recurrent pyogenic infection in boys with X-linked agammaglobulinemia. The gamma globulin is given as a 16% solution of immune serum globulin that is purified by alcohol fractionation from plasma pools obtained from two thousand blood donors. The dose is 0.6 ml or 100 mg per kilo of body weight every four weeks by intramuscular injection. This dose provides complete prophylaxis against pyogenic infections.

Common, Varied Agammaglobulinemia (Acquired or Late-Onset Agammaglobulinemia). The etiology of the acquired form of agammaglobulinemia is unknown. The onset may be at any age. Both sexes are affected equally. In contrast to the X-linked form of the disease, most patients with this disease have B cells, but these B cells fail to mature into Ig secretory cells. The following abnormalities have been observed: a) the B cells are unresponsive to antigen and T cell mitogenic factors. They fail to divide and synthesize and secrete Ig as do normal B cells in response to these stimuli. b) The B cells are responsive to antigen and T cell mitogenic factors. They divide and synthesize Ig but fail to secrete the newly synthesized Ig. This defect is associated with the failure of heavy chain glycosylation and an absence of Epstein-Barr virus receptors on the B cells. c) In rare patients, the B cells are normal but do not differentiate because of lack of helper T cells, or excessive suppressor T cells or rare autoantibodies to T or B cells.

The T cell function in patients with the common, varied form of agammaglobulinemia tends to slowly deteriorate over a long period of time. This is noted particularly in those patients with an associated tumor of the thymus gland, a thymoma.

The serum usually contains less than 250 mg per dl of IgG and less than 50 mg per dl of IgA and IgM. Susceptibility to infections is the same as in the X-linked form of the disease. Recurrent pneumonia prior to diagnosis results frequently in chronic progressive bronchiectasis (i.e., dilatation of the bronchi as a result of the persistent infection), the most common presenting finding in this disease. Associate autoimmune disease is common, particularly pernicious anemia. Hypertrophied collections of B cells in the lamina propria of the gut result in nodular lymphoid hyperplasia. This is frequently associated with chronic diarrhea, symptoms of sprue, and infection of the gut with the protozoan *Giardia lambdia*. The treatment for this disease is the same as that outlined for X-linked agammaglobulinemia.

Congenital Thymic Aplasia (DiGeorge Syndrome). Congenital thymic aplasia is not hereditary and results from an intrauterine insult to the third and fourth pharyngeal pouches between the fifth and sixth week of human gestation. Affected babies have no or very few T cells in their blood, lymph nodes, and spleen. Germinal centers are normal in lymph nodes and spleen. Plasma cells are also present in normal numbers. Delayed hypersensitivity and allograft rejection are absent. The thymus gland usually cannot be found at autopsy, or only tiny microscopic remnants are seen on serial sections in the neck. The serum immunoglobulin is normal. Weak primary antibody responses can be elicited, but no secondary responses can be made. Infections start early with opportunistic organisms (microbes which are ubiquitous but are pathogenic only for the immunosuppressed). Typically, patients get infected with yeast (*Candida albicans*) on the tongue and skin; they develop pneumonia, particularly due to the ubiquitous protozoan *Pneumocytis carinii*, and cannot terminate viral infections so that measles, chickenpox, vaccinia, or herpes can be rapidly fatal. Associated findings in this syndrome involve other congenital anomalies of the heart and face. Since the parathyroid glands have the same embryonic origin as the thymus, affected infants have no parathyroids, thus hypocalcemia and tetany. Effective treatment so far has been to transplant a fetal thymus. This causes prompt appearance, within seven days, of T cell function in recipients.

Severe Combined Immunodeficiency (SCID) (Alymphocytosis, Hereditary Thymic Dysplasia, Swiss-Type Agammaglobulinemia). The etiology is always genetic. The disease may be transmitted by X-linked or autosomal recessive inheritance. The male-to-female ratio of affected infants is 3:1. All patients with SCID lack T cells and have profound lymphopenia. The majority have no B cells. They are thus agammaglobulinemic and also have no delayed hypersensitivity and cannot reject grafts. The thymus gland is embryonal, lacking lymphoid elements and containing only endodermal cells arranged in small islands or clusters.

This finding in the thymus gland is pathognomonic of the disease. The patients have extreme susceptibility to opportunistic infections and usually do not survive more than two years of life. They are very susceptible to viral infections, particularly with herpes, cytomegalovirus, and varicella. Vaccination with attenuated tubercule bacilli (BCG) or smallpox may result in fatal infection. Patients with SCID are also very sensitive to graft-versus-host disease; in fact, many patients are born with a skin rash attributed to maternal lymphocytes that have crossed the placenta.

SCID is now treated successfully by bone marrow transplantation. The transplanted stem cell will grow and develop into mature T and B cells which reconstitute the immunological deficits. Extreme care has to be taken, however, to eliminate mature T cells from the bone marrow (in case of mismatched donors). Very few T cells will result in severe graft-versus-host disease since the patient has no mechanism for eliminating the foreign T cells.

SCID is a genetic disease that comprises different variants. In about 50% of the patients with the autosomal recessive form, a defined biochemical defect has been identified, and this is a deficiency of the enzyme adenosine deaminase (ADA). The gene for ADA has been localized to chromosome 20. ADA is normally found in all cells and is absent in the cells of the patients. (There is limited evidence that lymphoid lines derived from patients have a messenger RNA for ADA—these patients may have defective products or may rapidly degrade ADA.)

Despite the ubiquitous absence of ADA in all cells, ADA deficiency is manifested only as a defect in the lymphoid system. The thinking is that the defect in ADA results in a marked cellular accumulation of ATP as well as deoxyATP (dATP). The dATP is very toxic to lymphoid cells since it inhibits the enzyme ribonucleotidase reductase, shutting off DNA synthesis.

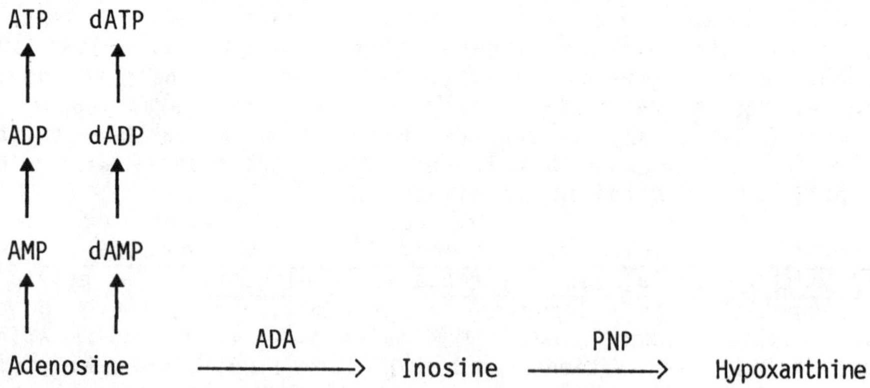

(ADA is adenosine deaminase; PNP is purine nucleoside phosphorylase.)

It is also possible that ADA results in problems with methylation reactions; adenosine in excess results in accumulation of S-adenosylhomocysteine (a product of s-adenosylmethionine) which inhibits methyltransferases.

The following is a case of ADA deficiency seen by Dr. F. S. Rosen at Children's Hospital Medical Center in Boston. A French-Canadian girl was admitted to the Center with chronic pneumonitis. The diagnosis of SCID was suggested by profound lymphopenia and absent thymus shadow on X-ray study. A male sibling had died at the age of three months and was found at autopsy to have SCID. Peripheral blood leukocytes failed to respond to phytohemagglutinin stimulation. The patient was placed in an Isolette and nursed under sterile conditions. Histocompatibility typing of the family showed that her only living sibling, a four-year-old brother, was HL-A identical. Mixed lymphocyte cultures between them were non-stimulatory; his erythrocytes were of blood group A, and the recipient's were O. The patient received 5×10^7 nucleated marrow cells per kilogram intravenously (total cells, 25×10^7) immediately after their aspiration from the donor. Eleven days later a maculopapular rash was first noted on the neck and behind the ears and then spread peripherally, but the patient remained afebrile. The rash faded after five days, when the skin began to desquamate over large areas, particularly the volar surfaces of the hands and feet. The desquamation continued for three weeks. A skin biopsy revealed only minimal round-cell infiltrates under the epidermis, and fluorescent antibody to all immunoglobulins and C3 were unreactive. A marked peripheral blood eosinophilia persisted during this time. The patient had developed a graft-versus-host reaction.

Fourteen days after transplantation peripheral blood leukocytes responsed weakly to phytohemagglutinin, and mitotic figures with a male karyotype were seen. Karyotype analysis of several bone-marrow aspirates contained only dividing female cells. The baby began to gain weight, and palpable lymph nodes appeared in the cervical, axillary, and inguinal regions. No thymus shadow was seen on X-ray study. Increasing levels of serum immunoglobulins appeared ten weeks after transplantation. Salivary IgA was 3 mg per 100 ml. After two boosters of fluid diphtheria and tetanus toxoids, an anti-tetanus and an anti-diphtheria antibody developed. Anti-B isohemagglutinin titer was 1:32; anti-A remained undetectable despite the fact that only Type O cells (recipient) were found. Ten weeks after transplantation, a full-thickness skin graft showed gross and microscropical evidence of rejection at seventeen days after placement.

Before discharge, the peripheral blood eosinophilia was decreasing, immunoglobulin levels were normal, and a bone-marrow aspirate revealed the presence of plasma cells. The peripheral blood lymphocytes showed a normal proliferative response to phytohemagglutinin and candida antigen. Moreover, the patient responded positively to an intradermal injection of candida antigen with a typical delayed hypersensitivity response of erythema and induration.

Now thirteen years after transplantation she is in good health. Erythrocytes are all Type O and no red-cell chimerism has been demonstrated.

A deficiency of the enzyme purine nucleoside phosphorylase also results in SCID. This is a rare enzyme defect now identified in several families. In most patients, the enzyme, localized to chromosome 14, is absent. NP-deficient patients have a high level of inosine, guanosine, deoxyguanosine, and GTP deoxyGTP. It is thought that the dGTP stops cell proliferation by inhibiting ribonucleotide reductase.

SECONDARY IMMUNODEFICIENCY

Specific immunodeficiency may be secondary to other disease states which result in loss, or destruction, of immunoglobulins or T and B cells. For instance, there may be gastrointestinal loss of immunoglobulin as a result of intestinal diseases. Loss of immunoglobulin may occur through the skin as in burns or eczema or due to other skin diseases. Increased catabolism of immunoglobulin occurs in the nephrotic syndrome and multiple myeloma, and this may result in profound hypogammaglobulinemia. The most common cause of secondary and specific immunodeficiency results from the use of cytotoxic drugs or irradiation or glucocorticoid therapy. All these modalities of therapy are highly destructive to T and B cells.

Acquired Immunodeficiency Syndrome (AIDS). An outbreak of AIDS has now developed in the male homosexual communities of the large cities in the United States. AIDS patients suffer from severe infection with opportunistic pathogens. As mentioned previously, these are microbes that are not infective in the normal individual but which become pathogenic in the absence of T cell immunity. Included among them are cytomegalovirus and *Pneumocystis carinii*, both of which can produce a severe lung infection. Patients with AIDS have no T cell immunity; they are severely lymphopenic and have inverted ratios of T4/T8 cells (Chapter 5). Their level of serum immunoglobulin is normal or elevated, implying no major defect in B cells. Patients with AIDS may also develop tumors, in particular, a rare form of skin cancer termed Kaposi's sarcoma. AIDS appears to be transmitted by sexual contact and by blood contact. Cases have been reported in hemophiliacs, possibly resulting from blood transfusions. The thinking at present is that AIDS is caused by an infective agent, possible a virus, that selectively affects the T cells.

COMPLEMENT DEFECTS

Genetic defects are known for most complement proteins, C1q, C1r, C1s, C2, C4, C3, C5, C6, C7, C8, and C9. They are all inherited as autosomal recessive traits, and heterozygotes can be readily detected by half normal levels of the components. C2 deficiency is common in humans; one in one-hundred people are heterozygous for the defect. C1q deficiency is common in the Japanese. About one per fifty individuals are heterozygous for the defect. The common symptoms associated with defects of early acting component (C1, C2, C4) are those of immune complex disease, whereas the late components (C5 through C8) defects are associated with recurrent Neisserial infection. C3 deficiency is associated with pyogenic infection (Table 15.1). These clinical associations point out the importance of complement in: 1) the elimination and/or solubilization of immune complexes; 2) the bactericidal reaction; and 3) opsonization (Table 15.1).

Clinically, the most important complement defects are those of the inhibitors of the system, C1 inhibitor and C3b inactivator (I). A few cases have now been reported of Factor H and Properdin deficiencies. C1 inhibitor deficiency is associated with the common genetic disease hereditary angioneurotic edema. It is inherited as an autosomal dominant trait. In 85% of affected kindred patients lack the C1 inhibitor. In the other 15%, patients have a non-functional, antigenically normal protein. Patients are subject to recurrent attacks of subcutaneous swelling in any part of the body or to intestinal swelling which causes colic (severe cramps), nausea, and vomiting or sometimes watery diarrhea. Swelling of the larynx may be fatal, and patients choke to death from this involvement. Activated C1 can be found in the blood of patients with the disease. They consume C4 and C2 *in vivo* at a very rapid rate so that their serum levels of C4 and C2 are low. C3 and the later-acting components are unaffected. Attacks of angioedema are provoked by trauma, menses, violent exercise, extremes of temperature, and anxiety. There is no specific treatment for attacks. Patients with laryngeal edema must be treated with tracheostomy. Complete prophylaxis against attacks can be achieved with androgens which induce synthesis of C1 inhibitor.

C3b inactivator (I) deficiency is inherited as an autosomal recessive trait. It is a very rare defect. Patients have recurrent infections with pyogenic bacteria as they cannot generate opsonically effective C3. The defect is associated with rapid *in vivo* catabolism of C3. There is no treatment for the disease save appropriate antibiotic therapy for intercurrent infections.

Acquired Complement Defects. The measurement of C3 is readily available in clinical laboratories, and its depression below 100 mg per dl is significant. This occurs principally in systemic lupus erythematosus due to increased C3 consumption and in acute post-streptococcal glomerulonephritis due to depressed C3 synthesis. Also C3 is low in

Table 15.1

Clinical Problems Associated with Complement Deficiencies

Complement Protein	Clinical Problems
C1q	High incidence of immune complexes disease
C1r	High incidence of immune complex disease
C2	High incidence of immune complex disease
C4	High incidence of immune complex disease
C3	Recurrent pyogenic infections
C5	Recurrent Neisserial infection, high incidence of systemic lupus erythematosus
C6	Recurrent Neisserial infection
C7	Recurrent Neisserial infection
C8	Recurrent Neisserial infection
C9	Asymptomatic
C1INH	Angioneurotic edema
Factor (C3bINA)	Recurrent pyogenic infections
Factor H	Recurrent pyogenic infections
Properdin (P)	Recurrent Neisserial infections

membranoproliferative glomerulonephritis, a severe form of immune complex-mediated nephritis, usually due to an antibody to C3bBb. This autoantibody stabilizes this C3-converting enzyme and causes increased consumption of C3.

PHAGOCYTIC DEFECTS

Polymorphonuclear leukocytes and monocytes are the most important effector cells in immunologically mediated reactions. Both cell types have receptors for C3 and IgG that facilitate the ingestion of antibody and complement-coated bacteria and thus the intracellular destruction of bacteria. These receptors have been discussed in Chapters 5 and 12. In Chapter 5 we also discussed the changes in oxidative metabolism that accompany phagocytosis. Phagocytosis activates membrane-bound NADPH oxidase which is needed to generate intracellular peroxide. These reactions do not occur in a genetic defect of NADPH oxidase called chronic granulomatous disease.

The disease is transmitted as an autosomal recessive or X-linked recessive trait. Affected children have persistent infection with bacteria that produce catalase, *Staphylococcus aureus*, *Serratia marcescens*, and certain coliforms. These bacteria, once ingested, luxuriate and multiply in the defective phagocytes, causing a granulomatous reaction. Usually microabscesses develop in lymph nodes, lung, and liver. The disease is readily diagnosed by the failure of affected leukocytes (both polys and monocytes) to reduce the dye nitrobluetetrazolium (NBT) from its normally colorless state to a deep purple formazan dye:

$$O^-_2 + NBT^+ \longrightarrow NBT + O_2$$

REFERENCES

Gottlieb, M. S., *et al*. *Pneumocystis carinii* pneumonia and mucosal candidiasis in previously healthy homosexual men: evidence of a newly acquired cellular immunodeficiency. N. E. J. Med., 305: 1425, 1981.

Hirschhorn, R., G. F. Vawter, J. A. Kirkpatrick, and F. S. Rosen. Adenosine deaminase deficiency: frequency and comparative pathology in autosomally recessive combined immunodeficiency. Clin. Immunol. Immunopathol., 14:107, 1979.

Janeway, C. A. Syndromes of diminished resistance to infection. J. Ped., 72:855, 1968.

Klebanoff, S. J., and L. R. White. Iodination defect in the lymphocytes of a patient with chronic granulomatous disease in childhood. N. E. J. Med., 280:460, 1969.

Rosen, F. S. Immunodeficiency. In: *Immunogenetics and Immunodeficiency*. B. Benacerraf, editor. MTP, Lancaster, England, 1975.

Rosen, F. S. Primary immunodeficiency disease. Clin. Immunol. Immunopathol., 28:450, 1983.

Glossary of Immunology Terms

ADCC: antibody-dependent cellular cytotoxicity—the ability of non-sensitized cells (i.e., cells from an unimmunized animal) to lyse other cells that have been coated by specific antibody.

Adherent Cells: cells from lymphoid tissues or inflammatory exudates that adhere strongly to glass or plastic surfaces—usually macrophages.

Adjuvant: any of many foreign materials introduced with an antigen to enhance its immunogenicity. These include killed bacteria (*B. pertussis*, mycobacteria) or bacterial products (endotoxin) or emulsions (Freund's adjuvant, alum).

Adoptive Transfer: the transfer of the ability to respond to antigen by transplanting immunocompetent cells into a host made immuno*in*competent, usually by irradiation.

Affinity: the thermodynamic quantity defining the energy of interaction of two molecules, usually that of an antibody with its corresponding antigenic determinant (see Avidity).

AI: anaphylotoxin inhibitor.

Alloantibody: antibody raised in one individual and directed against an antigen (usually cells) or another of the same species. When experimental animals of an inbred strain are immunized with cells of another strain, the antibodies are usually directed against histocompatibility antigens.

Alloantigen: an antigen obtained from another individual or inbred line of the same species. Such antigens are the result of genetic polymorphism. Histocompatibility antigens are common examples.

Allogeneic: originating from a different individual or a different inbred cell line of the same species (see Isogeneic and Xenogeneic).

Allogeneic Effect: the non-specific enhancement or suppression of an immune response by allogeneic T lymphocytes (specific for antigens controlled by the I-region of the major histocompatibility complex) can take the place of helper T cells under some conditions.

Allotype: a structure on the heavy chain of a particular immunoglobulin class or on the light chains that are different from other individuals or inbred lines of the same species. Can be used as a marker for genetic studies.

Alternative Pathway: a mechanism of complement activation that does not involve the binding of C1, C4, C2 by antigen-antibody complexes.

Anamnestic Response: same as Secondary Immune Response.

Anaphylaxis: a systemic immediate hypersensitivity reaction resulting in respiratory distress or vascular collapse.

Anaphylotoxin: a small fragment of C3 (C3a) or C5 (C5a) capable of degranulating mast cells and liberating vasoactive amines.

Antibody: an immunoglobulin molecule capable of combining specifically with antigen (see Immunoglobulin).

Antigen: a molecule capable of stimulating an immune response. It may have many determinants (see Determinants).

Arthus Reaction: a local immune reaction mediated by antigen-antibody complexes and resulting in vascular injury, thrombosis, hemorrhage, and acute inflammation.

Autologous: originating from the same individual (see Isologous).

Avidity: an imprecise measurement of the strength of binding of antibody and antigen molecules—usually involving multiple different molecular interactions (see Affinity).

B: symbol for a component of the Alternative Pathway—also C3 proactivator or GBG.

B Cell: one of the two major classes of lymphocytes. B cells derive from the Bursa of Fabricius in birds or the bone marrow of mammals and respond to antigen by differentiating into antibody-producing cells.

Bence-Jones Protein: a low molecular weight protein found in urine and consisting of light chains—frequently due to the presence of a malignant overgrowth of one clone of lymhocytes or plasma cells (e.g., multiple myeloma).

Beta-2 Microglobulin: a 12,000-dalton polypeptide found in association with the heavy chain of Class I molecules.

Bovine Gamma Globulin (BGG): a common antigen in experimental work, frequently used as a carrier for hapten.

Bovine Serum Albumin (BSA): a common antigen and carrier for experimental work.

Bursa of Fabricius: a lymphoid organ in the hind gut of birds that influences B cell development.

C1INH: symbol for an inhibitor of activated C1.

C3bINH (or I): symbol for an inhibitor of activated C3 (C3b).

C3 Receptor: a site on the surface of B cells and phagocytes able to bind activated C3.

Capping: the coordinated movement of membrane molecules to one region of the cell surface after binding by a multivalent ligand such as an antibody or an antigen.

Carrier: a molecule to which haptens are bound—usually immunogenic proteins (see **Hapten** and **Immunogen**).

Cellular Immunity: immune phenomena mediated by immune T cells and not by antibody, such as delayed hypersensitivity or cytolytic T cell lysis.

Complete Freund's Adjuvant (CFA): an oil-based adjuvant containing mycobacteria.

CH Region: the region of the heavy chain of immunoglobulins with constant amino acid sequence in different antibodies of the same class.

CL Region: the region of the light chain of immunoglobulins with constant amino acid sequence in different antibodies of the same class.

Class: the major molecule types of immunoglobulin, i.e., IgG, IgM, IgA, IgE, IgD.

Class I Molecules: refers to one of the two major sets of molecules coded by the Major Histocompatibility Gene Complex. HLA A, B, and C loci code for Class I molecules.

Class II Molecules: the other major set of molecules encoded in the Major Histocompatibility Gene Complex (see **Ia Antigens**).

Classical Pathway: the mechanism of complement activation by antigen-antibody complexes involving the binding of C1, C4, C2 to activate C3.

CML: cell-mediated lymphocytotoxicity—the ability of sensitized T cells (i.e., T cells from an immunized individual) to lyse other cells bearing membrane antigens to which they are sensitized.

Complement: a set of serum proteins activated in sequence by antibody-antigen complexes or by bacterial products (Alternative Pathway) and responsible for many biological defense mechanisms such as lysis, opsonization, leukocyte chemotaxis, inflammation, etc.

Concanavalin A (Con A): a plant substance that binds to sugar residues on cell surfaces and stimulates T cells to proliferate—a lectin.

Cortex: the peripheral region of lymph node or thymus.

Cytolytic T Lymphocytes (CTL): a subset of T cells that have specificity to cell surface antigens displayed on various target cells (virally infected, tumors, allogeneic cells). The CTL adhere to the target cells and lyse them.

D: symbol for a component of the Alternative Pathway.

Delayed Hypersensitivity: specific inflammatory immune reaction elicited by antigen in the skin of immune individuals. It takes twenty-four to forty-eight hours to develop and is mediated by T cells and macrophages, not by antibodies.

Determinant: that part of the structure of an antigen that binds to the antibody-combining site (see Hapten and Epitope).

Dinitrophenyl (DNP): a common hapten

E: symbol for erythrocyte.

EA: symbol for an erythrocyte coated by specific antibody.

EAC: symbol for an erythrocyte coated by antibody and complement.

Eosinophil Chemotactic Factor of Anaphylaxis (ECF-A): a molecule released immunologically during immediate hypersensitivity reactions and able to attract eosinophils.

Endotoxin: a lipopolysaccharide derived from cell walls of gram-negative bacteria that has multiple biological effects: it stimulates the immune response non-specifically, stimulates mouse B lymphocytes, and activates the alternative complement pathway.

Enhancement: a prolongation of allograft or tumor survival by specific antibodies against the foreign tissue.

Epitope: a determinant, usually one that occurs many times on the same antigen (see **Hapten, Determinant,** and **Antigen**).

Fab Fragment: a product of papain digestion of immunoglobulins with one intact light chain and part of one heavy chain. Fab fragments have one combining site for antigen.

Fab'2: a product of pepsin digestion of immunoglobulin with two intact light chains and parts of two heavy chains and two combining sites for antigen but lacking the Fc region.

Fc Fragment: a product of papain digestion of immunoglobulin with parts of two heavy chains and no combining sites for antigen. This fragment has sites for activation of complement and for the binding of immunoglobulins to macrophages, lymphocytes, and mast cells and is responsible for many biological functions of antibodies.

Fc Receptor: a protein on the surface of most lymphocytes and phagocytes able to bind the Fc portion of immunoglobulins of the IgG class.

Follicle: a circumscribed region in lymphoid tissue, in the superficial cortex of lymph nodes, containing mostly B cells.

Gamma Globulin: globulins with slow electrophoretic mobility in the gamma region, includes most of the immunoglobulin molecules. This term is sometimes used to refer to all immunoglobulins of various classes.

Globulin: any of a large number of serum proteins distinct from albumin and insoluble at high salt concentrations.

Graft-versus-Host Reaction (GVH): the pathological reactions caused by transplantation of immunocompetent T lymphocytes to an incompetent host. The host is unable to reject the T lymphocytes and becomes the target of attack by them.

H-2: the major histocompatbility complex in the mouse.

H-2K and H-2D: loci in the MHC coding for Class I histocompatibility molecules that are responsible for the rapid rejection of allografts and that serve as targets for T cell cytolysis in physiological interactions.

Hapten: chemically defined determinant that, when conjugated to an immunogenic carrier, stimulates the synthesis of specific antibody. It is capable of binding to antibody but cannot by itself stimulate an immune response.

Heavy Chain: the higher molecular weight polypeptide chain in an immunoglobulin molecule and the one determining the class of the immunoglobulin.

Helper Cells: a class of T cells that are necessary to help B cells produce antibody to thymus-dependent antigens.

Heterologous: originating from a different individual or a different inbred line; sometimes applied to a different carrier molecule (see Isologous).

Histocompatibility Antigens: cell surface antigens characteristic of an individual or an inbred line that regulate the interactions of T lymphoyctes and also stimulate the rejection of tissue allografts.

HLA: the major histocompatibility complex in man.

HLA-A, HLA-B, HLA-C: three distinct genetic loci in the MHC of man coding for Class I major histocompatibility antigens.

HLA-D: a region of the MHC of man coding for Class II antigens expressed primarily on B cells and macrophages.

Humoral Immunity: immune phenomena involving the production of specific antibody.

Hypersensitivity: a poor term yet widely used, usually applied to those immune phenomena that are damaging in some way to the host animal.

Hypervariable Region: defined portions of the variable region of either heavy or light immunoglobulin chains having extreme variability in amino acid sequence in different molecules. The antibody-combining site is made of the hypervariable regions.

Ia Antigens: histocompatibility antigens found on B cells, macrophages, T cells, and Langerhans cells of the skin. They are coded for in the I region of the MHC. The Ia antigens are the Class II molecules.

Incomplete Freund's Adjuvant (ICFA): Freund's adjuvant without mycobacteria.

Idiotype: an antigenic determinant on a specific antibody that is characteristic of that antibody and different from others even of the same **Isotype** and **Allotype**; idiotypes are usually located in or near the combining site.

Immediate Hypersensitivity: a specific immunological reaction mediated by antibodies that takes place in minutes to hours after administration of antigen (see **Arthus Reaction** and **Anaphylaxis**).

Immunogen: a molecule that elicits an immune response (see **Antigen**).

Immunoglobulin: the various classes of gamma globulin molecules having antibody activity.

Interferon: proteins that confer an anti-viral state to many tissue cells. There are three types of interferon: alpha, beta, and gamma. **Interferon-alpha** is produced by macrphages after their interaction with various stimulants. **Interferon-beta** is produced by cells infected with viruses. **Interferon-gamma** is produced by T cells following antigen stimulation.

Interleukin-1 (IL-1): a 15,000-dalton protein elaborated by macrophages and serving as a potent stimulator for thymocytes and T helper cells.

Interleukin-1 (IL-2): a protein elaborated by T helper cells capable of promoting the growth of other T lymphocytes.

IL-2 Receptors: structures on the membrane of activated T cells responsible for binding IL-2. This is the initial step in the stimulation of T cell growth.

Ir Genes: genes located in the I region of the MHC that control the ability to develop specific immune responses to thymus-dependent antigens. Ir gene products = Ia antigens = Class II molecules.

I Region: a region of the MHC where Ir genes are located and Ia molecules are encoded.

I-A, I-B, I-C, I-E, I-J: subregions of the I region of the mouse H-2 complex.

Isogeneic: originating from the same individual or the same inbred strain (see **Isologous**).

Isologous: originating from the same individual or a member of the same inbred stain (see **Autologous**).

Isotype: the class or subclass of an immunoglobulin, common to all members of that species.

J Chain: a small polypeptide found in IgM and IgA polymers and responsible for maintaining the polymeric forms of the immunoglobulins.

K Cell: a class of cells able to mediate ADCC (synonymous with Natural Killer Cells).

Kinin System: an activity in serum responsible for many biological effects of antibodies and composed of many proteins acting in sequence.

Keyhole Limpet Hemocyanin (KLH): a strong thymus-dependent antigen often used in hapten-carrier conjugates.

Lymphocytic Choriomeningitis (LCM): a disease induced by the LCM virus but dependent on the immune system to produce tissue damage.

Lectin: any of a number of plant products that bind to cells, usually by nature of a combining site for specific sugars.

Leukotrienes: a family of molecules derived from arachidonic acid and having potent effect on smooth muscle and vascular permeability (see SRS-A).

Light Chain: the lower molecular weight polypeptide chain present in all immunoglobulin molecules.

Lipopolysaccharide (LPS): the active component of endotoxin derived from bacterial cell walls; a B cell mitogen in the mouse.

Ly: a system of antigens found on murine T cells that distinguish different functional classes of T cells.

Lymphokines: a group of substances produced by lymphocytes having diverse effects on other cells.

M-Component: a large amount of homogeneous immunoglobulin detected in urine or serum frequently due to the presence of a malignant overgrowth of one clone of lymphocytes or plasma cells.

Macrophage: a ubiquitous phagocytic cell found in tissues and blood.

Medulla: the central region of a lymph node consisting of lymphatic sinuses and medullary cords.

Memory: the ability of the immune system to mount a specific secondary response to an immunogen that was previously introduced.

Major Histocompatibility Complex (MHC): a large region of genetic material containing genes coding for histocompatibility antigens.

Migration Inhibition Factor (MIF): a protein produced by lymphocytes upon interaction with antigens that inhibits the motility of macrophages in culture.

Mitogen: a substance that stimulates lymphocytes to proliferate independently of any specific antigen.

Mixed Lymphocyte Reaction or Culture (MLR or MLC): the proliferative response of allogeneic lymphocytes when cultured together.

Monocyte: a phagocytic blood leukocyte that is the precursor of most tissue macrophages. Monocytes originate from cells in the bone marrow.

Natural Killer Cells (NK Cells): cells having the capacity to kill undifferentiated cells, tumor, or virally infected cells. NK cells have an Fc receptor and can also kill by way of an ADCC mechanism.

Non-Adherent Cells: those cells in suspensions of spleen and other lymphoid tissue that do not adhere to plastic or glass, in contrast to macrophages. Usually include lymphocytes.

Null Cell: a class of lymphocyte that does not bear markers for either T cells or B cells.

Opsonization: the enhacement of phagocytosis of a particle or a cell (especially bacteria) by virtue of its being covered by antibody.

Platelet-Activating Factor(s) (PAF): a molecule released immunologically and able to aggregate and degranulate platelets.

Passive Cutaneous Anaphylaxis (PCA): the induction of a local, immediate-type immune reaction by injecting antibody into the skin and later injecting antigen intravenously or locally. This reaction is caused by the release of vasoactive amines from mast cells and is manifested by a large increase in vascular permeability.

Plaque-Forming Cell (PFC): an antibody-secreting cell releasing sufficient antibody against red cells to form an area of hemolysis in a layer of agar filled with red cells when complement is added, usually plasma cells. Antibody reactions are often quantitated by counting the number of PFC's. Cells making antibodies to protein antigens can be estimated by a modified PFC method in which the protein antigen is bound to an indicator red cell.

Phytohemagglutinin (PHA): a plant lectin that agglutinates animal cells and stimulates lymphocytes, mostly T cells, to proliferate.

Plasma Cells: a cell of the B cell lineage actively secreting large amounts of immunoglobulin.

Pokeweed Mitogen (PWM): a plant substance that stimulates lymphocytes to proliferate.

Primary Immune Response: the response occurring on first exposure to an immunogen.

Primed: refers to an animal or cell population that has been exposed previously to an immunogen and that is capable of making a secondary response.

Properdin: a component of the Alternative Pathway.

Rejection: the destruction of foreign tissue or tumor due to an immune reaction against it.

Secondary Immune Response: the accelerated response occurring on the second and subsequent exposure to an immunogen (memory).

Serum Sickness: a syndrome resulting from the localization of circulating immune complexes in small vessels and especially in the kidney glomeruli.

Specificity: the ability of antibodies to distinguish between different determinants.

SRBC: abbreviation for Sheep Red Blood Cells, a common antigen in experimental work.

SRS-A: Slow-Reacting Substance of Anaphylaxis—initial name used to describe molecules released immunologically and responsible for some of the effects of anaphylaxis. The Leukotriene is the name now given to these molecules.

Ss: a region of the MHC of mice coding for a serum substance that has been indentified as the C4 complement component.

Subclass: immunoglobulins of the same class but different in electrophoretic mobility or in an antigenic determinant detectable in the CH region, e.g., IgG1, IgG2, IgG3, IgG4.

Suppressor Cells: a class of T cells that is able to suppress the immune response to an antigen.

Systemic Lupus Erythematosus (SLE): an autoimmune disease characterized by the production of autoantibodies to different autoantigens and especially to DNA.

T4: a protein found in human helper T cells recognized by a specific monoclonal antibody.

T8: a protein found in human suppressor and cytolytic T cells identified by a monoclonal antibody.

T Antigens: antigens found in virally induced malignant tumor cells that are characteristic of the oncogenic virus, although they are not viral proteins. Different tumors induced by the same virus have the same T antigens. Different viruses produce tumors with different T antigens. T antigens are found in the nuclei of tumor cells, elicit antibody responses, but do not stimulate specific tumor rejection.

T Cell: a class of T lymphocytes derived from the thymus capable of responding to thymus-dependent antigens and MHC gene products. T cells do not produce antibodies; they mediate cellular immunological reactions and regulate immune responses.

T-Dependent Antigen: an immunogen that is able to elicit an antibody response without a major participation of T cells.

Theta: (also called Thy-1) an antigen found on T cells in the mouse, but best T cell marker in the mouse.

Thy: a system of T cell antigens (see **Theta**).

Thymus-Dependent Area: a region of peripheral lymphoid tissue such as lymph nodes and spleen containing mostly T cells that atrophies after thymectomy, e.g., the deep cortex of lymph nodes and the periarteriolar sheath of the spleen.

Thymus-Independent Area: a region within peripheral lymphoid tissue containing mostly B cells, e.g., the follicles of lymph nodes found in the superficial cortex.

TL: a system of mouse T cell antigens originally found on T cell leukemia cells and expressed in some mouse strains on normal thymocytes.

Tolerance: the failure of the immune system, as the result of previous contact with antigen, to respond to the same antigen, while reamining capable of responding to others. Tolerance is best established by neonatal injection of an antigen.

Transfer Factor: a small molecule extracted from sensitized leukocytes and able to transfer specific delayed hypersensitivity to antigens to which the donor of the leukocytes is sensitized.

Transport Piece: a polypeptide found associated with secreted IgA but not with serum IgA.

TSTA: Tumor-Specific Transplantation Antigens—antigens found on the cell membrane of tumors against which tumor rejection reactions are directed.

VH Region: the variable amino acid sequence region of the heavy chain.

VL Region: the variable amino acid sequence region of the light chain.

Xenogeneic: originating from a different species (see Isogeneic and Allogeneic).

Index

732-0615